Birth controlled

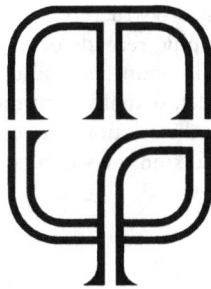

Manchester University Press

Governing Intimacies in the Global South

About the series

Governing Intimacies in the Global South deploys the categories of intimacy and governance to offer novel insights into the subjects, politics, cultures and experiences of the global south. The series showcases work that speaks to the affective and intimate worlds of communities located in Asia, Africa and Latin America while remaining attuned to governmental, social and other regulatory frames that undergird these worlds.

It seeks to bridge the gap between developmental analyses of the 'rest of the world', which theorise macro structures to the exclusion of the intimate, and historical and ethnographic records of micro-settings, allowing these to speak to larger structural conditions and constraints. Emphasising the postcolonial making of gender, sexuality and race as categories of meaning and power, this series views the relation between intimacy and governance from a position of theorising from the south, contributing to a reimagining of the idea of global south itself.

Birth controlled

Selective reproduction and neoliberal eugenics in South Africa and India

Edited by Amrita Pande

MANCHESTER UNIVERSITY PRESS

Published by Manchester University Press
Oxford Road, Manchester M13 9PL
www.manchesteruniversitypress.co.uk

British Library Cataloguing-in-Publication Data
A catalogue record for this book is available from the
British Library

ISBN   978 1 5261 6054 6   hardback
ISBN   978 1 5261 7890 9   paperback

First published 2022

Typeset
by New Best-set Typesetters Ltd

For Bratati and S. K. Pande
For being Ma and Baba
Piglet: 'How do you spell love?'
Pooh: 'You don't spell it, you feel it.'
(A. A Milne (1979). Winnie-the-Pooh. *New York: Dell)*

Contents

Notes on contributors

Kezia Batisai is Associate Professor in the Sociology Department at the University of Johannesburg and holds a PhD in Gender Studies from the University of Cape Town. Her research gaze is on gender, sexuality, political change, questions of being different and politics of nation-building in Africa – a theoretical standpoint that informs her current and forthcoming publications. Beyond academis, Kezia has more than ten years' working experience as a senior researcher for local and international organisations. She is an active member of: the International Sociological Association (Language and Society; and Women and Society working groups); the South African Association for Gender Studies; and the South African Sociological Association (Gender working group coordinator: 2015–present).

Rachelle Chadwick, PhD, is Senior Lecturer in Sociology at the University of Pretoria. She has published widely on childbirth, obstetric violence, feminist theory, and qualitative methodologies, with her work appearing in journals such as: *Health, Risk and Society*, *Qualitative Research*, *Feminist Theory*, and *Feminism and Psychology*. Her book, *Bodies that Birth: Vitalizing Birth Politics*, was published in 2018 by Routledge.

Sushmita Chatterjee is Associate Professor and Director of Gender, Women's, and Sexuality Studies in the Department of Interdisciplinary Studies at Appalachian State University. Her research and teaching interests include transnational gender and sexuality studies, postcolonial theory, animal studies, and visual politics. Her recent publications include a co-edited volume titled *Meat! A Transnational Analysis*, with Banu Subramaniam (Duke University Press, 2021).

She is currently working on a book project that brings animal studies and plant studies in conversation about their (dis)similar stakes.

Sreeparna Chattopadhyay is an Associate Professor of Sociology in the School of Social Sciences at FLAME University, Pune, India. She has an MA and a PhD from the Department of Anthropology and the Population Studies Training Centre at Brown University and a BA in Economics (Honours) from St. Xavier's College, Bombay. Her research has focused on the ways in which gender disadvantages interact with socioeconomic inequities, shaping women's life trajectories including impacts on health, education, and exposure to violence. Her work has been supported by the Harry Frank Guggenheim Foundation, the National Science Foundation, and the Mellon Foundation. Her most recent research has focused on maternal health in two regions of India – rural north-east India and Karnataka in south India – with an emphasis on understanding the institutional drivers of disrespectful and abusive care that pregnant women receive in hospitals. Sreeparna's research has been published by *Social Science and Medicine, Culture, Health and Sexuality, Reproductive Health Matters*, and the *International Journal for Equity in Health* among others. Her first book, *The Gravity of Hope*, which unravels the links between domestic and structural violence and weaves the personal with the political, will be published by Crossed Arrows Publication in 2022. Sreeparna has worked in the US, the UK and with non-profits and the government and writes for the popular media to make her research accessible to a wider audience.

Johanna Gondouin is Assistant Professor in Gender Studies at Linköping University, with a background in comparative literature and film studies. Her areas of expertise are postcolonial feminist theory and critical race and whiteness studies, with a specific focus on reproduction and reproductive technologies. She has recently completed the research project *Mediating Global Motherhood: Gender, Race and Sexuality in Swedish Media Representations of Transnational Surrogacy and Transnational Adoption*, funded by the Swedish Research Council, and is currently leading the research project *From Waste to Profit: Gender, Biopolitics and Neoliberalism in Indian Commercial Surrogacy*, also funded by the Swedish Research Council. She has published her research in journals such as *Critical Race and Whiteness Studies, Catalyst* and *Economic & Political Weekly*.

Manitza Kotzé is Senior Lecturer at the Faculty of Theology at North-West University, South Africa, where she teaches Dogmatics and Christian Ethics. She received her PhD at Stellenbosch University in bioethics and systematic theology. Her research interest focuses on the interplay between doctrine and bioethics, in particular questions raised by biotechnology, including assisted reproductive technologies and human biotechnological enhancement.

Vasudha Mohanka is an independent researcher interested in reproductive politics (repro)nationalism, phenomenology, transformation of the body and eugenics.

Tessa Moll is a medical anthropologist and Postdoctoral Research Fellow at the School of Public Health at the University of the Witwatersrand. Her research interests include reproduction, assisted conception technology, and postgenomics, with a focus on the circulation of knowledge and technology in South Africa. She is currently involved in a project on cross-border reproductive travel in sub-Saharan Africa and working on a monograph about fertility care and race in South Africa.

Rufaro Moyo is a PhD candidate in the Sociology Department of the University of Cape Town (UCT). She has presented the findings of her research at the Sociology Seminar Series of UCT and at the RINGS Conference and Annual Meeting at the University of Tallinn as part of a panel on Reproducing Feminist (dystopic) Futures. Her work sought to examine the role of race in the process of selecting an egg donor in Cape Town, South Africa.

Meghna Mukherjee is a PhD candidate at University of California Berkeley in the Department of Sociology. Her main research interests revolve around the social inequalities arising alongside emerging fertility and genetic technologies. Meghna's research is comparative between the US and India, and interrogates how medicalised spaces in both sites are reinforcing social hierarchies and reconstituting health and family-building. Prior to her PhD, Meghna worked in the non-profit and social development field in New York City, and pursued research related to commercial reproductive labour policies in India. Meghna graduated Magna Cum Laude from Columbia University with a BA in Sociology (honors) and Human Rights (2015) and holds an MA in Sociology from UC Berkeley (2019).

Verena Namberger completed her PhD in Gender Studies at Humboldt University Berlin, Germany. In her PhD research she explored the relations between value production, labour and the body in the South African bioeconomy of egg donation as a site of the transnational industry surrounding assisted reproductive technology.Her research interests include feminist science and technology studies, new materialisms, body studies, Cultural Studies of ARTs, biopolitics, philosophy and history of the life sciences. Currently, she is Vice Central Women's Representative and Project Coordinator for Gender Equality at Humboldt University Berlin.

Malika Ndlovu's words and productions have appeared on pages and stages across South Africa, in Austria, Uganda, the US, the UK, Holland, Ireland, Germany, Spain, Ethiopia, India and the Philippines. As a poet, playwright, performer and arts administrator Malika's contribution to South African arts and culture, via writing groups, numerous workshops, festivals and mentorship spans over twenty years. Her poetry collections include *Born in Africa But* (Van Schaik Publishers, 1999) *Womb to World: A Labour of Love* (self published, 2001), *Truth is both Spirit and Flesh* (LoTsha Publications, 2008), *Invisible Earthquake: A Woman's Journal through Stillbirth* (Modjaji Books, 2009), and *CLOSE* (Thousand Hands Press, 2017). Her published plays are *A Coloured Place* (Junkets Publisher, 1998) and Sister Breyani (Junkets Publisher, 2010).

Amrita Pande, author *of Wombs in Labor: Transnational Commercial Surrogacy in India* (Columbia University Press, 2014) is Associate Professor in the Sociology Department at University of Cape Town. Her research focuses on the intersection of globalisation and the intimate. Her work has appeared in *Signs: Journal of Women in Culture and Society, Gender and Society, Critical Social Policy, International Migration Review, Qualitative Sociology, Feminist Studies, Indian Journal of Gender Studies, Anthropologica, PhiloSO-PHIA, Reproductive Biomedicine* and in numerous edited volumes. She is also an educator-performer touring the world with a performance lecture series, *Made in India: Notes from a Baby Farm* based on her ethnographic work on surrogacy. She is currently writing a monograph on the 'global fertility flows', of eggs, sperms, embryos and wombs, connecting the world in unexpected ways.

Devika Prakash is a PhD candidate at KTH Royal Institute of Technology, Stockholm, Sweden. Her current research focuses on the intersection of infrastructure studies, urban digitalisation, and Science and Technology Studies (STS). She is particularly interested in postcolonial and feminist approaches within STS and the politics of knowledge production.

Mohan Rao was, until recently, a Professor at the Centre of Social Medicine and Community Health (CSMCH), School of Social Sciences, Jawaharlal Nehru University, New Delhi. A medical doctor specialising in public health, he has written extensively on health and population policy, and on the history and politics of health and family planning. He is the author of *From Population Control to Reproductive Health: Malthusian Arithmetic* (Sage, 2004) and has edited *Disinvesting in Health: The World Bank's Health Prescriptions* (Sage, 1999) and *The Unheard Scream: Reproductive Health and Women's Lives in India* (Zubaan/Kali for Women, 2004). He has edited, with Sarah Sexton of Cornerhouse, UK, the volume *Markets and Malthus: Population, Gender, and Health in Neo-liberal Times* (Sage, 2010). With Sarah Hodges, he has edited *Public Health and Private Wealth: Stem Cells, Surrogacy and Other Strategic Bodies* (Oxford University Press, 2016). His latest work is the edited volume *The Lineaments of Population Policy in India: Women and Family Planning* (Routledge, 2018). He has been a member of the National Population Commission, and several Working Groups of the National Rural Health Mission of the Government of India. He has worked on the Committee established by the National Human Rights Commission to examine the two-child norm in population policy. He is on the Executive Committee of the Centre for Women's Development Studies. He is also actively involved in the *Jan Swasthya Abhiyan* (People's Health Movement). He is currently an independent researcher based in Bangalore.

Deboleena Roy is Senior Associate Dean of Faculty for Emory College of Arts and Sciences and Professor of Neuroscience and Behavioral Biology (NBB) and Women's, Gender, and Sexuality Studies (WGSS) at Emory University. She also serves as Associate Faculty in the Neuroscience Program, Graduate Division of Biological and Biomedical Sciences at Emory. Roy received her PhD in reproductive neuroendocrinology and molecular biology from the Institute of Medical Science at the University of Toronto. Her research and teaching explore interdisciplinary exchanges between the natural sciences and humanities, and she has dedicated her career to creating new conversations between feminism, postcolonial studies, philosophy of science, reproductive justice, molecular biology, and neuroscience.

C. Sathyamala is a public health physician and an epidemiologist. Since the early 1980s, she has been active in both the health and women's movement in India. In 1982, she coordinated the first successful all India drug campaign against the Hormonal Pregnancy Tests (high fixed dose estrogen-progesterone combination drugs). She was one of the main architects of the case against the injectable contraceptive NET-EN (Norethisterone enanthate; Schering AG) filed in the Supreme Court of India, which questioned the safety of this contraceptive and raised ethical/legal concerns on human experimentation. As part of the initiative of the Medico Friend Circle and as an independent researcher, she coordinated two population based epidemiological studies on the people exposed to the toxic gases from the American Multinational Union Carbide Corporation factory in Bhopal, central India, in December 1984. She is a long term member of the Medico Friend Circle, an all India network of socially sensitive health professionals and worked as the editor of the organisation's bimonthly journal. She has authored and co-authored several books. She adapted David Werner's *Where There is No Doctor* for India (adaptation for India, New Delhi: Voluntary Health Association of India, 2014), co-authored *Taking Sides: The Choices Before the Health Worker* (Madras: Asian Network for Innovative Training Trust, 1984), a book on the political economy of health for field workers, internationally djudged as one of the top ten books in primary healthcare (see J. J. Macdonald (1987) 'Ten best books in ... primary health care', *Health Policy and Planning* 2:4, 352–4), authored *An Epidemiological Review of the Injectable Contraceptive, Depo-Provera* (Medico Friend Circle (Pune) and Forum for Women (Mumbai), 2000), co-edited *Securing Health for All: Dimensions and Challenges* (Institute for Human Development, 2006), and co-authored *From the Abnormal to the Normal: Preventing Sex Selective Abortions through the Law* (The Lawyers Collective, 2007).

Banu Subramaniam is Professor of Women, Gender, Sexuality Studies at the University of Massachusetts, Amherst. Trained as a plant evolutionary biologist, Banu engages the feminist studies of science in the practices of experimental biology. Author of *Holy Science: The Biopolitics of Hindu Nationalism* (University of Washington Press, 2019) and *Ghost Stories for Darwin: The Science of Variation* *and the Politics of Diversity* (University of Illinois Press, 2014), Banu's current work focuses on decolonising botany and the relationship of science and religious nationalism in India.

Suruchi Thapar-Björkert is docent and senior lecturer at the Department of Government, University of Uppsala (Sweden). She researches on gendered discourses of colonialism and nationalism, gendered violence and suburban vulnerabilities, ethnicity, social capital and social exclusion, empowerment and anti-poverty initiatives, transnational commercial surrogacy and qualitative feminist research methodologies. She has published widely in these research areas in journals such as *Ethnic and Racial Studies*, *NORA*, *Feminist Review*, *Feminist Theory*, *Sociological Review* and *Interventions*. She is the recipient of several research awards including the university research award (*Kraftpaket för Jämställdhet*) at Uppsala University in 2012. She is currently collaborating in the research project *From Waste to Profit: Gender, Biopolitics and Neoliberalism in Indian Commercial Surrogacy*, funded by the Swedish Research Council.

Foreword

Betsy Hartmann

This anthology on reproductive politics in India and South Africa is in the fine feminist tradition of international, interdisciplinary engaged feminist scholarship and activism. It pushes the boundaries of current understandings of the nexus between population policies, new forms of eugenics, assisted reproductive technologies, neoliberal markets, and persistent and perverse socio-economic, gender, and health disparities. It reveals the underlying structural violence that allows actual physical violence against women's bodies in healthcare settings in India and South Africa, and the global south more generally. Implicated are powerful state, international agency, and financial interests seeking to expand control over who can give birth and how.

The book arrives at a critical time. The COVID-19 pandemic, still raging in many global south countries as I write, has shone a stark light on the gross national and international inequalities that shape who lives and who dies, who receives life-saving treatment and vaccines and who is denied them. It has exposed the brutality and incompetence of right-wing ethnonationalist regimes as well. For example, India's tragic second surge of COVID deaths cannot be separated from Prime Minister Narendra Modi's Hindutva regime, quite literally in terms of the superspreading mass campaign rallies and Hindu festivals that he encouraged to take place.

The pandemic has also given rise to new iterations of populationism. Although 'population control' as a term has lost favour, populationism – blaming social and environmental ills on human numbers – is all too alive and well. Bhatia et al. (2019) identify the three main forms it takes. The first, *demopopulationism*, refers to the attempt to engineer human populations to achieve both 'optimal' population size and composition through curtailing the fertility of some and enhancing the fertility of others. The second, *geopopulationism*, entails the control of certain populations in terms of space and mobility. It produces specific geographies of displacement and containment and employs both direct and indirect forms of violence. Border walls, prisons, and the forced dispossession of poor communities by commercial agriculture, extractive industries, and special conservation zones are cases in point. The third, *biopopulationism*, is the enhancement of life itself through technoscientific means, including new reproductive and genetic technologies and services that are traded in global markets. Biopopulationism promotes a eugenic, neoliberal, and individualistic vision of the 'quality life'. Often these three forms of populationism work in tandem to reinforce each other.

In the present moment populationism has a pandemic twist. For some the virus is a Malthusian boon, a way to rid the world of 'surplus' population and thus save and cleanse the environment. Even if the racism is not overtly stated, the fact that black and brown people are dying in much higher numbers is treated as an inevitable if not welcome consequence. On the other side is an almost obsessive attention to the impact of covid on birth rates and women's fertility decisions, especially in the US, where the media is drumming up alarm about the economic effects of declining family size. Beneath the surface lurk fears that a shrinking, aging labour force may require more immigration.

Populationism frames the other global crisis, climate change, in similarly problematic ways. In many environmental circles, conventional wisdom holds that 'overpopulation' is a major cause of global warming and thus contraception is an important technology to mitigate it. The proponents of such views range from those who favour coercive means, such as one-child families, to more liberal approaches that call for individual self-regulated women to manage their sexuality and fertility voluntarily for the good of the planet (Sasser, 2018). Alongside these discourses are apocalyptic, highly racialised claims that climate change will set loose millions of dangerous climate refugees from the global south. Rather than staying in their own overpopulated countries, they will trespass northern borders and threaten 'our' security and way of life (Hartmann, 2017).

The double crises of climate change and the pandemic have produced a narrative about science with potential biopopulationist significance. To counter denial and inaction on both fronts, science has been popularised as a uniformly positive source of truth and technical fixes. For example, even though the pandemic calls into grave question neoliberal approaches to health, big pharma is often positioned as saviour of the day. This is not to downplay the important role of scientific research in producing life-saving medicines, vaccines and in the case of climate change, alternatives to fossil fuels, but to point out the dangers of reading science as Science writ large, ignoring its diversity of fields, practices, and ethical standards.

Unfortunately, this reification of science, if left unchallenged, could provide impetus for even more uncritical acceptance of the biomedical research and markets that presently drive selective reproduction and the control of births. This book offers a much needed counterpoint. Deftly combining theory, history, and on-site research at the clinical level, it provides a complex yet clear picture of reproductive injustices from population control, to obstetric violence, to the fertility industry's marketing of body parts. The comparative experiences of India and South Africa illustrate how powerful political and economic forces, nationally and globally, profit from and deepen inequalities of gender, race, caste, and class. The result is the further distortion and neglect of reproductive healthcare and the routinisation of violence against low-income women's bodies.

Editor Amrita Pande has done an excellent job organising the volume into three parts – Birth projects, Birth violated, and Birth assisted, which together form a coherent whole. Her introduction and first chapter provide the reader with an important historical overview of eugenics and population control and a theoretical framework with which to approach the ensuing chapters. As she writes in the introduction, '*Selective* reproduction has always been the cornerstone of national and global population campaigns, wherein eugenics and individual choice form an uneasy but convenient alliance around both anti-natalist and pro-natalist technologies and policies.' She also locates her analysis in the present moment, not only of the pandemic but of current anti-racist struggles that cast into sharp relief the ugly legacies of eugenics. In both its development through binational dialogue and the rich content that lies within, this book shows the value of international feminist solidarities in revealing and resisting reproductive injustice and violence. While we can take heart from the renewed strength of progressive social movements in many countries, the rise of the Far Right globally poses an enormous challenge. Defenders of present-day neoliberal eugenics often claim that the Nazi era of eugenics is long past and soundly discredited, and now the goal of selective reproduction is solely the enhancement of individual choice. But are we really so far from fascist and authoritarian applications of eugenics and population control? The forced sterilisations of Uighur women in Chinese concentration camps and India's mass repression of Muslim populations in Kashmir and Assam are but two examples of a frightening global trend.

This book shows us that in the face of reproductive violence of whatever kind, we should not stand idly by and watch.

References

Bhatia, R., Sasser, J. S., Ojeda, D., Hendrixson, A., Nadimpally, S., Foley, E. E. (2019). A feminist exploration of 'populationism': engaging contemporary forms of population control, *Gender, Place and Culture*, DOI:10.1080/0966369X.2018.1553859.

Hartmann, B. (2017). *The America Syndrome: Apocalypse, War and Our Call to Greatness*. New York: Seven Stories Press.

Sasser, J. S. (2018). *On Infertile Ground: Population Control and Women's Rights in the Era of Climate Change*. New York: New York University Press.

Editor's acknowledgement

An edited volume always has a life of its own. Most chapters in this volume were conceptualised in two, related, workshops – 'Reproductive Politics in India and South Africa' and 'New Reproduction and (Old) Stratifications' – that I organised at the University of Cape Town, South Africa in 2017 and 2018. I am grateful to the sixteen participants, who travelled across borders and continents to our tip of the African continent, for the passionate debates and discussions on reproductive justice and reproductive politics in South Africa and India. I am particularly grateful to those who contributed their work to this volume. Thank you for your commitment and engagement. The first workshop culminated in a public lecture 'Fertile Extractions: Women and Birth in the Global South', co-hosted by the Department of Sociology, African Gender Studies and Sexual and Reproductive Justice Coalition (SRJC). Thank you, Malika Ndlovu, South African feminist poet and performer, for pushing us beyond the comfort zone of academic dialogue and bringing the joy and tears of poetry, dance and movement to this project. A special thanks to Dr Jessica Rucell for her more than able assistance in brainstorming with me about the content and planning of the workshop, and to Tinashe Kushata for managing the logistics and budget. I would also like to thank the National Institute for the Humanities and Social Sciences (Grant: NIHSS/ICSSR201509) and the National Research Foundation (NRF) of South Africa (Grant 116345 & 118573) for generously funding the workshop and this research in such a way that we could include scholars and activists from India and other parts of South Africa. This book attests to the importance of funding transdisciplinary research, and the work and mobility of independent scholars and activists. The second workshop, part-funded by the NRF (grant 118573) and in part by the NIHSS-BRICS ThinkTank, focused specifically on the continuum of stratifications between technologies for population control and assisted fertility in the two countries. I would like to extend my thanks to the eight workshop participants for the two days of passionate dialogue and debate. A big thank you to Sepideh Azari for managing the complicated logistics of a transcontinental workshop with her usual charm, wit and camaraderie.

I am grateful to Thomas Dark, Humairaa Dudhwala and Lucy Burns, Manchester University Press, for their efficiency and generosity throughout the production process, series editors Srila Roy and Nicky Falkof for enthusiastically supporting the book proposal, and to the anonymous reviewers for their constructive comments. I express deep appreciation for Emma Arogundade's copy-editing skills. South Asian multidisciplinary artist Santosh Jain generously agreed to contribute her provocative and powerful artwork for the book cover. The artwork adds another affective dimension to the book. The artist's repertoire can be viewed at www.artbysantoshjain.com.

It is not customary to thank the family in edited volumes. Yet this book was written and compiled during a global pandemic, and without kin support we would have all floundered. So, thank you, cheers, chin-chin and sahtein:

To my Cape Town kin, Asanda Benya, Jasmina Brankovic, Ruchi Chaturvedi, Tracy Cook, Sumangala Damodaran, Shari Daya, Elena Moore, Ari Sitas and Rike Sitas, for their patience and generosity as I provided detailed updates of this book during our lockdown permitted runs and hikes.

To my family in Kingston: Ishita Pande and Chris Bongie for being my academic gurus (and for stocking the fridge with bubblies), and our Ishu, for frown-smiling at me and allowing me to sleep on the couch.

To Mataji and Papa for their enthusiastic praise for all my little achievements. Love and so much more. Ma and Baba, I made piglet say it for you.

To my daughter, Zaira (9) for asking astute and awkward questions about contraception and eugenics, and Sanaa (4), for piling inspirational artwork on my desk.

Always last to be thanked, the one and only, Adi Kumar:
For providing love, guidance, and nurturance like no man can
A salute, a bow and a double dose of Sam I am.

Prologue

Malika Ndlovu

In the sanctuary of my body
Under the cover of my ancestral skin
Within the layers of my womb
A sacred potential, inherent power
Innate possibility, a voice from my core
Is silenced, its story twisted
Manipulated, coerced or erased

Swinging the breadth of a pendulum
Between the right to exist, to belong
A packaged choice to give life, let live, let die
Where natural, economical and technological drives
Meeting ancient yet still morphing narratives
Of gene, bone, of worthiness or kin, are excavated
For contextual, demographical, political purpose

Sold as population strategy, essential industry
Ecological solution, bio-scientific evolution
In the soil of my own birthplace, right here in this body
I am made alien, violated, told I am being liberated
Under the penetrating glare of clinical or statistical light
In my most intimate of rituals, I am deprived of the right
To have, to hold, to decide, to reclaim, to breathe, to be

Introduction

Amrita Pande

In 2020, as I started compiling this edited volume, Black Lives Matter protesters, following the killing of George Floyd, toppled confederate statues across the US. In South Africa, the Rhodes Must Fall movement, which started with a student activist emptying a bucket of human faeces on a statue of Cecil John Rhodes, continued with the beheading of another Rhodes statue and the removal of other colonial and apartheid symbols. At Cambridge University, an as historic, but far less dramatic, removal took place with students demanding that a commemorative window, in honour of geneticist and evolutionary biologist Ronald Aylmer Fisher be removed because of Fisher's 'endorsements of colonialism, white supremacy and eugenics' (Donlon-Mansbridge, 2020). Fisher was a practising eugenicist, a firm believer in the intertwining of evolutionary biology and politics, and a proponent of breeding for genetic superiority (Johnson, 2020). Fisher was inspired by Charles Darwin's theory of evolution by natural selection but was far more unambiguous about the exact mechanisms of heredity. Yet another eugenicist believer is Darwin's cousin and the now controversial, Francis Galton. The cousins influenced each other in the founding of origin of the species, eugenics and selective breeding. When supporters of these, once iconic, scientists tussle with protestors over whether they were racists or not (Coyne, 2021; Roberts, 2020), they overlook the critical point that eugenics and selective reproduction have always underlined theories that surmise the limits of population. Darwin and Galton, for instance, were also keenly influenced by the work of the classic population pessimist Thomas Malthus and his eighteenth-century essay on the 'Principle of Population'. Although many critical scholars have since debunked Malthusian concerns connecting population to poverty, the 'Malthus effect' continues to shape contemporary debates and policies around reproduction, especially in and for the global south (Connelly, 2008; Rao and Sexton, 2010).

The connection between economic prosperity and population, and hence reproduction, may well be proven scientifically tenuous, yet it has inspired a long history of blatant and 'back door' eugenics (Duster, 2003). Early twentieth-century state-sponsored eugenic projects, based on assumptions of biological difference, attempted to manage futures by encouraging and/or preventing desirable and undesirable traits, and were notorious for their violent and blatant racism (Murphy, 2017). As the language of differential human evolution and racial biological inferiority became politically untenable, the focus shifted to more 'unconventional eugenics', where (racialised) bodies could be assigned differential worth based on their assumed economic potential. In the second half of the twentieth century, biologists' framing of differential and heritable traits amongst individuals from different races conveniently morphed into economists' calculations of surplus populations and disposable lives, particularly in the global south. Well-funded calculations about 'averted birth' announced that, for most countries in the global south, the worth of every child born is negative for the national economy (Murphy, 2017: 47). The violent racism of earlier decades morphed into violent control over women's bodies. National and global concerns about rapid population growth in the global south led to programmes that were singularly focused on reducing birth rates, and women became the primary site of intervention. What was remarkable about this new form of global racism and selective reproduction was not just its scale, but also its ability to target and manipulate entire populations, and at the same time make invisible the end users – the women in the global south who had been coerced and/or induced into accept long-term injectables, contraceptives, and irreversible methods of sterilisation (Chatterjee and Riley, 2001; Murphy, 2017).

In the twenty-first century, eugenics took another interesting turn – what some scholars have optimistically labelled grassroots eugenics (Tober, 2019) and liberal eugenics (Agar, 2004) – a new era of biopolitics led by individual consumer choice, which is assumed to be innocuous and starkly different from the race-based eugenics of the past. For example, in the book *Politics of Life Itself*, Nikolas Rose (2007) asserts that there is a concise break in the eugenic tendencies of the first four decades of the twentieth century and what we are witnessing in contemporary biopolitics. The term liberal eugenics is an attempt to shift focus from the usual, often negative, interpretations of biopolitics to a more life-affirming version, with a firm belief in a 'new regime of self' wherein prudent and enterprising individuals are expected to take greater responsibility towards the biological by making the right choices (Rose, 2007, 2009). The shift from a focus on the state to the individual is fundamental to the argument being made. While genetic make-up of the population still remains a political concern, Rose (2007: 69) argues, political obsession with race-based enhancements, and negative eugenics, is a thing of the past, or of countries with 'different rationalities'. The way forward, for Rose (2007) and the scholars of liberal eugenics, is to envision reproductive selection as an *individual, voluntary* and *state neutral* practice. Liberal eugenics scholars urge us to seek a balance between private freedom and public welfare to make the most of the benefits of having genetic science and technologies to improve the health of our populations. In sum, the belief is that with good science, good ethics, and a neutral state, individuals will choose to pursue both private and public good without coercion or abuse (Russell, 2018). But are these practices, modes, and technologies of selective reproduction that we witness today merely a reflection of individual autonomy and choice? This book looks at the history and presence of eugenics and its interactions with the various practices, modes, and technologies that allow selective reproductions. In the use of the term selective reproduction we go beyond the more recent biomedical definition that limits it to technologies, for instance, selective abortion, prenatal genetic diagnosis in vitro fertilisation (Wahlberg and Gammeltoft, 2018). We use the term to refer to any intervention that influences reproductive outcomes and allows only some pregnancies to be borne to fruition. Although selective reproduction is not new and has been observed for decades, we live in an ostensibly 'post population control' world, with lowered total fertility worldwide. Given this reality, we ask the following specific questions. Is the international campaign to control birth over? Is selective reproduction, and the managing of reproductive futures, an individual choice, unhindered by state control and notions of eugenics?

The premise is that as fertility rates decline worldwide, the fervour to control fertility, and fertile bodies, does not dissipate; what evolves is the preferred mode of control. Although new technologies, for instance those that assist conception and/or allow genetic selection, may appear to be an antithesis of the violent versions of population control, both are part of the same continuum and need to be unpacked as such in order to understand their mechanics and effects on existing structures of stratification, based on gender, race, class, and caste. Much like all population control policies target and vilify (Black) women for their over-fertility, and coerce/induce them into subjecting their bodies to state and medical surveillance, assisted reproductive technologies (ARTs) and repro-genetic technologies have a similar gendered and racialised burden of blame and responsibility (Pande, 2014; Pande and Moll, 2018). These practices, instead of being mere reflections of individual autonomy and choice, are shaped by, and embedded within, power relations. The focus on intimacy and privacy of choices around kinship, familial and racial identity depoliticises questions of inequalities, based on race, class, caste, and gender and nationality.

To empirically and historically ground the analysis, this volume gathers together chapters on two postcolonial nations, South Africa and India, where the history of colonialism and the economics of neoliberal markets allow for some parallel moments of selecting who gets to legitimately reproduce the future. The chapters have grown from presentations at two related workshops at University of Cape Town, South Africa in 2017 and 2018. In the first workshop, we discussed and highlighted the common grounds in reproductive politics in South Africa and India. The second workshop, which focused specifically on the continuum of stratifications between technologies for population control and assisted fertility, connected emerging forms of repro-genetic technologies in the two countries to broader questions of politics, (repro)nationalism and belonging. The discussions for this publication have evolved since these initial workshops. These, along with some commissioned work, aim to offer new directions for thinking about selective reproduction and the modes of controlling birth.

This volume emerges from an interdisciplinary dialogue around the critical issues that shape current reproductive politics in the two countries. While the literature around population control and global governance is rich and interdisciplinary, the conversations have not made the necessary connections to other forms of interconnected birth projects that are shaped by global politics. The contributors bring their disciplinary foci, ranging from gender studies, sociology, medical anthropology, politics, science and technology studies (STS), to theology, public health, epidemiology, women's health, and performance studies, with the aim of facilitating an interdisciplinary dialogue around the interconnected modes of controlling birth in the global south. The domain of reproductive research and policy making is enmeshed in the hierarchies of knowledge production – between patients/consumers, experts (scientists and academics), civil society, and the state. By bringing together this diverse group of feminist scholars and activists, the book attempts to address some glaring gaps in the existing debates: a disjunction between academic and activist conversations, international policy making and local realities, as well as between disciplines.

The entanglements between biology and politics are central to each contribution and bind together Part I of the volume – Birth projects. The first chapter provides a brief overview of the birth projects underlying each of the contributions that follow. I specifically analyse three such birth projects – population control, reproductive violence, and assisted reproduction – in these two countries. These three modes of controlling birth continue to connect the volume thematically. This chapter provides context to the rest of the volume but, just as critically, underlines the main argument – that *selective* reproduction has always been the cornerstone of national and global population campaigns, wherein eugenics and individual choice form an uneasy but convenient alliance around both anti-natalist and pro-natalist technologies and policies. In the next piece, science and technology studies (STS) scholars Sushmita Chatterjee, Deboleena Roy, and Banu Subramaniam focus on how such birth projects are unfolding in a Hindu nationalist state. In this dialogic piece they attempt to decolonise their disciplines, and the descriptions of biopolitics in South Asia, which remain largely western and Euro-centric. Mohanka continues this process of decolonising the theoretical entanglements of biology and politics in the South Asian context by analysing nationalist projects, which deploy non-biomedical Ayurvedic procedures to allegedly reproduce desirable biogenetic and phenotypic characteristics in the future generation to serve the project of Hindutva nation-building. While Mohanka analyses eugenics through Ayurveda, in the next contribution Prakash examines ways in which genetic evidence and DNA have been mobilised by the Hindutva state in India to classify certain populations as superior and 'indigenous' in order to create arguments against those who 'do not belong'. This chapter extends our dialogue around biomedicalisation of reproduction to the biomedicalisation of national belonging. We close Part I with South African theologian Kotzé's chapter, which brings her disciplinary perspectives to demonstrate the importance of the Universal Declaration on Bioethics and Human Rights in understanding questions of biopower and its intersections with vulnerability, justice and right to belong.

The next part of the book features works that represent new takes on violent modes of controlling birth. The chapters are each about forms of violence that women experience due to stratified access to reproductive healthcare. In the first chapter of Part II, Sathyamala, a veteran member of the health and women's movement in India, writes about the active promotion of inherently hazardous and life-threatening anti-natal technologies by the state as an indication of the reversal from a biopolitical project of 'letting die' to one of 'making die'. In a paradoxical interplay with Sathyamala's focus on forced contraceptives imposed on low-income women in India, Batisai highlights the violence experienced by young Black women in southern Africa due to *limited* access to contraceptives and legal reproductive health services. In the next chapter, Chadwick asks 'whether a vocabulary rooted predominantly in a critique of medicalised birth and technology is sufficient to theorise the systemic, normative, and multidimensional violence associated with birthing under global racial capitalism'. In conversation with Chadwick's reflections on the usefulness of the term obstetric violence in South African contexts, Chattopadhyay interrogates the utility of the term in the Indian context using ethnographic insights from two geographically distinct areas of India.

Part III offers an array of critical engagements with ARTs, with particular focus on the stratifications and new forms of eugenics that are emerging in the fertility market. Mukherjee explores how commercial egg provision is organised in unregulated fertility markets in India and the implications this has for the egg providers to take ownership of their bodily labour. In the next chapter, Gondouin,

Thapar-Björkert, and Rao draw on interviews with Dalit feminists to highlight the tensions within Indian feminist discourses on reproductive technologies, reproductive labour, rights and justice. Namberger draws on her ethnography of the South African egg provision market to highlight the new forms of eugenics emerging in the global business around fertility-related services, often couched in the positive frame of choice. In the next set of chapters, Moll and Moyo explore the racialisation of the South African egg provision market. While Moll highlights how the egg providers situate themselves within markets that commodify and racialise their reproductive tissues, Moyo argues that the desire for racial matching, by agencies and recipients, and the routinised reinscription of race is a clear indication of neo-eugenics.

As I write this introduction, the COVID-19 pandemic rages on, wreaking havoc in all parts of the world, through its various strains and surges. It highlights the biosocial nature of such diseases and their contagion and exposes the inadequacies of and inequities within global healthcare systems. While the pandemic has been labelled an 'equaliser' – no one is immune to the virus – the reality is that it has disproportionately affected the poor. Much like other epidemic diseases, for instance HIV-AIDS, tuberculosis, and Ebola, the structural violence of this pandemic cannot go unnoticed, wherein the deleterious effects are not just of the virus on an individual, but its interaction with poverty, discrimination, marginalisation, and lack of access for particular communities to basic resources (Farmer, 2003). At the same time, the pandemic intensifies related debates around the politics of belonging with recurring incidents of migrant and refugees finding themselves stranded during pandemic emergencies due to their non-citizenship, and the onset of what is being labelled vaccine nationalism. The COVID-19 pandemic and the consequent structural violence brings up questions of belonging and right to exist, much like the tensions raised by several contribution in the parallel sphere of reproductive justice and right to exist.

With the pandemic, we are witnessing an extraordinary event and global experiment, a kind of 'perfect storm' for us to reflect on the world order. With her metaphor 'pandemic as a portal', Arundhati Roy (2020) talks of the current situation as a gateway between one world and the next, as the virus brings 'the engine of capitalism to a juddering halt', it exposes the fault lines of our systems. In this so-called 'war zone', the healthcare and essential workers in farms, mines, shops become soldiers and martyrs, and war becomes a convenient metaphor for capitalism's lack of care, where debilitating demands can be made on workers without an ounce of reciprocity, collateral damage in a perennial war zone. War allows for tanks, rubber bullets, surveillance, and policing of lockdowns, in countries like India and South Africa, to be prioritised over provision of healthcare, basic income grants, and food security (Ramushu, 2020). The war metaphor also makes invisible the fact that the majority of pandemic 'warriors', whether healthcare workers, nurses, sanitary workers, farm workers, teachers, or parents, are not 'masculine' soldiers but women. It exposes not just the deficiencies of the market and state systems but affirms that these deficient systems have been limping along because of the unpaid and unrecognised labour of women. The pandemic is being written down in history as a crisis in capitalism and production, but in all its true colours, it is ultimately a crisis of social reproduction (Fraser, 2017).

Unarguably, the burden of the pandemic is gendered. How does the pandemic affect our world of (stratified) reproduction? As the virus spreads, governments and professionals are forced to ask: 'Is assisted reproduction an essential service?' In March 2020, the American Society for Reproductive Medicine (ASRM) and the European Society for Human Reproduction and Embryology, its European counterpart, the world's leading bodies in the field of reproductive medicine, recommended stopping all new fertility treatment. This did not go unchallenged by either investors or clients of such services. A public petition with thousands of signatories asked the ASRM to reconsider its recommendations, and the New York Department of Health issued guidance to explicitly include these treatments as essential. South Africa witnessed a similar trajectory. In 2020, the professional body in South Africa, SASREG issued guidelines suspending all non-urgent fertility treatments but a few weeks later published a legal opinion allowing new fertility treatments for almost all categories of patients, in essence classifying fertility treatment as an essential service. Apart from the very pragmatic question as to whether one should pursue any kind of treatment that is not life threatening when there is a deadly virus making its rounds, there are other ethical dilemmas. For instance, should we be diverting resources towards fertility treatments during a pandemic that threatens to be debilitating for health infrastructures in all parts of the world? One can argue that fertility treatment, especially in the global south and countries like India and South Africa, falls primarily under private healthcare, with minimal investments by the government, and hence anxieties around diverted public resources are unfounded. But any argument built on the public/private binary underplays the overlaps between the two, and the ways in which private healthcare is subsidised by the government in these two countries. Such treatments are affecting critical and scarce resources, which include: personal protective equipment such as masks and gloves; hospital beds; operating rooms; and the time, and effort, of physicians and support staff – all of which could be meaningfully diverted towards emergency care (Pande, 2020).

These dilemmas go beyond the pandemic context, especially in countries with limited resources and many competing (reproductive) health priorities. For instance, what are the social consequences of classifying infertility as a disease? On the one hand, in India and South Africa, where the burden of 'failed fertility' falls almost exclusively on women and causes extreme socio-psychological and even physical harm, recognising infertility as a treatable problem may reduce the gendered stigma. But on the other hand, does the prevailing setting of offering high cost and high-tech fixes, primarily via private healthcare, even meet this 'essential' need? The causes of infertility (especially among low-income and Black women), such as sexually transmitted infections, poor medical treatment during an earlier birth/abortion, or workplace and environmental toxins require relatively affordable preventable measures rather than the ex-post facto technological interventions that such patients cannot afford.

What the pandemic is forcing us to ask is this: can we continue to legitimise the investments in cutting-edge technology and five-star luxury fertility clinics when our reproductive health sector is riddled with systemic inequalities and violence? Can we justify ARTs as essential if they continue to serve just a privileged few? Can we continue to look for individual-based biomedical solutions to these 'diseases' when our health system is in a permanent state of crisis? This is the perfect storm to challenge the neoliberal approach to reproductive healthcare, where individually accessed technological solutions have effectively depoliticised structural inequalities. This volume, much like the pandemic, provides us with the prism to reflect on what and who is deemed 'essential', and at what cost.

References

Agar, N. (2004). *Liberal Eugenics: In Defense of Human Enhancement*. Malden, MA: Blackwell Publishing.

Chatterjee, N. and Riley, N. E. (2001). Planning an Indian modernity: the gendered politics of fertility control, *Signs* 26:3, 811–45.

Coyne, J. (2021). Assessing Ronald Fisher: should we take his name off everything because he espoused eugenics? 18 January, 2021. https://whyevolutionistrue.com/2021/01/18/assessing-ronald-fisher-should-we-take-his-name-off-everything-because-he-espoused-eugenics/. Accessed 17 November 2021.

Donlon-Mansbridge, L. (2020). Remove the window in honour of R. A. Fisher at Gonville and Caius, University of Cambridge. www.change.org/p/gonville-and-caius-college-remove-the-window-in-honour-of-ronald-aylmer-fisher-in-gonville-and-caius-hall. Accessed 17 November 2021.

Duster, T. (2003). *Backdoor to Eugenics*. 2nd ed. London: Routledge.

Farmer P. (2003). *Pathologies of Power: Structural Violence and the Assault on Human Rights*. Berkeley, CA: University of California Press.

Johnson, E. M. (2020). Ronald Fisher is not Being 'Cancelled', but his Eugenic Advocacy Should Have Consequences. https://thisviewoflife.com/ronald-fisher-is-not-being-cancelled-but-his-eugenic-advocacy-should-have-consequences/#_ftnref9. Accessed 17 November 2021.

Murphy, M. (2017). *The Economization of Life*. Durham, NC: Duke University Press.

Pande, A. (2014). *Wombs in Labor: Transnational Commercial Surrogacy in India*. New York: Columbia University Press.

Pande, A. (2020). Are surrogate and IVF babies 'essential' in a pandemic? *Mail and Guardian*, 22 May. https://mg.co.za/coronavirus-essentials/2020-05-22-ivf-surrogacy-south-africa-race-class/. Accessed 17 November 2021.

Pande, A. and Moll, T. (2018). Gendered bio-responsibilities and travelling egg providers from South Africa, *Reproductive Biomedicine & Society Online* 6, 23–33.

Ramushu, K. (2020). Feminise the pandemic: covid-19 and gender inequality in South Africa. www.coronatimes.net/feminising-the-pandemic-covid-19-hypermasculinity/. Accessed 17 November 2021.

Rao, M. and Sexton, S. (2010). *Markets and Malthus: Population, Gender, and Health in Neo-liberal Times*. New Delhi: Sage Publications India.

Roberts, P. C. (2021). Western civilization has surrendered to barbarians. TheAltWorld.com, 12 October 2020. https://thealtworld.com/paul_craig_roberts/western-civilization-has-surrendered-to-barbarians. Accessed 29 November 2021.

Rose, N. (2007). *A Politics of Life Itself*. Princeton, NJ: Princeton University Press.

Roy, A. (2020). The pandemic as portal. www.ft.com/content/10d8f5e8-74eb-11ea-95fe-fcd274e920ca. Accessed 17 November 2021.

Russell, C. (2018). *The Assisted Reproduction of Race*. Bloomington: Indiana University Press.

Tober, D. (2019). *Romancing the Sperm: Shifting Biopolitics and the Making of Modern Families*. New Brunswick, NJ: Rutgers University Press.

Part I

Birth projects

1

Birth projects, selective reproduction and neoliberal eugenics

Amrita Pande

See Taj Mahal by the moonlight while your embryo grows in a petri-dish. (A reproductive travel website, India, 2006)

The young doctor doesn't remember the first time he slapped someone in the [public] labour room [in Kolkata, India]. Everyone slaps patients, all his MBBS classmates did, and the postgraduate students do, too. It is almost a rite of passage. 'There was one guy, he was so shy. He never lost his cool. The day he slapped his first patient, that was an event. We made him treat us to biryani,' he chuckles. (Chattopadhyay, 2015)

South Africa, for a variety of reasons, especially its stratified health care and racial composition of the population, has emerged as a node for global egg provision in the Global South. (Pande and Moll, 2018)

[In South Africa] The routine administration of injectable contraceptives immediately following childbirth has resulted in them being referred to facetiously as the fourth stage of labor. (de Gruchy and Baldwin, 2005)

Social scientists have convincingly demonstrated that population control and related matters have never been restricted to biomedical interventions or patient–doctor relationships. They have always been deeply political. In his seminal work, *Fatal Misconception*, Mathew Connelly surmises that the global campaign for population control, although not a conspiracy theory, is a neo-colonial attempt to control the world, 'a transnational network of population experts taking over where the empires left off (2008: 11). What are these neo-colonial projects that attempt to control the world? What shape do these projects take in an era where population control has become a taboo phrase in policy making? This chapter draws on the concept of birth projects to demonstrate that as fertility rates decline worldwide, the fervour to control birthing bodies, especially of low-income and Black women in the global south, does not dissipate. The twentieth-century top-down population control projects, embedded in state propaganda and policies, were easily identifiable because of their starkness and brutality. What we have today are birth projects that are diffuse and couched in the frame of individual choice, which absolve the state of its responsibility. These neo-eugenic birth projects are based on a subtle form of eugenics that depoliticises issues and justifies systemic inequalities by couching them in the frame of choice. The following sections compare the history and presence of population control policies in South Africa and India to two other modes of delimiting the fertility of a certain demography – that of obstetric violence and to emerging repro-genetic technologies.

I argue that forced contraceptive, limiting (legal) access to contraceptive, exposing women to violence during pregnancy and birthing, and the inherent stratifications of new repro-genetic technologies, although seemingly contrasting, belong to the same neo-eugenic continuum.

Population control in India and South Africa

India has been declared the 'first' in many aspects of the global campaign for population control. It attracted the first sustained efforts by British and American birth control activists to establish clinics abroad. It invited the first United Nations advisory missions in demography and family planning. It hosted the funding conference of the International Planned Parenthood Federation, and together with Bangladesh and Sri Lanka, the Indian subcontinent was the testing grounds for new contraceptive techniques as well as the recipient for an outpouring of international assistance around the same. The population 'problem' of India had become a colonial focus as early as the nineteenth century, in effect, before any real data existed to establish population growth (Rao, 2004a). This colonial anxiety had enthusiastic support from the Indian elite. The National Planning Commission (NPC), established by the Indian National Congress, framed birth control as a way to keep the reproductive machinery 'fresh and vitalized' for a healthy nation, as well as to advocate for an explicitly eugenic programme that ensured a physically and mentally healthy race (NPC 1948, quoted in Rao, 2004b: 20). As expected, the burden of this imagined healthy state fell on the shoulders of Indian women. The Indian woman was the primary target of nationalist reformist agendas such as the population control campaigns, partly because 'archaic' practices like *sati*, child marriage and polygamy had been used by British colonisers to legitimise their civilising mission. But 'modernity' needed to be defined cautiously. The modern Indian woman had to be distinguished, not only from the archaic woman but also from the westernised, 'individualistic' woman. This is what Nilanjana Chatterjee and Nancy E. Riley (2001: 819) call the 'nationalist leadership's selective appropriation of modernity'. For instance, nationalist reformers and activists supported the use of contraception for improving maternal and child health and not as a means to greater female autonomy. Autonomy was seen as a 'distinctly Western notion and therefore not necessarily desirable' (Chatterjee and Riley, 2001: 821).

This continues to be the underlying philosophy of the government's agenda, which frames its anti-natalist policy as 'family welfare planning'. Such framing avoids the association of contraceptive use with so-called western notions of sexual freedom and autonomy and at the same time reaffirms the state's initiative in upholding the 'traditional' institution of the family (Pande, 2014). Post-independence, India became the first country to have an official population control programme. Unlike China, the democratic state of India had to maintain its liberal stance, but these liberal principles have been constantly eroded by numerical targets, financial (dis)incentives, and sometimes aggressive promotion of sterilisation (Ram, 2001). In general, the sterilisation programme was implemented with coercion and, not surprisingly, the illiterate, economically disadvantaged, Dalits and members of other disadvantaged castes, and Muslims were the primary targets (Karkal, 1998).

While the population control policies had caste, religious and ethnic underpinnings in India, in South Africa the conversation around population control is deeply embedded in racial politics and apartheid policies. But, much as the chequered history of contraception in India does not start and end with the British impetus, the history of birth control in South Africa starts before the National Party's (NP – Afrikaner ethnic nationalist party that designed and implemented the apartheid state) preoccupation with apartheid and population control. An emphasis on selective reproduction, by race and class, can be observed as early as the 1930s, and during the time of the Great Depression. The starkness of these programmes of (selective) birth control allows comparisons between birth control and other instances of reproductive violence. In the 1930s, a eugenic take on population control influenced one set of policy makers to take policy measures of a surprising, racialised nature – targeting the population of low-income whites in urban areas in order to prevent a 'national decline of the entire white race' (Klausen, 2004). Although such eugenicists (for instance, the Race Welfare Society) were responsible for the first birth control clinics, they were not as successful as the 'maternalists', mostly middle-class and elite anglophone white women troubled by the high mortality rates related to botched abortions amongst low-income white women, but also the threat this posed to 'white prestige' in South Africa (Stoler, 2002). Though the concerns of the two differed, they were, in effect, together in the campaign for white supremacy and a modern white nation. The campaign to increase access to birth control was to prevent poverty amongst white people, with little regard for the poverty simultaneously being imposed on Black South Africans.

With the NP and the apartheid state, there was a shift in population control policies, with the singular focus of limiting the population of Black South Africans. The fertility of Black South Africans was unambiguously portrayed as a problem and a threat to white dominance. The policy efforts to curb population growth went hand in hand with the promotion of a white South Africa. Even without an official population control programme targeting the Black population, the agenda of a white South Africa was maintained through other related policies, for instance encouraging large white families and white immigration, sometimes through active recruitment and at other times though government subsidies to white immigrants (Brown, 1987). In its blatant form, the NP made free contraception (and hardly any other reproductive health service) available to Black women, sometimes in coercive ways, so as to curb the growth of their families (Klausen, 2004). For instance, controversial hormonal long-acting contraceptives, like the Depo Provera injections, were made freely available to the Black population (Gruchy and Baldwin, 2005). While in India the feminist and women's health movement were able to prevent the government from including Depo Provera in its contraceptive programme because of its dangerous side-effects (see Chapter 6, this volume), this long-term contraceptive continues to be promoted by the government in South Africa. Although these attempts were a clear indication of the state's priority, an overt official population programme was avoided, in part because the apartheid state was convinced that the Black population was not 'sufficiently developed' to use contraceptives and, in part, to avoid any accusations of racially motivated population control (Kaufman, 1996). To avoid any political backlash, the government chose to increase funding to non-governmental Family Planning Associations instead. It was only in 1974 that a formal state-run family planning programme was announced, which was given top priority and allocated an ever-increasing budget, despite far more critical and competing reproductive health needs.

Although race and eugenics have always been central to the provision of contraception in South Africa, this national imperative has been greatly abetted by an international agenda that provided legitimacy to even the most oppressive measures of contraceptive provisions in the global south. In effect, even though population control programmes may have their distinct local trajectories in India and South Africa, they cannot be discussed merely as nationalist agendas. The population control movement has been recognised as one of the most unprecedented global campaigns, underlined by two, often contradictory, philosophies – of nation states in competition (or the survival of the fittest) on the one hand, and the notions of social responsibility and global family, on the other. In fact, many of the leaders of the population control movement, for instance Annie Besant and Margaret Sanger, did not identify themselves in national terms; the slogan of population control was embedded in philosophies of a global family and of responsibility towards humankind. This had resonance with the eugenicists, who believed themselves to be of 'a secular religion, a faith handed down to save humanity from degeneration' (Connelly, 2008: 13). But eugenicists and Malthusians were not always on the same side. The history of their slow (and sometimes reluctant) alliance over the global population control campaign is critical for understanding the connections between the birth projects highlighted in this chapter and the rest of the volume. For instance, early national eugenicist organisations attacked Malthusians for 'endangering the future of the supreme race' or what was colourfully labelled 'race suicide' (Connelly, 2008: 43). While eugenicists and some Malthusians, like Annie Besant, agreed on the need to reduce the fertility of the unfit, they disagreed on the need for the fit to control their fertility. The inter-war period of the 1920s and 1930s saw a move towards reconciliation of this relationship between birth control and eugenics by emphasising selective birth control. The first Rockefeller-funded study in 1927 made this distinction clear by developing contraceptive measures that could be accessed by 'the wife of the slum dweller, the peasant or the coolie, though dull of mind' and Margaret Sanger called for 'constructive birth control' which promised 'to fill the comfortable cradles and empty the gutters' (quoted in Connelly, 2008: 61). Interestingly, one of the only factors to have consistently been correlated with lower fertility rates is women's education, but little effort has ever been made to invest in women's education. Instead, the convenient solution has been to promote simple and cheaper contraceptives to the uneducated, especially those that do not require the cooperation of individuals – methods adapted to the so-called 'dullest of minds'.

Although one might have expected that the mass genocide caused by Nazi eugenics would put an end to selective reproductive policies, there was instead a post-war resurgence of the population campaign with the involvement of United Nations agencies, which effectively established a direct connection between population campaigns and global governance. Now, small family size was to be imposed not just on poorer families but also poorer nations, through media, education and even food aid. The post-war population movement was shaped by a group of public and private organisations including the Rockefeller Foundation, the Population Council, the US Agency for International Development (USAID), the United Nations Population Fund and the World Bank. These foundations not only invested in fertility control programmes in countries like South Africa and India but also in the training of administrators and students in these countries (Chatterjee and Riley, 2001). This was also the time when anti-colonial movements in Asia and Africa had started revealing the instability of colonial rule. Demographers connected population growth in the colonies to independence movements and fuelled the fear that rapid population growth was an imminent sign of these colonies posing a threat to the global order. As the debate about 'population quality' broadened, eugenics shifted from more blatant negative eugenics to more politically savvy forms, for instance reform eugenics, the successful manipulation of that segment of society that is unfit for parenthood (Connelly, 2008: 106). There was a concomitant shift in the language of reproductive policy making, and a move away from population control to family planning. The more comprehensive slogan of 'family planning', where each child is a wanted child, was adopted quickly by governments as an antidote to the rising discontent with the campaign that explicitly emphasised 'control'. However, family planning was not that different from population control – it just gave poor nations and poor people the illusion that they were choosing and planning their families, while their preferences were actively being shaped through incentives and disincentives. As Sathyamala argues in Chapter 6 below, the active promotion of anti-natal technologies such as the long-acting injectable contraceptives, though built around notions of reproductive choice and freedom, in fact indicates the biopolitical intention of 'making die' at the national and global level. The legacy of the global population control campaign outlined above is to produce an unwavering image, whether in media, popular discourses or our popular imaginations: of Black (and Brown) women as recklessly reproductive and to blame for not just their own poverty but that of their families and their nations.

Reproductive violence in India and South Africa

The official justification for much of the global campaign around population control has been women's right to choose and have control over their reproductive options. Much of the history outlined above indicates that, in many parts of the world, the consequences might well have been the exact opposite. This paradoxical interplay of choice and coercion are as stark in the second mode analysed in this volume, that of 'reproductive violence'. Scholars and activists have used a range of terms – birth violence, reproductive violence, and most recently obstetric violence – to capture the many kinds of violence faced by women while giving birth. These include a host of dehumanising physical, psychological and health-access related practices that affect pregnant women and women giving birth, verbal and physically violent acts like slapping women in labour, non-consensual contracepting, and unnecessary medical interventions such as caesarean sections. Reproductive violence, in turn, contributes to maternal and neonatal deaths, as well as the short and long-term illnesses women suffer relating to pregnancy and childbirth. According to the World Health Organization (WHO, 2019) the rate of a woman's risk of maternal death is twenty-seven times higher in so-called developing compared to developed countries. The maternal mortality rate (MMR) in South Africa rose dramatically after 1998 (because of the HIV epidemic) and although it has been declining steadily in India, it still accounts for 17% of the burden of global maternal deaths (WHO, 2014). The conversations around reproductive violence cannot merely be about statistics, however alarming these statistics may be, but need to be connected to debates around state policies, private and public healthcare systems and the power and vulnerabilities embedded in birth and delivery. As Shabot (2016: 231) has convincingly argued, obstetric violence is gendered and embodied violence, 'directed at women because they are women'. Violence against women while they give birth is an effective gendered mechanism of disciplining bodies of women when they are closest to nature and hence most threatening. But is reproductive violence just a manifestation of *gendered* forms of power?

The term obstetric violence might be new but discussions about birth violence have been going on for decades. In fact, in the North American context, birth activism in the 1950s was a direct response to such violence, which was often associated with the medicalisation of childbirth. In the 1950s, an article titled 'Cruelty in maternity wards' had nurses and women expose the horrific and inhumane treatment of women during childbirth (Schulz, 1958). As the world heard stories about a labouring woman being tied down while her doctor ate dinner, and of a doctor administering episiotomies without anaesthetic while a nurse stifled the birthing woman's cries with a mask, there was outrage, activism and demands for birth reforms. As a response to this violent biomedical model of birth, Euro-American birth activists advocated for a return to a more natural, and woman-centred experience of birth. They argued that technological interventions serve primarily to shift control over the birth process from the mother to the (often male) doctor. This argument, although profoundly critical, emerges from a specific socio-cultural context and can be traced back to the Enlightenment era, where female midwives gradually came to be replaced by male doctors (Davis-Floyd, 1990; Van Hollen, 2003). Pregnant women were constructed as potentially pathological and as 'patients' who needed constant surveillance. But, as southern scholars and activists have recently demonstrated, this narrative of reproductive violence is predominantly a white middle-class northern-centric one (see Chapters 8 and 9, this volume). While white women in the north might have been forced towards biomedicalised birth, often by male doctors, the history of reproductive injustices in the global south is quite the contrary. Reproductive experiences and reproductive violence need to be unpacked and analysed in very different terms in the southern contexts of India and South Africa, with an understanding of how gendered forms of power intersect with other axes of power, for instance race, class, caste and religion.

In late nineteenth- and early twentieth-century India, the management of childbirth emerged as a key issue in colonial and nationalist discourses in India. The growing interest in maternal and infant mortality was partly the result of 'pronatalist fears of depopulation' and colonial anxiety about a 'shrinking labor pool' in the colony (Van Hollen, 2003: 36). The colonial state's 'concern' for maternal and infant mortality was partly also designed to legitimise colonialism as necessary for the emancipation of the vulnerable subaltern women. The state thus promoted professionalisation of obstetrics as the solution to the problem of high mortality during childbirth. Despite these early attempts by the colonial state, medicalisation of childbirth remained relatively low in most parts of India, and hospital births did not become the norm. Masculinised professionalism is also not a historical feature in India, where cultural restrictions against women being examined or touched by a male doctor, especially during childbirth, meant that one could find many more female obstetricians during the early history of obstetrics than in Europe and the US (Van Hollen, 2003). In the late nineteenth century, for instance, there were hospitals called '*zanana* hospitals', reserved for women and run by female nurses (Mavalankar and Vora, 2008). Biomedicalisation in India has many related complexities, which highlight the uneasy alliances and occasional ruptures between the local/global, and reproductive rights/ reproductive justice. In rural India, trained professionals, or auxiliary nurse midwives (ANMs) are expected to interact directly with the community and provide basic medical care (Mavalankar and Vora, 2008). In theory, the ANMs are expected to provide a variety of regular services to pregnant women – medical check-ups, distribution of essential medicines and vitamins, administration of injections – as well as to assist in their deliveries whenever required.

But over the years, the focus of ANMs has undergone a shift from basic community health and delivery services to targeted family planning (Mavalankar and Vora, 2008). They are also expected to maintain a network of *dais* (midwives), with some basic training in home delivery (Shariff and Singh, 2002). But in practice, as a result of corruption and/or inadequate support systems, *dais* seldom establish contact with pregnant women. Arguably, the low utilisation of institutional delivery services is not only a result of limited access. Even when professional nurses or *dais* are available, women in rural areas rarely consult them during pregnancy. In general, pregnancy is looked upon as a condition that does not require medical attention (Shariff and Singh, 2002). Home delivery is preferred to institutional delivery, especially in large multigeneration families where the older women can provide traditional maternity and childbirth information and advice as well as assistance at the time of delivery (Munjial et al., 2009; Shariff and Singh, 2002).

Since 2000, the focus of maternal health related policies in India has been on increasing institutional births, often by providing (cash) incentives to health workers and/or mothers for hospital births. While institutional deliveries and access to emergency obstetric care may reduce maternal mortality, experience of childbirth, especially in public hospitals, can be marred by verbal and physical birth violence. Writing from the north-east Indian state of Assam, a state with the highest maternal mortality rate in India, Chattopadhyay et al. (2018) demonstrate that while the expansion of institutional deliveries and access to emergency obstetric care is likely to reduce maternal mortality, institutional deliveries continue to be characterised by the 'paradox of safe but violent births', and since the public healthcare system is mostly used by the poor, these violent experiences are another instance of embedded inequities in reproductive experiences. Obstetric violence, then, is not just gendered but often a classed and racialised form of disciplining women assumed to be the 'problematic others', that is not conforming to middle-class norms of femininity and motherhood (Smith-Oka, 2015).

In South Africa, biomedicalisation of obstetrics had its own local manifestations, with explicitly racial underpinnings. Much like in colonial India, debates around biomedicalised reproduction, and the scientific management of hygiene and motherhood, were interlinked with the quest for modernity in South Africa. In early nineteenth-century South Africa, German doctors had an effective professional mechanism of demeaning the work of Black midwives, and indigenous medicine and practices, in the name of 'training' and 'certification' of midwives (Deacon, 2000). By the early twentieth century this marginalisation of midwives was systematically included in laws and legal frameworks, which directly targeted (Black) African people (Burns, 1995). Despite this systematic marginalisation, Black women in South Africa who were trained in midwifery and nursing formed the largest group of professional women on the African continent.

Currently, birth in South Africa is highly institutionalised, with 93% of women giving birth in a medical facility: only 6% of these births are in private hospitals (Chadwick and Foster, 2013). Much like the rest of the health system, obstetric services are riddled with debilitating inequities based on race and class – a legacy of the colonial state's policy of catering to the health of 'European soldiers, civil servants, and settlers', reaffirmed by the apartheid state's racist ideology, which guided all health action between 1973 and 1994 (Pande and Moll 2018). If we compare India and South Africa, the total healthcare expenditure in South Africa is much higher: 8.7% of Gross Domestic Product (GDP), as compared to only 1% of GDP spent on healthcare in India. But of the amount allocated towards healthcare in South Africa, nearly 60% goes directly towards the private sector, which only services 16% of the population (Daniels, 2021). The two countries have remarkable similarities in the shifting priorities between private and public health investments. Although both countries have a long history of public policy in healthcare (including reproductive health), there has been a persistent presence of a parallel stream of private medical care. In both countries economic liberalisation significantly changed the priorities of public policy as well as the character of the private sector in health and medicine. The focus on economic growth and reduction of social subsidies has led to a neglect of public healthcare provision (Qadeer, 2008). With liberalisation, medical care has become an industry exposing health of the people to the logic of big private capital.

The business of healthcare and the insurance-led model have led to a consistent transfer of public resources to the corporate sector in medical care. Even though the public sector still plays a role in healthcare provision, the sector itself has become commercialised, out-of-pocket expenditure has increased exponentially, and this affects all stakeholders involved in public healthcare, not just the client/ consumers (Hodges and Rao, 2016). One of the consequences is that public sector services and workers, including doctors, nurses and hospital midwives, are under-resourced, stressed and overworked, leading to 'compassion fatigue' and adding to the systemic reasons for reproductive violence in such settings. As Rachel Chadwick summarises in the context of obstetric violence in South Africa: 'Rather than problematic individual perpetrators responsible for "causing" violence, nurses are themselves intersectional subjects positioned in multiple ways in the birth assemblage. They are often overworked, stressed, and left to work in difficult and under-resourced conditions' (Chadwick, 2017: 505). In both South Africa and India, the maternal health outcome that has been singularly emphasised is the rate of maternal mortality, without any focus on the quality of maternal healthcare, or labouring women's access to a dignified and supportive treatment. In both countries, while women on low income and in rural areas struggle to get biomedical interventions in time, middle-class women often undergo unnecessary technological interventions because of commercialisation and corporatisation of healthcare, and the push for the insurance-led model (Daniels, 2021; Ghosh, 2010; Humphrey, 1998).

The troubling reproductive history of forced contraception, controversial contraceptive trials and reproductive violence outlined above, and its effects on women in the global south, have become the focus of several academic and activist works (Chapter 8, this volume; Connelly, 2008; Qadeer, 2010; Rao, 2004a). This history, and its current forms is intertwined with structural factors of race, religion, class and gender. In the next section, I juxtapose this colonial history and postcolonial presence of the state's obsessive anti-natalism as well as the commonplace reproductive violence with its seemingly paradoxical counterpart – booming markets in fertility and assisted reproduction in both India and South Africa.

Fertility markets in India and South Africa

There is limited literature that addresses assisted reproductive technologies (ARTs) in the global south, partly because of the assumption that such technologies are unsuitable for and unavailable in low-resource settings. Fertility-control, rather than assisted fertility, is assumed to be more relevant for southern contexts. However, while these postcolonial states tend to be anti-natalist, their cultures are explicitly pronatalist, with a high demand for fertility fuelled by social, economic and religious imperatives to reproduce. Additionally, many African and South Asian countries with high fertility rates continue to have high (secondary) infertility rates especially due to untreated post-abortion and postpartum infections. In South Africa and India, although demand-side factors, for instance, increased incidence of infertility and the societal stigma of remaining childless, are critical (Dyer et al., 2005), the booming market in ARTs is primarily driven by supply-side factors. Much as with contraceptives, where supply of birth control in its various forms to women in the global south was rarely driven by demand, scientists, pharmaceutical companies, professionals and brokers involved in ARTs do not wait for the demand to be high to inundate markets and nations with new ways of conceiving a baby. This supply-side bias can be sustained in emerging economies like India and South Africa because of the historically stratified infrastructure, neoliberalisation of healthcare and the rise of private-sector corporate hospitals, all of which have allowed the countries to become hubs for medical travel (Mazzaschi, 2012; Pande, 2014; Sengupta, 2011). While the public healthcare system flounders in both countries, there is an increasing investment in cutting-edge technology, and 'five-star luxury hospitals' that often aim to cater primarily to the national elite and international clients, mostly from the global north. The emergence of high-tech investments in assisted reproduction services in South Africa and India – countries that are simultaneously struggling with minimal health resources in the public sector – is a striking example of such a shared paradox. Both countries are established hubs of medical and reproductive travel from across the world.

Reproductive travel, or repro-travel – clients travelling for various forms of infertility treatment – is a practice that has been going on for decades. Historically, wealthy elites from the global south travelled to the global north in search of the best technologies and treatment, not available or not reliable at home. Now we witness a reverse traffic – clients from all over the world are heading to the global south to get treatment at bargain prices and to get access to reproductive resources in ways that they cannot at home. My interest in this intriguing world of repro-travel started in 2006 and culminated in a monograph on gestational surrogacy in India (Pande, 2014). I argued that despite warnings by radical feminists that this service is akin to baby farms, where low-income Black women are breeding white babies, there is much more to debate. In their narratives the gestational mothers, the surrogates, made it clear that surrogacy was exceptionally hard labour, but it was also work where they produced something of value, and instead of glass bangles or shirts in a factory, they were now (re)'producing' a priceless baby. Yet I highlighted the paradox of this temporary valuation of their bodies and celebration of their contribution – their fertile bodies were being taken care of, fed and pampered for the first time in an anti-natal state like India. For decades these women had been told that their excessive fertility was what was making their families, and in fact the entire nation, poor. Through long-term injectables and sterilisation, they had been coerced into 'choosing' not to reproduce. Even when they needed to, they could not afford proper medical care for their own pregnancy and birth. Suddenly, this same class of women was being treated to the most sophisticated biomedical technologies because they were birthing children for other, richer, and often whiter parents to keep. This is what I called 'neo-eugenics', the new, subtle form of eugenics whereby the neoliberal notion of consumer choice justifies promotion of assisted reproductive services for the rich and, at the same time, by portraying poor people (often in the global south) as a strain on the world's economy and environment, justifies aggressive anti-natal policies.

Between 2005 and 2015, the surrogacy industry boomed in a legal vacuum in India, with minimum state interference and few laws regulating the procedures, the contract or the surrogate-client relationship. But this has changed dramatically since 2015, when an affidavit was placed before the Supreme Court of India, which, in a nutshell, declared that the Indian government 'does not support commercial surrogacy' and the scope of surrogacy would be now limited to needy Indian married couples only. The Indian government seems convinced that the underlying problems with surrogacy will be erased by restricting the clientele to couples who the government deems legitimate – namely heterosexual married nationals of India. This Bill is another clear indication of the conservative hetero-normative ethics of the current right-wing government. The intersection between reproductive politics, birth projects and Hindutva nationalism is highlighted by other contributors to this volume (Chatterjee, Roy and Subramaniam in Chapter 2, Mohanka in Chapter 3 and Prakash in Chapter 4). At the same time, the bill and the surrogacy ban ignore the inherently unequal and stratified nature of the ART industry, and its reaffirmation of existing reproductive stratifications, based on race, class, caste and not just gender.

While India is the controversial hub for paid gestation, South Africa is the preferred destination for 'egg safaris', where (gamete) recipients from Europe, Australia and North America are matched with white South African gamete (ova and sperm) providers, as they combine this medical procedure with sunshine and game safari (Namberger, 2019; Pande and Moll, 2018). There is a deep irony that the demand for whiteness within the transnational fertility industry is filled by women from South Africa, a country that is majority Black and where, more than two decades after apartheid has ended, racial classifications remain the foundation of society. Within the healthcare sector, public healthcare systems flounder, yet there is increasing investment in new technology and five-star luxury hospitals to cater for international clients, mostly from the global north (Crush et al., 2012). Reproductive travel, a growing portion of this industry, has similar paradoxes and is riddled by debilitating inequalities, based on race and class (Coovadia et al., 2009). For the majority of South Africans, who cannot afford basic healthcare and are not covered by any insurance system, assisted reproduction remains a 'luxury' (Namberger 2019: 41), but as a global hub for reproductive travel, South Africa maintains a thriving industry in IVF, and, relatedly, egg provision. What is most striking about the industry of egg provision in South Africa is its racial underpinnings.

Race has always underlined the fertility industry. With the advent of ART, especially third-party reproduction through surrogacy and egg provision, the 'natural' basis for establishing kinship has been disrupted. These relationships have to be constructed and legitimised through a process that Charis Thompson (2005) labels strategic naturalising. Race and racial matching, in the hunt for gametes become 'resources' for intended parents and clinics in this racialising and naturalising process, and in establishing which contribution to the child's birth can be claimed as authentic parental status (Russell, 2018). Within the gamete provision industry, in India and South Africa, racialised imaginaries and notions of race are manipulated, transformed and put to new use (Chapters 12, 13, 14 this volume; Pande, 2021).

Several scholars have highlighted the paradoxical and, often, contentious role of race in genetic technologies and assisted reproduction in the twenty-first century (Kaufman and Hall, 2003; Roberts, 2009; Russell, 2015). In these discussions around race and reprogenetic technologies in the twenty-first century, there are emerging debates around the role of 'reprogenetics in ensuring or preventing the inheritance of particular genes in a child' (Silver, 2000: 375). In my previous discussions of gestational surrogacy, my concept of neo-eugenics was, in part, a critical response to a strand of scholarship around such reprogenetics, or what some science and technology studies (STS) scholars have labelled 'liberal' eugenics (Agar, 2004; Blencowe, 2011; Rose, 2007) – a new era of biopolitics led by individual consumer choice, where the only role that the state plays is to 'foster the development of a range of technologies of enhancement' (Agar, 2004: 5). The scholars acknowledge the possibility of controversies and conflicts in decisions about the 'worth of different human lives', and emphasise the need for 'biological responsibility', by 'a prudent yet enterprising individual, actively shaping his or her life course through acts of choice (Rose, 2007: 134). The way forward, for the scholars of liberal eugenics, is to envision reproductive selection as an individual, voluntary, state-neutral and, often, empowering practice. But are these practices merely a reflection of individual autonomy and choice, or are they also shaped by, and embedded within, power relations?

As the fertility industry grapples with nationally restrictive laws, for instance the surrogacy ban in India, and shifts scale from national to transnational, crossing borders to access ART and third-party reproductive services becomes a legitimate way to reimagine racialised desires about our next generation. In my work with the fertility industry, gamete provision and surrogacy, I have observed that as intended parents and fertility professionals 'co-produce' racialised desires about eggs and babies, the industry naturalises choices that reaffirm an explicit hierarchy in bodies: those of certain races and classes of women are valued more highly than others. At the same time, the industry naturalises the desire for whiteness – whiteness that is fluid, travelling, and yet hyper visible as a heritable privilege (Pande 2020, 2021). Several chapters in this volume unpack such complex intersections between racialisation of gametes (and providers) and notions of desirability and enhancement of the next generation, in India and South Africa.

As ART becomes a means to 'invest' in a child, intended parents and fertility professionals become co-producers in designing desires. These discussions bring out the paradoxical nature of ART, which has the potential to be a harbinger of radical change, but often replicate social inequities. As Jennifer Parks noted: 'It is still an open question whether ART will eventually bring about radical change or whether radical change is required before ART can be liberating' (Parks, 2009, quoted in Russell, 2018). As we move towards an allegedly post-population control and post-eugenic world, birth projects aimed at curtailing the reproduction of a certain demography continue. We cannot let a focus on intimacy and privacy of choices around kinship, familial and racial identity depoliticise urgent questions of inequalities, stratifications and reproductive justice.

References

Agar, N. (2004). *Liberal Eugenics: In Defense of Human Enhancement.* Malden, MA: Blackwell Publishing.

Blencowe, C. P. (2011). Biology, contingency and the problem of racism in feminist discourse, *Theory, Culture and Society* 28:3, 3–27.

Brown, B. B. (1987). Facing the 'black peril': the politics of population control in South Africa, *Journal of Southern African Studies* 13:2, 256–73.

Burns, C. (1995). Reproductive labors: the politics of women's health in South Africa, 1900–1960, Northwestern University. ProQuest Dissertations Publishing. 9537400.

Chadwick, R. (2017). Ambiguous subjects: obstetric violence, assemblage and South African birth narratives, *Feminism and Psychology* 27:4, 489–509.

Chadwick, R. J. and Foster, D. (2013). Technologies of gender and childbirth choices: homebirth, elective caesarean and white femininities in South Africa, *Feminism and Psychology*, 23:3, 317–38.

Chatterjee, N. and Riley, N. E. (2001). Planning an Indian modernity: the gendered politics of fertility control, *Signs* 26:3, 811–45.

Chattopadhyay, S. (2015). The horrifying sights and sounds from the labour room of an Indian public hospital, 12 June. https://qz.com/india/422338/in-horrific-indian-hospitals-women-in-labour-are-slapped-when-they-scream/. Accessed 18 November 2021.

Chattopadhyay, S., Arima, M. and Jacob, S. (2018). 'Safe', yet violent? Women's experiences with obstetric violence during hospital births in rural Northeast India, *Culture, Health and Sexuality* 20:7, 815–29.

Connelly, M. (2008). *Fatal Misconception: The Struggle to Control World Population.* Cambridge, MA: The Belknap Press of Harvard University Press.

Coovadia, H., Jewkes, R., Barron, P., Sanders, D. and McIntyre, D. (2009). The health and health system of South Africa: historical roots of current public health challenges, *Lancet* 374:9692, 817–34.

Crush, Jonathan, Chikanda, A. and Maswikwa, B. (2012). Patients without borders: medical tourism and medical migration in Southern Africa. Cape Town: Southern African Migration Programme. SAMP Migration Policy. Series No. 57.

Daniels, N. (2021). *Obstetric risk worlds: a multi-site, feminist ethnography of private-sector obstetric, maternal and unborn caring concerns in Cape Town.* Unpublished PhD Dissertation, University of Cape Town.

Davis-Floyd, R. E. (1990). The role of obstetrical rituals in the resolution of cultural anomaly, *Social Science and Medicine* 31:2, 175–89.

Deacon, H. (2000). The politics of medical topography: seeking healthiness at the Cape during the nineteenth century. In R. Wrigley and G. Revill (eds), *Pathologies of Travel*, 279–98. Amsterdam: Rodopi.

de Gruchy, J. and Baldwin, L. (2005). Apartheid and health professional accountability: violations of the reproductive rights of women. In O. Nnaemeka and J. Ezeilo (eds), *Engendering Human Rights: Cultural and Socio-Economic Realities in Africa*, 39–59. New York: Palgrave Macmillan.

Dyer, S. J., Abrahams, N., Mokoena, N. E., Lombard, C. J. and van der Spuy, Z. M. (2005) Psychological distress among women suffering from couple infertility in South Africa: a quantitative assessment, *Human Reproduction* 20, 1938–43.

Ghosh S. (2010). Increasing trend in cesarean section delivery in India: role of medicalisation of maternal health. In S. Ghosh (ed.), *Working Paper 236*. Bangalore: The Institute for Social and Economic Chang, 1–16.

Hodges, S. and Rao, M. (2016). *Public Wealth and Private Wealth: Stem Cells, Surrogates and Other Strategic Bodies.* New Delhi: Oxford University Press.

Hollen. C. V. (2003). *Birth on the Threshold: Childbirth and Modernity in South India.* Berkeley, CA: University of California Press.

Humphreys, K. (1998). *Medicalised Maternity: An Investigation into Women's Experiences of Medicalised Childbirth.* Unpublished Masters Thesis. University of Cape Town.

Karkal, M. (1998). Family planning and the reproductive rights of women. In L. Lingam (ed.), *Understanding Women's Health Issues: A Reader*, 228–44. New Delhi: Kali.

Kaufman. C. E. (1996). *The politics and practice of reproductive control in South Africa: a multilevel analysis of fertility and contraceptive use.* Unpublished Doctoral Dissertation. Ann Arbor: Department of Sociology, University of Michigan.

Kaufman J. S. and Hall, S. A. (2003). The slavery hypertension hypothesis: dissemination and appeal of a modern race theory, *Epidemiology* 14:1, 111–18.

Klausen, S. M. (2004). *Race, Maternity, and the Politics of Birth Control in South Africa, 1910–39.* Basingstoke, Palgrave Macmillan.

Mavalankar D. and Vora, K. (2008).The changing role of auxiliary nurse midwife (ANM) in India: implications for maternal & child health (MCH). Ahmedabad: Indian Institute of Management, Working Paper 2008-03-01.

Mazzaschi, A. (2012). Surgeon and safari: producing valuable bodies in Johannesburg, *Signs* 36, 303–11.

Munjial M., Kaushik, P. and Agnihotri, S. (2009). A comparative analysis of institutional and non-institutional deliveries in a village of Punjab, *Health and Population* 32: 131–40.

Namberger, V. (2019). *The Reproductive Body at Work: The South African Bioeconomy of Egg Donation.* Oxford: Routledge.

Pande, A. (2014). *Wombs in Labor: Transnational Commercial Surrogacy in India.* New York: Columbia University Press.

Pande A. (2020). Visa stamps for injections: traveling biolabor and South African egg provision, *Gender and Society* 34:4, 573–96.

Pande, A. (2021). 'Mix or match?' Transnational fertility industry and white desirability, *Medical Anthropology*, 40:4, 335–47. DOI:10.108 0/01459740.2021.1877289.

Pande, A., and Moll, T. (2018). Gendered bio-responsibilities and travelling egg providers from South Africa, *Reproductive Biomedicine & Society Online* 6, 23–33.

Qadeer, I. (2008). Health planning in India: some lessons from the past, *Social Scientist*, 36:5/6, 51–75.

Qadeer I. (2010). *New Reproductive Technologies and Health Care in Neo-liberal India: Essays.* New Delhi: Centre for Women's Development Studies.

Ram, K. (2001). Rationalizing fecund bodies: family planning policy and the modern Indian nation-state. In M. Jolly and K. Ram (eds.), *Borders of Being: Citizenship, Fertility, and Sexuality in Asia and the Pacific*, 82–117. Ann Arbor: University of Michigan Press.

Rao, M. (2004a). *The Unheard Scream: Reproductive Health and Women's Lives in India.* New Delhi: Zubaan.

Rao, M. (2004b). *From Population Control to Reproductive Health: Malthusian Arithmetic.* New Delhi: Sage Publications.

Roberts, D. (2009). Race, gender, and genetic technologies: a new reproductive dystopia? *Signs* 34, 783–804. DOI:10.1086/597132.

Rose, N. (2007). *A Politics of Life Itself.* Princeton, NJ: Princeton University Press.

Russell, C. (2015). The race idea in reproductive technologies: beyond epistemic scientism and technological mastery, *Bioethical Inquiry* 12, 601–12.

Russell, C. (2018). *The Assisted Reproduction of Race.* Bloomington: Indiana University Press.

Schultz, G. D. (1958). Cruelty in maternity wards, *Ladies' Home Journal* 44–5, 152–5.

Sengupta, A. (2011). Medical tourism: reverse subsidy for the elite, *Signs* 36, 312–19.

Shariff, A. and Singh, G. (2002). Determinants of maternal health care utilisation in India: evidence from a recent household survey. New Delhi: National Council of Applied Economic Research.

Silver, L. M. (2000). Reprogenetics: third millennium speculation. The consequences for humanity when reproductive biology and genetics are combined, *EMBO Reports* 1:5 375–8.

Smith-Oka, V. (2015). Microaggressions and the reproduction of social inequalities in medical encounters in Mexico, *Social Science and Medicine* 143, 9–16.

Stoler, A. L. (2002). *Carnal Knowledge and Imperial Power: Race and the Intimate in Colonial Rule.* Berkeley, CA: University of California Press

Thompson, C. (2005). *Making Parents: The Ontological Choreography of Reproductive Technologies*. Cambridge, MA: MIT Press.

WHO (2014). Trends in maternal mortality: 1990 to 2013. http://apps.who.int/iris/bitstream/handle/10665/112682/9789241507226_eng.pdf?sequence=2. Accessed 30 November 2021.

WHO (2019). Maternal mortality. www.who.int/news-room/fact-sheets/detail/maternal-mortality. Accessed 30 November 2021.

2

Spectres of biological politics: conversations within and across South Asia

Sushmita Chatterjee, Deboleena Roy, Banu Subramaniam

In tracing the history of the term biopolitics, the editors of a recent reader on the subject, Timothy Campbell and Adam Sitze (2013: 1) write:

> No such singular moment comes to mind when charting the history of biopolitics. No defining interval offers itself as the lens able to superimpose the past and the future, allowing us to look back and say, 'ah, yes, it was precisely then that biopolitics was born, exactly then that politics gave way to biopolitics, power to biopower, and life to *bios*, *zoë*, and the forms of life that characterize our present.'

As the editors argue, a singular genealogy of the term biopolitics is difficult. The first analysis of 'biopolitics' comes from Michel Foucault, in a short piece, 'Right of death and power over life', in his 1976 book, *La Volonté de Savoir*. The short thesis seemed more an appendix than a central part of the text. While not taken up immediately, the concept slowly gained traction. Over the years, many theorists, including Donna Haraway, Etienne Balibar, Paul Gilroy, Agnes Heller, Anne Laura Stoler, Giorgio Agamben, Achille Mbembe, Michael Hardt and Antonio Negri, Paolo Virno, Roberto Esposito, Slavoj Zizek, and Gilles Deleuze among others have all contributed to the 'biopolitical turn', helping establish biopolitics as a critical term for the twentieth and twenty-first centuries.

There is no doubt that biopolitics is an important and influential concept, one that has fundamentally shaped each of us in our work. The three of us have been in conversation for many years regarding our overlapping interests in postcolonial studies, feminist theory, and science and technology studies and while each of our academic engagements with South Asia is varied, in our emerging collaborations on South Asia, biopolitics has loomed large. We each feel a debt of gratitude to this term and its many interlocutors. We also recognise that biopolitics has emerged as a veritable industry in its intellectual proliferation – with theorists critiquing, substantiating, modifying, and expanding its intellectual terrain. Drawing on a South Asian metaphor, we would suggest that biopolitics has many 'avatars', each useful in its many ways.

In this short piece, we are less interested in chronicling its varied treatments but rather make the observation that the many descriptions of biopolitics in South Asia remain largely western and Eurocentric – in their historicity, genealogy, application, and analyses. What has emerged for us is not only a recognition of the importance of the nexus of biology and politics, but also a gnawing suspicion and discomfort on the sufficiency of 'biopolitics' as a conceptual terrain for transnational South Asian biological politics. With colonialism's deep impact, it is certainly the case that legacies of Eurocentrism remain in the South Asian imagination, but there is something about South Asia that at once escapes and exceeds the western biopolitical imagination. In each of our work, the varied genealogies of biopolitics do not always 'fit'. In what follows, we want to elaborate on these ruminations, signalling the deep imbrications of biology and politics in transnational circulations. We also use the term 'India' when we refer to the nation that formed since 1947, and the term 'South Asia' to signal the shared geographies and histories with neighbouring nations before independence.

We use a conversational mode of inquiry in this chapter. This helps delineate the intricate nuances that frame 'biopolitics' within specific disciplines and transdisciplinary conversations. The method also allows us to nudge at the contours of our own thinking and enables a generative intellectual process. We want to centre and highlight the tensions that emerge when thinking about biopolitics in South Asia – ruminating all the while on the political framings of each of the terms. Style and content play off each other, in this chapter, to showcase the impurity and dialogical construction of the theories and issues per se. Together, and individually, we think about our own intellectual journeys with the term, our collaborations, and more importantly the varied intellectual and political motivations that profoundly shape our interventions. What emerges are the many ironies and limits to language and imaginations that underpin thinking about biopolitics. This dialogical style, and content, is explicitly useful for a project that seeks to undo the many meanings in biopolitics, and also for the overall volume, which centres the urgency of understanding reproductive politics, neoliberal landscapes, rights, health, markets, eugenics, and social hierarchy, within continually changing landscapes.

Our conversation persistently returns to the impossibility of framing biopolitics within a singular logic and showcases the inevitability of translations and re-translations as bodies and theories cross borders. Just as India spills forth from any frame that contains it, whether in terms of markets or history, biopolitics takes on new meanings as we ponder together 'birth politics' and the need for impure prisms to understand power regimes that determine conditions of life, birth, death, and measures of recognition. Through different narratives, we collectively emphasise the futility of universalising biopolitics as a theory that travels the world unconnected or uncluttered with varied resonances and meanings. By stressing impure theories, impure bodies, and impure worlds, we emphasise the need to anchor impurity as a resonant lens to understand the workings of biology and politics. Alexis Shotwell's words, 'we are not, ever, pure' resounds through our conversation and amplifies the urgency to understand the specific nuances of biopolitics in South Asia (2016, 7).

An emphasis on the differential resonances of theories and bodies, physical and territorial, is an attempt towards a decolonial science and technology studies (STS), one that engages with our classificatory mechanisms of life and birth, for instance, all the while noting entanglements within power structures. Like a biopolitics that takes on varied nuances as it travels the world, attempts at decolonising STS cannot work with a universal solution. For instance, South Asia and South Africa are joined by histories of colonialism and different realities of caste, race, gender, and political economies. And yet they are not the same, and yield different genealogies of caste, race, gender, and political economies. Without homogenising a decolonial solution and keeping our attention on power structures, we think together about laws, markets, modernity, and tradition and note its messy confluences. Engaging with messiness and impurity is as much an attempt to un-contour biopolitics, as it is a yearning to decolonise STS.

Deboleena: The concepts of biopower and biopolitics have been extremely valuable to me, particularly in making sense of the role that the institutions of science play in how we come to know our bodies and our biologies. I came to learn about biopower while I was a graduate student in a molecular biology and reproductive neuroendocrinology lab, working with an in vitro neuronal cell line derived from a transgenic mouse. How, you might ask, did Foucault's work make its way to my lab bench? The answer is through Donna Haraway's figuration of the oncomouse, prominently featured in her 1997 book *Modest Witness@Second_Millenium.FemaleMan©_ Meets Onco_Mouse™: Feminism and Technoscience*. As a graduate student in the natural sciences, I was grappling with understanding my own kinship with the neurons, hormones, contraceptives, cancer-causing SV40 DNA tumour viruses, PCR machines, radioactive isotopes, and animal model-based laboratory practices, when a copy of *Modest Witness* made its way into my hands. There on in, Haraway's (1997: 129) idea of technobiopower and her iterative naming of the 'stem cells of the technoscientific body' found at the end of the second millennium such as the 'seed, chip, gene, data-base, bomb, fetus, race, brain, and ecosystem' (Haraway, 1997: 12) loomed large in my scientific training. It was my kinship with oncomouse that led me to Haraway's (1997) definition of technobiopower, which in turn, led me to Foucault's (1976) concept of biopower.

My work has since attempted to combine feminist, queer, and postcolonial studies with scientific knowledge making practices in neuroscience, molecular biology, and reproductive endocrinology research (Roy, 2018). The questions that have interested me the most have primarily been grounded in the philosophy of science, with special attention to the ontological, ethical, epistemological, and methodological assumptions made by feminists, scientists, and feminist scientists in producing knowledges on and of the body. However, in 2008, my attention was drawn to an article titled 'Reproductive tourism soars in India' (Sehgal, 2008). Through this article, I found out that commercial surrogacy services were starting to come under severe scrutiny in India. This scrutiny was due, in part, to a high profile international case in 2008 (referred to as the 'Baby Manji' case) involving a Japanese couple who commissioned the birth of a child through surrogacy services in the Indian province of Gujarat, and then later divorced. The husband still wanted to raise the child, but his ex-wife wanted no part. The biological mother who donated the egg was anonymous and not in the picture, and the Indian surrogate mother who had carried the child held no legal responsibility following childbirth. I learned that this case was but one of many in what was to become a multi-billion dollar reproductive tourism industry, which had been growing steadily in India since 2002, when the country opened up its borders and economy to reproductive technology and reproductive tourism-based services. This industry was booming, not only due to foreign interest, but also due in large part to the fertility issues experienced by Indian nationals themselves and the demand for assisted reproductive technologies (ARTs), including in vitro fertilisation (IVF) and surrogacy services. What interested me the most, however, from this article was that it also reported that several hotspots for reproductive tourism in India had emerged, including the city of Bhopal in the province of Uttar Pradesh, where some of the cheapest surrogates (approximately US$4,500) in the entire world were available for hire.

As I read this article, I thought to myself, really? Bhopal? Where the Gas Tragedy of 1984 had occurred? Where a methyl isocyanate gas explosion at the Union Carbide (now Dow Chemical) pesticide plant had killed thousands of people overnight and had left many more thousands with serious long term health issues (International Campaign for Justice in Bhopal, 2020)? Where both women and men were reported to have incurred severe reproductive harm (Dhara, 1992)? Where women, who were pregnant on the night of the disaster, experienced spontaneous miscarriages? Where women who were of childbearing age suddenly entered the menopause? Where young girls exposed to the gas never got their periods? Where transgenerational health ramifications had been reported, indicating that the long-term effects of the methyl isocyanate gas were not only somatic but also gametic? The day I read that article, I started conducting research for what has now become a more than decade-long project to understand and untangle surrogacy and molecular biopolitics in Bhopal.

The concept of biopower and Haraway's (1997) idea of techno-biopower have been helpful for me to frame this event. The tech-noscientific body presented here, to name a few stem cells and sticky threads, is an ecosystem comprised of plants, pesticides, the Green Revolution in India, gametes, IVF technologies, reproductive organs, placentas, surrogates, and a bioeconomy of reproductive tourism entirely dependent upon a market made possible by 'in vivo human labor' (Cooper and Waldby, 2014: 7). Yet something about the specificity of this event occurring in India has made it ongoingly difficult for me to wrap my head around the full range of biological politics involved. I have been unable to find the appropriate theoretical tools and vocabulary to fully address my bewilderment at how a woman in Bhopal, where the world's worst industrial disaster occurred, and where severe reproductive health concerns have affected generations of women, could also come to serve as the cheapest surrogates in the world. Have people forgotten about Bhopal? Are couples willing to hire a surrogate in Bhopal because they believe that the surrogate body does not play a role in the development of the fetus? And/or are commissioning couples willing to risk biologi-cally transferred toxicity for the chance to have their own genetic/biological child? How does an event such as this occur?

Within a larger sense of biopolitics, India has been the poster child and the laboratory for Malthusian principles and population control. However, the hauntings of colonisation (the active pushback by many Indians to accept or emulate 'values' from the 'west'), the complications of Hinduism and caste (the idea that one can't touch women who are low caste but yet a woman from a lower caste can carry one's baby), and a number of mistranslations (both material and semiotic around definitions of life and surrogate/fetal biological 'mixing') have left me with more questions than answers. Other chapters in this anthology have raised similar questions, including, for instance, the piece by Gondouin, Thapar-Björkert, and Rao. Their chapter explores the tensions that exist within Indian feminist discourses on reproductive technologies, rights, and justice. In this case, by focusing on the sexual exploitation and socio-economic factors that impact the lives of Dalit women, the authors highlight how Dalit feminist voices can challenge our under-standing of biopolitics in the context of surrogacy and reproductive technologies.

Banu: For me, biopolitics has emerged as a term I cannot ignore, but neither can I embrace whole-heartedly. I engaged with this deep tension in my recent work on science and Hindu nationalism in India (Subramaniam, 2019). The central node of difficulty for me is one of language. The term biopolitics draws on its prefix 'bio'. As I argue in the book, in English, the root is the Greek *bios*, which refers to the form or manner in which life is lived, finite and mortal, contrasted with *zoē*, the biological fact of life, infinite and a general phenomenon of life. The concept of biopolitics and power emerges from Foucault (1976) who chronicles how western societies in the eighteenth century consolidated power into a new medical authority, and ushered in new forms of power that constitute life and death, that is, biopower. This shift in power marked the ascendency of the life sciences, giving them a central role in constituting life, the body, and health.

However, this constitution of a more scientific and medical conception of life does not fully translate into the Indian context. As I explored biological politics in India, I encountered many levels of incommensurability. Most importantly were the difficulties of translatability, between Indian languages and English and between various Indian languages. Indeed, given that India was constituted by the British in 1947 by consolidating various local rulers with diverse linguistic and cultural roots, I suspect there is considerable variation even between various Indian languages (an aspect I have not explored). For example, 'bio' evokes the word life. In Hindi, many words broadly translate into English *life*, such as *zindagi, jeevan, pran, atma, rahen, josh, jaan*, and *aayushya*, as do the Tamil words *vazhkai, uyire*, and *ayul*. In part, this is because the Indian words continue to incorporate and embody ideas of soul, spirit, energy, and other vitalist notions of life (potentially inhabiting different bodies across generations), ideas long purged from western definitions. In terms of biological politics on the ground, I trace a distinct biopolitics of Hindu nationalism, a politics that is incorporated in the body's physiognomy, in biology and in practices of bodily discipline, as well as a biopower that governs populations and governments in the Foucauldian sense. I would argue that this 'biopolitics' is not the same as the Foucauldian transformations in the nineteenth century in the west, and yet it is not unrelated; the Indian context embodies a different genealogy of life and time into its conceptions. To complicate the matter, colonial and postcolonial India have been thoroughly disciplined by a western biopolitics. Thus, the Indian state engages with world trade laws, patent laws, transnational health initiatives, and rules of the World Health Organization, necessarily adopted for western standards and transnational purposes. The census, biological variables of health and illness, population level indicators, and indices of national health all follow a western template. Thus, 'life' in India inhabits several registers, including untranslatable local understandings, various dimensions of biopolitics of Hindu nationalism, and a Foucauldian unfolding of western global biopolitics. The politics of life on the ground in India reveals multiple elisions and erasures, and one finds that much is lost in translation.

I have found such fissures, mistranslations, and incommensurability repeatedly in my work on South Asia. In short, English does not have an equivalent vocabulary for India, nor the biological sciences the ontologies for these concepts. Yet in wanting to engage with work on biological politics in feminist studies, postcolonial studies, and STS, rather than invent a new term that would most likely be lost in the tendency to proliferate vocabulary in western academia, I chose to retain the world 'biopolitics', while noting its capacity to underdetermine and overdetermine histories and geographies beyond the west.

Sushmita: I approach 'biopower' and 'biopolitics' as capacious and generative concepts that have inspired much critical inquiry on their meaning, limits, and applicability. I find it particularly intriguing that their meanings oscillate between 'administration of life', 'technology of life', 'confluence of life and power', and 'biological politics'. In so many ways, 'biopower' has become larger than life through the incredible attention it has received in trans-disciplinary conversations. I'll start with a few questions that I have always been intrigued by when reading about the use and critiques of the terms 'biopower' and 'biopolitics'. First, why does a term that is ostensibly so capacious with rolling meanings – think here about 'biopolitics' connoting the relation between life and power – elicit specific responses? In other words, when critiquing its inability to speak to specific scenarios, are we not entrusting it with a particular interpretation even while critiquing it for precisely that reason? Second, would taking seriously its erratic and confused genealogy inspire different conversations?

While the term 'biopower' is attributed to Foucault (1976), one can state that its origins cannot be restricted to a theorist or place and time. It may be useful here to think through the erratic genealogy of the term per se in terms of its extraction from multiple works of Foucault and its use in inspiring and provoking much critical debate about the limits of the Greek *zoē* and *bios*, meaning of life, and the framing of life and death in postcolonial studies, feminist studies, and critical race theory, amongst other conversations. Many indigenous societies, for instance, have varied theories of life and politics, and so does South Asia, as Banu draws out above.

Third, and following on from the above-mentioned question, if South Asia has its own specific biopolitics, does that also not open up the framing of 'South Asia' as a particular configuration of biopolitics from the global north? Let's note all the while vast differences in the area and heterogeneous proliferation of the meaning of life and power, for instance in Hinduism, Buddhism, Islam, Sikhism, and Jainism, multiplied by the necessary observation that meaning structures within any frame change through time and place? Thus, I begin by situating the capaciousness of the terms, biopower and biopolitics, its proclivity to inspire different questions about place and time, and resonances and dissonances through meaning structures in political-economic systems. Overall, I think it is impossible for biopower or biopolitics to be a 'thing' that can be applauded or dismissed as belonging to a singular origin. Rather, it is a seething presence and absence through place and time.

Trained as a political and feminist theorist in India and in the US, my interest and work with biopower has traversed through different projects that seek to situate framings of the body in politics, categories of human and animal in political discourse, and bodily practices that are involved within power structures and governmentality. My first foray in understanding biopolitics was reckoning holistically with the idea that even though we are trained to think in contained ways within specific disciplinary contours, life and death and areas in between seldom follow definitions, and 'politics' cannot be restricted to formal institutions of governance. When studying political science in India and in the US, I was amazed to see how biology, physics, literature, geography, sociology, and myriad other prisms intersect to frame an understanding of power and politics. Whether reading Kautilya's *Arthasastra* or Machiavelli's

Prince, I soon learnt that statecraft, politics, laws and rules are framed within trans-disciplinary conversations.[1]

Thinking within a specific Indian cosmology where kings and kingdoms sprung from the bodies of gods and goddesses, and gods and goddesses change shape into human, animal, water, or fire, an Indian biopolitics has fluid cartographies, and is heterogeneous, and infinite. Wendy Doniger (1975: 11) writes in *Hindu Myths*, 'each myth celebrates the belief that the universe is boundlessly various, that everything occurs simultaneously, that all possibilities may exist without excluding each other'. I remain inspired to think about how biopower and biopolitics take many configurations and reconfigurations and how 'the universe is boundlessly various' (Doniger, 1975: 11). Or even the imaginary of a *Leviathan* from seventeenth-century England where sovereignty is established when the bodies of many coalesce into one sovereign power. 'Bodies' in this schema connoted the bodies of white propertied men, while women and slaves were excluded from these power calculations or contractual agreements. Seldom have imaginations of bodies, life, and death been inclusive, even when they mutate and change shape. Thus, I am always inspired to ask: what are the parameters of our political imagination? What do we see, and when do we see that, and what are the exigencies of life and power that frame certain questions for specific periods of time?

Picking up on Banu's emphasis on translations and mis-translations, I wonder whether situating biopolitics and biopower as a persistent haunting would help us grapple with the theories' reach and prowess as it does appear everywhere and nowhere. It seethes through multiple conversations on production, reproduction, what constitutes life and who can die through national and transnational landscapes. It often appears in negation, for what it lacks or exceeds rather than something that *is*. Like a spectral presence, it provokes us to question what we see. As a haunting, biopower is always in translation and its traces seethe through conversations. Capacious and narrow, here and there, past and present, dead and alive, as a spectral presence, biopower haunts our categories of analyses.

Deboleena: I think you have both articulated the many dimensions involved in theorising biological politics in India today. I want to turn to three recent laws in India that were passed in early 2020 to ask if together we can theorise how reproductive politics are unfolding in a Hindu nationalist state. The project I describe above, on tracking the new genetic and reproductive technologies, surrogacy, and molecular biopolitics in Bhopal, began for me before the Bharatiya Janata Party (BJP) took over in India. While I have been trying to figure out how to ask the right questions, the BJP administration has been working on continuing paternalistic traditions in India by curtailing female sexuality and regulating surrogacy under the guise of protecting women from the west and elevating Indian culture. As I mentioned, as a result of the 2008 'Baby Manji' case involving the Japanese commissioning couple and the unclear legal status of the child who was produced through surrogacy services, the Indian government began reviewing its surrogacy laws. In 2016, under a relatively newly elected BJP government, the Union Cabinet passed the Assisted Reproductive Technology (Regulation) Bill 2016, which proposed to ban commercial surrogacy in India. In addition to proposing a ban of commercial surrogacy, this bill also proposed to bar 'foreigners, homosexual couples, people in live-in relationships, and single individuals' from accessing surrogacy services, in effect making it only possible for the 'straight Indian couple married for a minimum of five years' to be eligible for such services (*The Hindu*, 2016). The 2016 bill also outlined that only altruistic surrogacy performed by a close relative should be allowed, so that money does not serve as an incentive for a given surrogate. The Minister for External Affairs, Sushma Swaraj, a staunch proponent of the bill at the time defended the 2016 bill by saying 'each country has to make laws that are aligned with our values, as per a legal framework. Homosexual couples are not recognized by law in India' (*The Hindu*, 2016).

In early 2020, three separate bills designed to protect the reproductive welfare of Indian women were approved by the Union Cabinet, chaired by Prime Minister Narendra Modi. The newly structured Assisted Reproductive Technology Regulation Bill 2020, which primarily intends to regulate IVF clinics in the country, further proposes 'stringent punishment for those practicing sex selection, sale of human embryos or gametes, [and] running agencies/rackets/organizations for such unlawful practices' (BioVoice, 2020). A second bill, known as the Medical Termination of Pregnancy Amendment Bill 2020, was also recently approved and seeks to extend the period for the termination of pregnancy from twenty to twenty-four weeks. The intention of this second bill is to make it 'easier for women to safely and legally terminate an unwanted pregnancy' (Drishti, 2020). The third bill, specifically referred to as the Surrogacy Regulation Bill 2020, proposes to create a national board at the federal level and state boards to oversee surrogacy services around the country. The bill proposes to prevent all forms of commercial surrogacy and 'control the unethical practices' associated with surrogacy in India including the 'potential exploitation of surrogate mothers and children born through surrogacy' (Civilsdaily, 2020). The Rajya Sabha Select Committee in charge of drafting The Surrogacy Regulation Bill 2020 further recommended that the regulation of surrogate mothers not be restricted to close relatives (as was suggested in the 2016 proposal) but that any woman willing to serve could do so, as long as the arrangements does not involve the transfer of money between the commissioning couple and the surrogate. Additionally, single women of Indian origin, including widows and divorcees, will also now be permitted to access surrogacy services.

How are we to read the legislation of these three recent reproductive 'welfare' bills in this present moment of biological politics in India? How can we account for the mistranslations that emerge when we habitually frame biopolitics in India through what the editor of this volume have referred to as the 'Malthus effect?' What are the limits of our political imagination when we confine our understanding of biopower in India to simply the right over life and death? What meanings of life can be made operational here – *zindagi, jeevan, pran, atma* … and more, when our vocabularies and ontological moorings of what gets to count as 'life' itself are not knowable? What are the exigencies of life and power in this specific moment that can help us account for a multi-billion dollar bioeconomy that has been steadily growing in India and that has been built upon a growing market of in vivo human reproductive labour?

As surrogacy laws are now being made to conform with the values of the BJP government and Hindu right in India, the fact remains that a different set of values has always been placed, and will continue to be placed on which individuals get to reproduce and which individuals get to perform the labour(s) of reproduction. Recent work on 'fertility outsourcing' and transnational commercial surrogacy practices occurring specifically in India reveals the extent to which reproductive technologies have come to rely on the biological labour and capacities of bodies shaped by the histories of race, class, caste, gender, and more. Although it appears that with The Surrogacy Regulation Bill 2020 there will now be strict regulations on commercial surrogacy services offered in India, other ARTs involving non-surrogacy related forms of in vivo and in vitro reproductive labour will continue to be offered to both Indian citizens and international commissioning couples. In fact, there is a fear that once surrogacy services become so strictly regulated, it will drive commercial surrogacy underground, thereby opening the doors for further exploitation of women who participate in this form of labour. This is particularly relevant in the context of Bhopal, where ART and IVF clinics promoting 'test-tube' babies are growing, and where some of the cheapest surrogates in the world will continue to be found for hire.

Banu: The recent laws that Deboleena lists are good examples of the complexities of biopolitics in South Asia. But to understand this, we need a bit of a background on recent political shifts in the Indian subcontinent. India has seen the steady rise of an organised, aggressive, and political Hindu nationalism over the last few decades, culminating in a Hindu nationalist government in 2014 (Subramaniam, 2019). Their vision is an ideological Hindu nationalism that celebrates Hindutva or 'Hinduness'. In 2019, the party returned to power with an even greater and overwhelming majority. To understand contemporary India is to understand the potency of Hindutva politics – where the past and the future cohere in their vision of India as an 'archaic modernity'. Contemporary Hindu nationalists are our prophets who look 'backward', bringing a pride of ancient India seamlessly into a quest for India as a future global superpower. Religious nationalists in contemporary India have selectively and strategically used rhetoric from science *and* Hinduism, modernity *and* orthodoxy, western *and* eastern thought, to build an archaic modernity, a powerful but potentially dangerous vision for a Hindu nation. With Hindu nationalists at the helm, the secular origins of the nation have been remade – secularism as tolerance, and democracy as majoritarianism (Vinaik, 1997). Hindu dominance, intolerance of and supremacy over other religions, faiths, and traditions, and hatred and bigotry toward non-Hindus and those belonging to sexual minority groups and lower castes mark this nationalist vision. Rather than characterise Hinduism as ancient, non-modern, or traditional, Hindu nationalists have embraced capitalism, western science, and technology as elements of a modern, Hindu nation.

Hindutva is grounded in a deep-seated belief in the lost greatness of an ancient India, a greatness that the movement means to reclaim. The confluence of science and religion that has always coexisted in the fabric of India has now claimed a public stage. Science and religion here are not oppositional forces, but syncretic collaborators. I think Hindu nationalism is best understood as a thoroughly scientific bionationalism, and those theories, practices, and politics of the body are central to its imaginaries. An apt slogan encapsulates these sentiments – 'Be Modern, Not Western.' Contemporary India challenges us, as it professes another reason, another modernity, another enlightenment.

While I will discuss the syncretic aspects of science and religion in India shortly, it is important to reiterate how the politics of global development grounds a neo-Malthusian rhetoric of overpopulation. Early in postcolonial India, the spectre of overpopulation has made India the world's laboratory for birth control, long-term contraception coercive family planning and sterilisation ever since. As always, Malthusian logics play out on female bodies. Despite plenty of evidence that the number of children is guided by complex socio-economic rationalities, in practice, overpopulation has repeatedly translated into curtailing the reproductive futures of the uterus. This strain seems unchanged with the rise of Hindu nationalism.

Deboleena's juxtaposition of the three recent laws bring this starkly into view. The first law extends right to an abortion to twenty-four weeks. On the face of it, we could read this as a bolstering of the rights of women to bodily autonomy. There are two reasons we should not. Soon after winning his second term, the Prime Minister Narendra Modi expressed concern over India's 'explosive population growth' and again chanted the Malthusian mantra that it was 'small families' that contributed to the 'development' of the nation. Thus, this is more a continuation of what is by now the well-established ideology of Malthus in postcolonial India. Second, the other two laws demonstrate the increasingly paternalistic and patriarchal view of the state on women's bodies. In the two laws on ARTs and surrogacy laws, we see the state refusing to grant bodily autonomy to women. Before the BJP came to power, India had emerged as a global hub of gestational surrogacy. Scholars have argued that India proved to be an important site because it housed both high-tech reproductive technologies alongside a low-tech and economically marginalised workforce. In 2016, the new Hindu nationalist government proposed a complete ban on commercial surrogacy in The Surrogacy (Regulation) Bill 2016 by seeking to 'protect women from exploitation and ensure the rights of the child born through surrogacy'. The earlier entrepreneurial, neoliberal subjects of gestational surrogacy were transformed into the new victims of global exploitation – these have long been the two sides of patriarchal public policy – exploitation and protection. And feminists in India have long fought both these options – instead asking for regulation of ARTs and surrogacy so that the rights, resources, and recourse for women were enacted and enforced.

The Surrogacy (Regulation) Bill 2016 banned commercial surrogacy but allowed restricted altruistic surrogacy for needy infertile heterosexual married couples – but to avoid 'commercial exploitation', the surrogate mother had to be a 'close' relative (like a sister or sister-in-law) who is married with at least one child. No money could change hands. Several groups were barred from accessing surrogacy in India: foreigners, including diasporic Indians who were non-resident or Overseas Citizens of India or Persons of Indian Origin, Indian citizens who are 'homosexual', 'single', or 'live-in couples'. Couples who already have children (biological or adopted) are also barred. The bill proposes a hefty penalty of imprisonment of not less than ten years and a million rupees fine.

The reasons given by the BJP were revealing. In interviews, the government identified the infertile married heterosexual couples as the only deserving candidates. All others were undeserving because they were westernised, too fashionable, too casual about children, or not belonging to 'a true Hindu ethos'. Sushma Swaraj, the external affairs minister, specifically criticised several high profile cases of surrogacy by arguing that 'Surrogacy is not a fashion or a hobby, but we have surrogacy as a celebrity culture' (Dhar, 2016). 'What began as a convenience has become a luxury today', she argued. When asked about the exclusion of homosexuals, Swaraj said 'this is against our ethos'. Her reasons for barring nonresident Indians and foreigners were that 'divorces are very common in foreign countries' (Lakshmi, 2016). The minister declared that, 'banning commercial surrogacy was the duty of the state and a revolutionary step for women's welfare'.

Feminist critics in response raised some fundamentally troubling issues. Why was surrogacy linked to marriage? Would banning commercial surrogacy rather than regulating it only drive it underground, causing more exploitation than an outright ban? Can altruism within patriarchal structures ever be free of coercion? Is reproductive labour that undervalued not to merit payment? The law had paid no attention to surrogate mothers, there were no safeguards of any kind, making her 'another process in the chain of (re)production' (P. Bharadwaj, 2016). The 2020 legislation is the fruit of these earlier actions and subsequent discussions. Clearly, the benefiting individuals have been expanded beyond heterosexual married couples to include single, divorced, and widowed women, but the basic patriarchal and paternalistic bent of the policy has not changed.

Beyond government regulations, a second aspect of reproductive politics in India is worth noting. The ART recipient and 'gestational surrogate' are best viewed as figures of bio-nationalism, where science and religious work coalesce. Ethnographical work on ARTs and surrogacy in India have shown how science and religion cohere in the new clinics of surrogacy. For example, Aditya Bharadwaj's wonderful ethnography of IVF clinics (2016) in India shows how science and religion are everywhere, deeply imbricated in the practices of the clinics, the doctors, and their patients. Rather than adhere to ideological commitments to 'scientific rationality', we find that the divine, the spiritual and religious beliefs fill 'the vacuum of uncertainty' that underlies technoscientific practices. The doctors, Bharadwaj argues, are deeply committed to induce conception in the IVF clinics, and use their considerable cultural beliefs to provide successful outcomes. For example, in an interview, a doctor explains that ARTs are an 'incomplete science'. Success rates are low. As someone who believes in God, astrology, palmistry, Vastu shastra, the doctor engages the power of alternate medical practices to improve success rates. He encourages patients to engage with religion and alternative medicine. The doctor claims success. The irony is striking – reproductive technologies are ways to assist human reproduction when nature fails, but when technologies themselves need assistance, the divine is invoked!

Similarly focusing on surrogacy clinics in particular, Amrita Pande in her excellent *Wombs in Labor* (2014), demonstrates that the divine pervades surrogacy clinics. She argues that women understand their work largely in the language of gods, goddesses, and the divine. Stories from Hindu mythology are used to argue that surrogacy is not new and is in fact part of the Hindu religion. Pande's (2014) work reinforces the pervasiveness of the divine to the point of creating a mythical god of surrogacy, the 'surrodev' or 'surro-god' that has blessed women with the opportunity of surrogacy.

The new 2020 laws have now placed reproduction – family planning, ARTs and surrogacy – firmly in the politics of patriarchal families. Indeed, this confluence has come starkly into view with the rise of Hindu nationalism, and its promotion of the ancient Vedic Sciences as modern science. We have seen the rise of the ancient *garbha vigyan* (science of the womb) and *garbha sanskar* (education in the womb). These efforts at reproductive enhancements using Vedic and Hindu sciences draw from an older history. For example, Lucia Savary (2014) describes 'vernacular eugenics' in colonial India. *Santati-śāstra* (the 'science of progeny' or 'progeniology'), was based on the principles of Francis Galton's 'classical eugenics' but re-adapted as a form of Indian eugenics, using Ayurveda or *ratiśāstra*, as its knowledge base. This reinvigorated eugenic logic is being resurrected in workshops that promise *su-santan* (a superior child) or *uttam santan* (superior child). *Garbha sanskar* brings together 'sexology, eugenics, cultural practices, and maternal and child health' (Sur, 2018), through ritual practices of the corporeal and spiritual. It includes advice on diet, daily activities that regulate the mind and body, to create a child who is 'mentally, emotionally, physically, and spiritually superior to the rest'. Vasudha Mohanka's detailed chapter in this collection (Chapter 3) elaborates on this most recent 'neo-eugenic' incarnation of a long history of repronationalism in India.

We see all the key elements of an archaic modernity emerge in these new sciences. First, the ancient Vedas are seen as perfectly allied with modern biosciences. Second, the workshops stress nationalism. 'If you want a strong nation, you have to start with strong children' (Sud, 2018: 20). Third, are the eugenic promises that these practices will purify 'impure' wombs to produce 'fair, tall, intelligent, and perfect progeny' (Bharadwaj, 2017; Ghoshal, 2017). The desired traits are decidedly upper caste, upper-class, and male. The promotional material and pamphlets distributed are not from fringe groups, but often government funded and supported entities. In this effortless blending of the ancient and modern, the west and the east, we see the many elisions and erasures. Tracking *garbha sanskar* and its controversies allows us to see the epistemological contradictions inherent in *archaic modernities* (Ghoshal, 2017). Ayurveda and modern science have distinctly incommensurable epistemologies, ontologies, and methodologies. Yet, in promoting a *garbha vigyan*, such projects effortlessly elide the considerable differences between science and religion, scripture and science, ritual and experiment, and between western biomedicine and Ayurveda.

Sushmita: Banu coins the term 'postcolonial pregnancies' in her book *Holy Science* (Subramaniam, 2019), and I find it very useful to think with the irony of this nomenclature to sieve through some of the issues at hand. 'Postcolonial pregnancies' aptly draws out the reproductive logic at the core of structural transformations and tells us that even though we see an ostensible shift from colonialism to postcolonialism, patriarchal structures are reproduced and colonialism simply changes form under new conditions of global capital. Besides a reproduction of structural conditions, 'postcolonial pregnancies' also gestures towards the bodies that live through systems and labour under it, all the while dictated by the historical materialism of the present. Thinking with 'postcolonial pregnancies' and turning to the legislative examples delineated by Deboleena and Banu, what do we discern about reproductive decision making in contemporary India? We started in 2008 with the 'Baby Manji' case involving the Japanese couple. The baby's biological Japanese father was unable to adopt the baby as Indian law does not allow for single men to adopt children. Ultimately, the child was issued a birth certificate with the biological father's name on it, and allowed to leave the country. All of this was celebrated by the media as 'new' and a first occurrence. In 2016, we get the law that bans commercial surrogacy and prohibits foreigners and homosexual couples from hiring sur-rogates in India. The 2020 laws regulate IVF clinics, extend the term-limit for termination of pregnancies, and put in place new surrogacy regulations to prevent exploitation of mothers and children. Interestingly, single women can now access surrogacy services. First, I find it interesting that these laws, while pertaining to India, are directly linked with India's relation to the 'outside', such as foreigners, homosexual people, and those considered morally deficient. The intertwining of public, private, morality, sexuality, gender, class, nation is convoluted and persistent. Second, these laws showcase a broadening of juridical authority on questions of who and what deserves protection, guided all along by considerations of religion, class, gender, and sexuality. The deepening and broadening of the orbit for the state, and a specific Hindu nation is explicit. May we ask: what then is being birthed through 'postcolonial pregnancies'? Working with the reproductive logic of biopolitics, how do we envisage alternate political imaginations?

The invocation of 'Be Modern, Not Western' haunts with its insidious meanings through different periods of Indian colonial and postcolonial politics. This postcolonial modernity is the anchor for a spiralling diasporic Hindu family and nation. Transnational Hinduism is a strategic actor in the politics of globalisation. Saskia Sassen (2006: 1) notes that 'The epochal transformation we call globalization is taking place inside the national to a far larger extent than is usually recognized.' Rather than juxtaposing the local and the global or the national and the global, Sassen (2006) urges us to note the global within the national. These 'postcolonial pregnancies' and the rules for *garbha sanskar* travel rapidly through a growing transnational Hindu family along with the validity of Ayurveda and yoga to combat westernisation's maladies. The 'west' also eagerly consume these products as a remedy to itself; such is the marketability and resonance of global Hinduism. None of this is new though. Nationalism in its many forms has always conversed with transnationalism. Whether noting the many foreign trips of the current Indian ministry or thinking about nationalists in colonial India who travelled extensively abroad, and hosted international visitors in India, nationalism converses intimately with transnationalism and generates each other. Can we thus argue that the laws discussed above also showcase a transnational push and pull in framings of biopolitics, rather than a specific national control of biopolitics? What would we add to our analyses if we actively think with transnational entanglements that situate biopolitics and its governance? Biopolitics takes on many lives through spi-ralling communities, their inter-actions, and movement through history.

The questions of markets and a political-economy of Hinduism are central to this conversation. What is happening through this novel branding of 'archaic modernity'? When science, religion, and modernity are orchestrated in a seamless choreography, who profits in this marketplace of values, goods, and bodies? Hinduism serves many purposes and is bestowed with varied possibilities as religion, civilisation, political-economy, and morality structure. Tulasi Srinivas, for example, invokes the term 'experimental Hinduism' to write about 'a whole world of iterative, strategic, and creative improvisa-tions within and around Hindu rituals as they interact with modernity' (2018: 15). Working with the transnational logics of a consistently morphing Hinduism enables us to note the expanding markets in a globalised economy that are enabled through this specific branding. Who can escape the proliferation of Hindu iconography in most local markets, or even yoga studios, through the world as seen in images of Hindu gods and goddesses used to sell varied products with an other-worldly branding strategy? Conversations on biopolitics and religion spiral in many interesting directions when seen through the exchanges in a transnational market.

'Markets', while being a central economic anchor, are also het-erogeneous and have various histories. While 'north' and 'south' define geopolitics and international relations, they also constitute markets that interact through differences and similarities on multiple levels. The 'north' has many norths and souths within it, as does the 'south'. And many bodies remain invisible within geopolitical nomenclatures such as 'north' and 'south' even when they constitute its reproductive labour. Oftentimes markets are constituted by diasporas moving through different political territories, and common histories of colonialism. India and South Africa constitute one such south-south configuration, with increased attention being paid to strengthening bilateral relations. Food security, sharing infrastructure, and security ties often dominate conversations south-south. Also, intense pride with histories and cultural backgrounds inspire these political-economic bondings. It will be interesting to see how south-south relations configure and reconfigure under new economic realities shaped by global emergencies. How will markets reproduce and what exigencies will shape choices for 'markets in reproduction' under altered geopolitical realties? Competition and collaboration are often different faces to the same coin, and the logic of growing markets will fashion political choices on population growth and control.

A Malthusian logic of population control or a Foucauldian framing of biopolitics takes many shapes in transnational shifts and in contemporary India. Deboleena and Banu have described, through our conversation, how eugenics, religion, culture, and modernity work in multiple ways framing their own reproductive logic, that is, the reproduction of the Hindu nation. Seemingly opposite values as seen in anti-natal and pro-natal policies cohere when we pay attention to who exactly is allowed to reproduce. An overarching politics of purity frames official articulations about India, its inhabitants, and its rightful citizens. And thus, transnational India recreates its markets of reproduction. Transnational markets weave through disparate territories and even when selling a 'pure' logic, they are irreverently impure in terms of how they are intermeshed within global structures. Rationality and irrationality coalesce when it comes to thinking about profit margins and the economy of biopolitical exchanges. Thinking with impurity provides a way to discern these complex braiding and extend our political imagination towards a decolonial ethos.

Conclusion

As we share our different encounters of biological politics, what strikes us is that each of us has approached these questions from our varied interdisciplinary locations. As a result, what is subsumed within biological politics emerges as infinitely capacious, necessitating a methodological apparatus suitably ambitious. Feminist and postcolonial theories have provoked us to question what we see, and at the very least, to make accounts of what appears to us as incommensurable. Our interdisciplinary training and expertise allow us to conduct vibrant ecologies, acknowledge hybrid constitutions, and reveal impure formations. In our attempts to unravel biopolitical imaginations in and of South Asia, the hybrid, syncretic, and the impure reign supreme. We have found it most helpful to think about purity politics through impure theories that situate the interactive nature of structures.

Through this conversation we have collectively agonised about incongruent realities such as the demand for surrogates in Bhopal despite its history of biopolitical disaster. Laws and evolving parameters for surrogacy signal towards purity politics and containment, while broadening transnational markets showcase the uses of purity in global markets which are themselves impure, intermeshed, and evolving. Pure categories of east and west are muddied inextricably, and Malthus and Foucault travel within convoluted global structures, often as spectres denoting a haunting presence or absence. Purity schemas are seen as inherently impure and impurity helps us situate geopolitics and its markets in reproduction. Banu puts it best when she writes, 'What we need are impure politics, impure theories for impure time' (Subramaniam, 2019: 229).

Traversing through a global pandemic that has raptured our theoretical prisms and terms for classification, we emphasise the urgency for continual engagement with the politics (and impossibility) of purity and futile attempts at containment of bodies and theories. Classifications of private and public remain dislocated under rearranged work structures, and labour categorisations such as 'key workers' or 'essential workers' often relay the lowest in the pay chain. Animal, human, virus, plant, air, and place are jostled together in unimagined intimacies while we wonder about configurations of life-to-come. 'birth politics' under these new contexts are imbued in impurities, whether in terms of new structures for health and medicine or even more accentuated social stratifications. The spectre of biopolitics haunts our present regimes of life and death and instils anew the urgency to think with impure theories and incessantly work towards decolonising STS.

Notes

1 Kautilya, also known as Chanakya, was a minster in Chandragupta Maurya's court in fourth-century BC and the *Arthashastra* is usually seen as a treatise that informs a ruler on the pragmatics of power and

politics. Niccolo Machiavelli (1469–1527) was writing during the Italian Renaissance and his political text *Prince* carries advice about how to administer and perpetuate political power.

References

Bharadwaj, A. (2016). *Conceptions: Infertility and Procreative Technologies in India*. New York: Berghahn Books.

Bharadwaj, A. (2017). RSS wing has prescription for fair, tall 'customised' babies. *Indian Express*, 7 May.

BioVoice (2020). Cabinet approves the Assisted Reproductive Technology Regulation Bill. www.biovoicenews.com/cabinet-approves-the-assisted-reproductive-technology-regulation-bill-2020/. Accessed 2 September 2020.

Campbell, T. and Sitze, A. (2013). Biopolitics: an encounter. In T. Campbell and A. Stize (eds), *Biopolitics: A Reader*, 1–40. Durham, NC: Duke University Press.

Civilsdaily (2020). Surrogacy in India: Assisted Reproductive Technology Regulation Bill, 2020. www.civilsdaily.com/story/surrogacy-in-india/. Accessed 2 September 2020.

Cooper, M., and Waldby, C. (2014). *Clinical Labor: Tissue Donors and Research Subjects in the Global Bioeconomy*. Durham, NC: Duke University Press.

Dhar, A. 2016. India to Ban rent-a-wombs, limited surrogacy allowed but not for single women, gays. *The Wire*, 8 August.

Dhara, R. V. (1992). Health effects of the Bhopal gas leak: a review, *Epidemiologia e prevenzione* 14:52, 22–31.

Drishti (2020). Medical Termination of Pregnancy (Amendment) Bill, 2020. www.drishtiias.com/daily-updates/daily-news-editorials/medical-termination-of-pregnancy-amendment-bill-2020. Accessed 2 September 2020.

Doniger, W. (1975). *Hindu Myths*. London: Penguin.

Foucault, M. (1976). *Society Must be Defended. Lectures at the College de France, 1975–1976*, Vol. 1. Basingstoke: Macmillan.

Ghoshal, R. (2017). A few shades fairer, please, *Indian Journal of Medical Ethics* 3:3, 230–4.

Haraway, D. (1997). *Modest Witness@Second_Millenium.FemaleMan©_Meets Onco_Mouse™: Feminism and Technoscience*. Routledge: New York.

The Hindu (2016). Surrogate children only for married couples: bill. www.pressreader.com/india/the-hindu/20160825/textview. Accessed 2 September 2020.

International Campaign for Justice in Bhopal (2020). The death toll. www. bhopal.net/what-happened/that-night-december-3-1984/the-death-toll/. Accessed 21 May 2020.

Lakshmi, R. (2016.) India to propose a ban on commercial surrogacy. *Washington Post*, 24 August.

Pande, A. (2014). *Wombs in Labor: Transnational Commercial Surrogacy in India*. New York: Columbia University Press.

Roy, D. (2018). *Molecular Feminisms: Biology, Becomings, and Life in the Lab*. Seattle, WA: University of Washington Press.

Sassen, S. (2006). *Territory, Authority, Rights: From Medieval to Global Assemblages*. Princeton, NJ: Princeton University Press.

Savary, L. (2014). Vernacular eugenics? Santati-śāstra' in popuar Hindi advisory literature (1900–1940), *South Asia: Journal of South Asian Studies* 37:3, 381–97.

Sehgal, P. (2008). Reproductive tourism soars in India. *Alternet*. www. alternet.org/2008/11/reproductive_tourism_soars_in_india/. Accessed 2 September 2020.

Shotwell, A. (2016). *Against Purity: Living Ethically in Compromised Times*. Minneapolis, MN: University of Minnesota Press.

Srinivas, T. (2018). *The Cow in the Elevator: An Anthropology of Wonder*. Durham, NC: Duke University Press.

Subramaniam, B. (2019). *Holy Science: The Biopolitics of Hindu Nationalism*. Seattle, WA: University of Washington Press.

Sur, S. (2018). Garbha Sanskar and the politics of masculinity in West Bengal, *Economic & Political Weekly* 53:5, 20–2.

Vinaik, A. (1997). *The Furies of Indian Communalism: Religion, Modernity, and Secularization*. New York: Verso.

3

Ved Garbh Vihar: Hindutva's latest neo-eugenic repronational project

Vasudha Mohanka

American anthropologist Sarah Franklin's concept of 'repronationalism' refers to a country's reproductive policy shaping its 'national identity, while similarly expressing its national identity through its reproductive policy' (Franklin, 2016). Reproductive nationalism has been conceptually used by other scholars like Margaret Jolly and Kalpana Ram (2001: 10) who analyse the engendering of the 'natural' hierarchy of the family 'projected on the nation state, not just as familial metaphors but in bureaucratic practices and policies that impinge on sexed bodies'. I, however, use the concept more loosely to analyse a particular right-wing run programme (and not a policy), Ved Garbh Vihar (VGV), which overly endorses neo-eugenic ideals, through Ayurvedic procedures (non-biomedical) and disciplining of the body, aimed at the larger nationalistic project of expressing Hindutva[1] identity. Hence, identity and nationalism are crucial aspects reproduced through the birth of seemingly prodigious babies!

I argue that, historically, reproductive nationalism in India has thrived in a casteist, classist and gendered context, wherein certain already marginalised groups (read Muslims, Christians and the socio-economically underprivileged) have been perceived as fecund, hyperfertile bodies (Sarkar, 2002), as the Other, contributing to population growth. Such bodies have been conceived as a burden, aiding in population growth and as a stumbling block to achieving Hindutva (an ideology seeking to establish the hegemony of a conservative Hinduism) and economic nationalism as well. Repronationalism, in this context, elucidates on demographic anxiety (more specifically in the postcolonial period) and paranoia that most often lead to intervention, control, surveillance and influencing reproductive decision making of the population. It signifies encouraging certain marginalised groups to have fewer children in the name of population control. Population control 'linked national reproduction to modernity, positing population limitation as the means to jumpstart economic development' (Nadkarni, 2014: 7). The complexities and ambiguities of reproductive nationalisms in India during the colonial and postcolonial periods have been well documented (Ahluwalia, 2008; Hodges, 2010; Tarlo, 2003; Sarkar, 2002; Rao, 2010; Jolly, 1994, Nadkarni, 2014).

Population control through forced sterilisation may be conceived as a eugenic measure. In the more recent past, neo-eugenics includes both the use of biomedicine through new/assisted reproductive technologies and a simultaneous Ayurvedic neo-eugenics (VGV). Within the more recent drive toward building a Hindutva nation, Hindus are conceived as a pure-bred 'race' despite more recent linguistic and archaeological evidence suggesting India as having historically experienced an admixture of races (Thapar, 1996, 2014, Thapar et al., 2016). The Bhartiya Janata Party's (BJP) and Rashtriya Swayamsevak Sangh's (RSS) (two of the primary players pushing the Hindutva agenda, fully explored later in this chapter), cultural nationalism is transplanting cultural rights in place of political rights, in favour of 'primogeniture, racial purity and genetic ancestry' contained in the ideas of the homeland and motherland (Menon in Thapar et al., 2016). This in a country with a long history of Malthusianism during British colonial rule, and neo-Malthusianism in the postcolonial context. Within this history, particularly within the Hindutva movements of RSS since the 1920s, there has been a concern around Hindu emasculation by the coloniser, and a concurrent concern for the hyper virile Muslim man and the hyperfertile Muslim women Other (Sarkar, 2002). This, argues Sur (2018), saw the emergence of the 'anxious' (Anand, 2007) and 'corporeal' Hindutva masculinity that has stoked mass fear of being minoritised among the Hindu population in India.

It is within this context that the development of a programme such as VGV is located, in which the process of reproduction does not merely produce babies. A context where the industry of reproduction includes both biomedical markets for assisted reproduction and surrogacy, and a growing parallel reproductive enterprise, that of VGV, which deploys non-biomedical (read non-western) Ayurvedic procedures to beget the 'best progeny'. Much like the biomedicalised reproductive industry, this reproduces the desire to beget certain desirable biogenetic and phenotypic characteristics. VGV is thriving in a particular state in India (Gujarat), also popularly known as the 'Hindutva laboratory' (Sud, 2018). The BJP's political victory in Gujarat in 2002 saw the then VHP[2] President, Pravin Togadia, proclaim Gujarat as the 'Hindutva laboratory', expressing the intent to establish 'Hindu supremacy in India' with a promise to 'make a laboratory of the whole country' (HT Correspondent, 2002). Togadia asserted that Gujarat had turned out to be a 'graveyard for secular forces' (HT Correspondent, 2002). Academicians like Spodek (2010) and journalists like Dionne Bunsha (2006) have also outlined detailed accounts of communal violence and pogroms against Muslims and Christians, which left more than 2000 people dead due to the Godhra riots during Narendra Modi's Chief ministership at the time.

The Hindutva laboratory project, which has been gradually spreading in various states across the country, has as its aim to project all Muslims, Parsis and Christians as foreigners, to revere fascist dictators like Hitler and Mussolini through changing pedagogy and curriculum in schools and tracing the first ever human ancestry to India (Bunsha, 2006: 374–5).

Unsurprisingly, the VGV programme is run by a militant chauvinistic hard Hindutva nationalistic state propagating the use of alternative medical knowledge systems like Ayurveda combined with yoga and music in a predominantly reproductive-temple-corporate-industrial-complex.

The state of Gujarat has, since 2002, also seen a burgeoning gestational surrogacy industry (Pande, 2010, 2015), which promotes reproductive tourism and employs cheap reproductive labour (gestational surrogate mothers), which Nadkarni (2014) conceives as neo-eugenics of new reproductive technologies.

The proliferation of assisted reproductive technologies (ARTs) like IVF, and (often legal) arrangements like commercial gestational surrogacy, were legalised in India in 2002 and thrived in a non-regulated, globalised context. Dr Nayna Patel, who runs the Akanksha Fertility Clinic in Anand, Gujarat, shot to fame after delivering thousands of babies from 2002 till the mid-2010s through contracting with gestational surrogate mothers, primarily from financially marginalised groups, who delivered babies mostly for more privileged people (who were unable to conceive or bear children, or chose to opt for surrogacy) who could afford to pay for surrogacy. Gujarat gradually became a world-renowned 'surrogacy hub', a 'baby factory', offering cheap reproductive labour and English-speaking doctors (Carney, 2010; Nadimpally et al., 2011). A ban in 2015 for foreigners and gender non-binary people to avail of commercial gestational surrogacy led to a reduction in the number of surrogacy arrangements. This was due to numerous surrogacy cases being embroiled in legal battles and complexities. A bill remains pending in Parliament since 2016 to ban all forms of commercial gestational surrogacy (PRS India, 2020).

The film Google Baby also highlighted how globalisation and reproductive technologies have made possible the act of baby-making without sex.

This chapter focuses on how hard Hindutva conservative right-wing forces in India have orchestrated the spread of the neo-eugenic programme through promoting it among socio-economically privileged Hindu men and women – participating in an Ayurvedic eugenic programme through disciplining their bodies with yoga, exercise, music, non-consumption of meat, and the invocation and chanting of Vedic chants during the prenatal period to (re)produce superior and ideal progeny to contribute to the project of nation-building. The simultaneous projects of forced sterilisation of Muslim bodies and the control of pregnant Muslim bodies like Safoora Zargar's amidst the Citizenship Amendment Act (CAA) and National Registration of Citizens (NRC) Bills[3] reflects the reproductive landscape in the larger political and moral economy of the country.

Media narratives have revealed that the VGV programme thrives in a context of commercialising Ayurveda, validating it through the claims of RSS leaders who (apparently) met Germans who reminded them of the glorious Indian past and the techniques in Ayurveda to produce superior progeny for the ideal nation. The likening of VGV to Nazi idealogues has been prominent in numerous English print media narratives (Bhardwaj, 2017; Das, 2017; Gowen, 2017; Outlook Web Bureau, 2017).

The conception of Ved Garbh Vihar

VGV is a 'confluence of sexology, eugenics, cultural practices, and maternal and child health' claiming 'to produce su-santan or uttam santan (perfect child)' for the perfect nation (Sur, 2018). VGV thrives under a predominantly Hindutva dominant government with the agenda of advancing the Hindu 'race' to outnumber the Muslims and Christians who are seen as hyper virile and hyper fertile and posing a threat to Hindus. The VGV programme functions as part of a larger discursive apparatus of Hindutva nationalism at the intersection of law (for example the CAA-NRC), media (for example, Modi's histrionic televised yoga and pranayama) and the control and persecution of Muslim bodies (for example, the arrest of the pregnant Safoora Zargar, a Muslim woman who was protesting the CAA). The programme thrives in the larger context of perpetuating demographic paranoia through reproductive nationalism towards a larger project of homogenising India as a part of the Hindutva project's agenda of nation-building.

VGV promotes and markets itself as a centre for 'Vedic Motherhood facilitating Ayurvedic antenatal care through Panchkarma' dedicatedly working towards generating the best progeny. Earlier known as Garbh Vigyan Sanskar, VGV was established in 2003 in Jamnagar in Gujarat, India. The state of Gujarat is infamously known as the Hindutva laboratory in the country. Garbha sanskar is claimed to be 'a scientifically proven fact' and a way of interacting with the 'unborn baby in the womb during pregnancy' (Garbhasanskar website). It covers the prenatal, pregnancy and postnatal periods (Garbhasanskar website). The process of garbh samvad (dialogue with the foetus), along with other activities such as yoga and music are provided during the orientation programme to pregnant women at the Garbh Sanskar Kendra (Santoshi, 2015).

In the final section, I present an analysis of English-language print media articles, and the Twitter and Facebook pages of VGV. I argue that VGV produces not just babies, but reproduces neo-eugenic ideals creating a potential 'Made in India babies' industry, contributing towards the larger project of Hindutva nation-building. VGV locates itself in a globalised world, commercialising Ayurveda, and promising to produce prodigious children to serve the Hindutva project of nation-building.

Repropolitics and conceptions of eugenics

This section provides an overview of the varying nationalist sentiment around the conceptions of eugenics since the early 1900s. During the early 1900s, there were various groups of people in India, each with a different understanding of eugenics. One group not overtly engaged in voluntary organisations wrote and published on eugenics, focusing on specific cultural Hindu practices such as caste endogamy and arranged marriages based on astrological combinations. Eugenics in India, to them, predated the colonised India. They argued that ancient Indian scriptures and Indians themselves knew the secrets to 'national regeneration' and 'revitalisation' that the west was much later in discovering (Hodges, 2006, 2010).

The birth control agenda through the early decades of the twentieth century was dominated by the middle-class, upper-caste, English-speaking well-educated privileged men and women who conceived of eugenics, in terms of controlling the population and aimed at preserving a specific middle-class masculinity. Further, such privileged middle-class men and women aimed at achieving 'bourgeois nationalism'. Through bourgeois nationalism, they 'identified lower-caste and working-class Indian women as primary targets of contraceptive technologies – both chemical and mechanical (Ahluwalia, 2008: 4).

The male advocates of birth control through the 1920s and 1930s aimed at surveilling the reproductive practices of the middle class and managing reproductive practices of the subaltern groups such as the lower castes, lower classes and Muslims to ensure national wellbeing (Ahluwalia, 2008).[4] They were responsible for the setting up of voluntary organisations to promote eugenics through contraceptive distribution and knowledge dissemination (Ahluwalia, 2008; Hodges, 2010).

The Hindu Neo-Malthusian League, which was started in 1882 and re-emerged as the Madras neo-Malthusian League in 1928, was run by the English-speaking elite, who published in English and explicitly incorporated eugenics. Gopaljee Ahluwalia, who was instrumental in setting up the Indian Eugenic Society in Lahore and Simla in 1921, borrowed from Francis Galton's (1909) definition of eugenics[5] and added that Indian conditions and moral and spiritual components are crucial to 'racial improvement' projects. In 1922, Ahluwalia founded the Indian Birth Control Society and corresponded with British birth control activist, Marie Stopes.[6] Other eugenic societies were set up in Bombay (now Mumbai) and Sholapur in the late 1920s.

Most of the male birth advocates were deeply invested in safeguarding the interests of middle-class upper-caste Hindu men, and while some of them advocated for women's sexual needs, they believed that the ultimate expression of women's sexuality was in maternity (Ahluwalia, 2008). By the 1930s, the discourse on overpopulation moved to demographic control.

Maternalism and eugenics

Unlike their western counterparts, Indian middle-class nationalist feminists from the 1920s to 1947 (when India attained independence from British rule) furthered the 'maternalist eugenics' logic through a preoccupation with women's reproductive health by providing adequate resources for maternal and infant welfare as a part of nation-building (Hodges, 2010). Further, their concerns included varied notions of individuality, femininity, motherhood and sexuality in an emerging anticolonial Gandhian nationalist movement in 'an alliance with patriarchal nationalism and an engagement with modernity' (Ahluwalia, 2008: 87). Some of the prominent names were: Rameshwari Nehru, Dr Muthulakshmi Reddi, Margaret Cousins, Rani Laxmibai Rajwade, Lakshmi Menon, Begum Hamid Ali and Kamaladevi Chattopadhyaya.

Margaret Sanger, who was a staunch advocate of birth control – later called population control – was closely aligned to the eugenics movement and began to emphasise directing population control efforts towards women (Green, 2018).

Dhanvanthi Rama Rau's engagement with birth and population control led her to found the Family Planning Association of India and she also supported compulsory sterilisation during the Emergency declared by Indira Gandhi in 1975.

Eugenic feminism (Nadkarni, 2014) is but one strand among the many simultaneous coexisting complex strands of feminisms. In late colonial India, feminists who were a part of the nationalist movement focused less on contraception and more on women's and children's health as part of health and governance projects, in turn highlighting that only healthy mothers could produce strong children and a healthy race in order to oust foreigners or colonisers for swaraj or self-rule (Hodges, 2010).

After the Second World War, especially in postcolonial India, eugenics came to be replaced by population control and, from the 1940s till the 1960s, poverty alleviation through interventions in reproductive behaviour and decision making aimed at 'social engineering and improvement' (Hodges, 2010). From the mid-1950s to the 1970s, vasectomies were encouraged by the Indian government through mobile camps. However, one bureaucratic decision during the Emergency period in 1975, when all civil liberties were suspended, also saw the implementation of the forced male sterilisation programme, which has had a longstanding impact on vasectomies since.

Coercive male sterilisation during the Emergency

Continuing from earlier periods, sterilisation continued to be an important part of bureaucratic programmes. While most sterilisation had been conducted on women's bodies in the past, the period of Emergency witnessed coercive male sterilisation on a large scale.

An Emergency was declared in early 1975 in India by then Indian Prime Minister, Indira Gandhi (who was a member of the Indian National Congress Party). Her younger son, Sanjay Gandhi wielded 'extra-constitutional authority' and power, executing his five-point programme, one of the key agendas being population control through vasectomy camps (Dayal, 2015). Mass coercive male sterilisation revealed the government's 'demographic paranoia' and Islamophobia. The mass sterilisation is often compared to the Nazi regime in Germany (Biswas, 2014). Popular socialite, and a close aide to Sanjay Gandhi, Rukhsana Sultana, who was a Muslim woman, was asked to be instrumental in convincing Muslim men to be sterilised. She set up her 'infamous family planning clinic' in Dujana House, also one of the major locations for tension during the Emergency (Tarlo, 2003: 143). Deeply committed to the *Hum do hamare do* (one family, two children) slogan of family planning, Sanjay Gandhi was at the forefront of the incentive-disincentive coercive male sterilisation programme, not distinguishing between men of any age, especially the poor and the marginalised (Tarlo, 2003).

The coercive vasectomies were conducted alongside the town planning and beautification of certain areas in the capital city with the aim of creating resettlement colonies for the already marginalised that, included a large number of Muslims and other marginalised groups (Tarlo, 2003).

Since the Emergency, male sterilisation has been pushed aside and female sterilisation has become the dominant focus of control of reproductive bodies. Since the 1990s, right-wing Hindutva groups in India like the BJP along with the Vishwa Hindu Parishad (VHP), the Rashtriya Swayamsevak Sangh (RSS) and the Bajrang Dal (more on this in subsequent sections) have desired a 'saffron demography' (Rao, 2007: 1) due to their own demographic anxiety and paranoia expressed through the slogan, *Hum Do, Hamare Do; Woh Paanch Unke Pachees* ('We Hindus are two and have two children, while, they, the Muslims are five and have twenty-five children'). The slogan became popular at a time when the Sangh Parivar was engaged in fierce campaigns and violent communal acts such as the destruction of the Babri Masjid (a mosque) in the state of Uttar Pradesh. The demographic anxiety reinforced their fear of Muslims outnumbering the Hindus and their aspiration to build a 'theocratic state, a Hindu Rashtra' (Rao, 2007: 1) has continued to date. More recently, a neo-eugenic programme that aspires to build a perfect nation with perfect progeny is being run by the RSS, and is deeply problematic.

While the ruling BJP government in India at present has been overly critical of the opposition party, the Indian National Congress and especially the political decisions during the Emergency, the consistent othering of Muslims and Christians has continued since the BJP has been at the centre (earlier in the 1990s for five years, and more recently since 2014).

Hindutva nationalism and othering the Muslim

Gujarat, known as the laboratory of Hindutva (HT Correspondent, 2002; Spodek, 2010; Bunsha, 2006) witnessed violence in 2002 under the leadership of then Chief Minister of state, Narendra Modi. As mentioned above, the Hindutva laboratory has been the epicentre of violence and pogroms against Muslims, Christians and minorities.

An extreme RSS female member, Sadhvi Deva Thakur, also expressed her demographic paranoia (like many in her group) when she proposed that Muslims and Christians be forcibly sterilised because the Hindus were threatened by their growing population (Dayal, 2019). Echoing xenophobia and extreme right-wing sentiments with a disregard for minority communities, making them appear hyper fertile and encouraging Hindus to have more children to counter the rise of the other communities echoes eugenic measures such as coercive sterilisation.

The city of Anand in the state of Gujarat in India has seen the proliferation of one of India's largest fertility clinics, the Akanksha Fertility Clinic run by Dr Nayna Patel who shot to fame on the Oprah Winfrey Show, foregrounding India as a surrogacy destination in the early 2000s. Dr Patel deployed the use of assisted reproductive technologies (read western biomedicine) such as in vitro fertilisation (IVF) and non-traditional gestational surrogacy, more specifically appealing to foreign commissioning parents as well as economically upwardly mobile and privileged Indians who could afford to pay for such treatments (Pande, 2010).

The geopolitical and socio-cultural location and the simultaneity of two programmes, one biomedical and the other seen as traditional (read Ayurveda) began to thrive in the state of Gujarat with the latter gaining prominence after the mid-2010s, just when many foreign commissioning parents were restricted from gaining entry into India to access ARTs.

In 2014, as a part of a 'paid incentive programme aimed to control poverty through population containment' (Wilson, 2018), eleven low-caste women died due to blood poisoning or haemorrhagic shock after being sterilised in a government-run camp in the state of Chattisgarh, while eighty-three women were sterilised in less than six hours. Female sterilisation is the commonest form of contraception in India since the failed attempts at vasectomy in the 1970s and especially after the Emergency (Bhuyan 2018; Wilson, 2018). This new form of eugenics has targeted vulnerable and socially marginalised groups much like the eugenics of the past (Wilson, 2018).

As discussed previously, neo-eugenics has taken various forms in India – from Malthusian and neo-Malthusian concerns around population, leading to population control measures such as forced sterilisations, to a programme, more recently, that aspires to juxtapose identity and nationalism to create a perfect nation through creating prodigious children. The disciplining of the mind and body through Ayurvedic practices, Vedic chants, customs and rituals, yoga, abstinence from meat and alcohol, valorising motherhood and promising to create intelligent, fair and tall babies towards the project of nation-building is significant in understanding the Hindutva nationalistic project.

The following section provides a brief overview of the concept of Hindutva to provide a context to help elaborate further on the VGV programme, which signifies the Hindutva project of nation-building.

Caste and race in Hindutva neo-eugenics

The social stratification system of caste is a 'hereditary Hindu system of occupation, endogamy and social culture' (Hodges, 2010: 231) that emerged in colonial bureaucracy from the eighteenth century as the critical marker for understanding social organisation in India. Experts in the early twentieth century could not reach a consensus on distinguishing Indians through race as well as caste that 'might stand in for race as the taxonomy within which to undertake eugenic analysis' (Hodges, 2010: 232). Eugenic-racial theories found significant application in the Hindu reprimand of Muslims wherein Hindus were seen as India's supposed 'originary' inhabitants, while Muslims were cast as an invading race (Datta, 1993).

Sharma (2002) elucidates on the ambiguity in the terms, namely, Hindu, Hinduism, Hindustan and Hindutva. The Indian National Congress' aspiration represented *territorial nationalism*, wherein Gandhi's influence barred the rise of Hindu reactions and their move towards religious nationalism. Neo-Hinduism 'became somewhat revivalistic with the rise of the Arya Samaj' (Sharma, 2002: 21), and its 'ethnic streak' in the 1920s saw the growing popularity of Hindutva.

Chandranath Basu, a privileged Bengali literary scholar coined the term Hindutva in 1892, in his book, *Hindutva – Hindur Prakrita*

Itihas ('Hindutva – An Authentic History') defending traditional Hindu rituals, the caste system, maintaining patriarchy and restricting women's education and civil rights.

The term Hindutva was later popularised by a right-wing leader and member of the Akhil Bharatiya Hindu Mahasabha, Vinayak Damodar Savarkar, who while in prison wrote *Essentials of Hindutva*, published in 1923 under the pseudonym A. Maratha and later retitled *Hindutva: Who is a Hindu?* and reprinted in 1928. Savarkar argued through this foundational Hindu nationalist text, that while Hinduism is a 'derivative of Hindutva', Hindutva describes the quality of being a Hindu and a Hindu is one who claims India to be his motherland (*matribhu*), the land of his ancestors (*Pitribhu*) and his holy land (*Punyabhu*). He conceives of Hindus not just as Indian citizens, hence a nation (*Rashtra*), but also a race (*jati*), signifying common origin and common blood (*Sanskriti*). Savarkar thus elucidates on the essentials of Hindutva – 'a common nation (Rashtra), a common race (Jati), and a common civilization (Sanskriti)' (Savarkar, 1923).

Founded in 1925 by K. B. Hedgewar, the RSS is 'the most potent organised Hindu cultural group of the twentieth century in India' that emerged to unite Hindus to prepare India to be rid of colonial rule and to organise Hindus against Islam, Christianity and other creeds that the organisers felt posed a threat to and tended to 'denationalise Hindus' (Andersen, 1972: 589). Drawn from the Maharashtrian tradition, the RSS was a combination of 'a gymnastic and military tradition, and a Hindu *math* (i.e., monastery)' (Andersen, 1972: 589). While the Hindu Mahasabha (HM) was more loosely organised till 1937 with internal differences, Savarkar's leadership from 1937 made it into a political organisation that predominantly represented Hindus. The RSS propagated not just the Hindutva ideology but 'intended to infuse new physical strength into the majority community' (Jaffrelot, 2007: 16).

One of the ways that the ultranationalist and chauvinistic movement of Hindutva seeks to modernise India is by recovering the pristine Vedic-Hindu roots of Indian culture, simultaneously acquiring the most modern technology and putting it in the service of a religious-nationalist resurgence. The Hindutva movement also sees itself as the *Sangh Parivar* (literally, the family or *Rashtriya Swayamsevak Sangh* – RSS which roughly translates into National

Volunteers Association). RSS was not just paramilitary, it contained religious overtones of worshipping 'Mother India' as an avatar of the goddess (Banerjee, 1998; Basu et al., 1993; Nanda, 2003).

The following section provides a brief overview of the VGV programme and contextualises the socio-cultural location in which the programme thrives. It is important to note that the Ved Garbh Vigyan has different names on its website, Twitter and Facebook pages. With the recent proliferation of the programme within the state of Gujarat and across other states, there are various websites in circulation.

The representation of Garbh Sanskar

As a Hindutva nationalist project, the language register of the programme echoes neo-eugenic sentiments, garbed in neoliberal notions of 'choice', through the articulation of creating a superior race and a great nation. Exactly how this is achieved through online representation is explored in the next section.

VGV claims to have ensured the delivery of 450 'customised babies' through a 'scientifically proven fact' and a way of interacting with the 'unborn baby in the womb during pregnancy'. The programme covers antenatal and postnatal periods, and aimed to have a Garbh Vigyan Anusandhan Kendra (VGV centre) in every state of India by the year 2020. The process of *garbh samvad* (education in the womb), *shuddhikaran* (purification), and the importance of increasing karmic level will help in bearing superior, intelligent babies, more specifically sons. The programme aspires to create a *srestha vyakti – srestha samaj –srestha rashtra* (superior/great person – superior society – superior nation), using Ayurveda and the divinity of parenthood, more specifically motherhood.

The print media analysis showed an inconsistent narrative, with some articles mocking the programme through provocative titles and humourous images, likening the RSS representatives' narratives to the Nazi regime and invoking cultural knowledge exchange with Germany, related to Hindu mythico-religious characters such as Abhimanyu from the Mahabharata. Others seemingly endorse the programme through detailing success stories of prodigious children born, eliding the embedded elements of Hindutva nationalism. Most tweets draw upon the mother-as-god and mother-as-nation metaphors valorising biological motherhood. The Facebook posts demonstrate a metaphorical imagination to validate Ayurveda as science, claiming the inherent eugenic ideals within Ayurveda.

Garbh Sanskar website

VGV is expanding at a rapid pace across the state of Gujarat. The internet is replete with various websites, namely scientificgarbhsanskar. com and divyagarbhsanskar.com, vedgarbhsanskar, abhimanyugarbh-sanskar, ojasgarbhsanskar and many more. Even mobile phone applications have been launched on Google Play Store and App Store (iOS) with apps like Krishnacoming launched in the state of Maharashtra.[7] The expansion and digital presence of the programme beyond the state of Gujarat to other states like Maharashtra (which, as discussed earlier, had a significant role in the advent of the Hindutva project) is significant.

The website focuses on the significance of the prenatal stage, especially the intrauterine environment, which, according to Ayurveda, influences the mind, body and soul of the foetus. The evidence-based approach of the programme, in collaboration with Vidhya Bharati Educational Institution, through pilot studies, observational studies, literary research and clinical trials at Jamnagar as well as other places in Gujarat, demonstrates the need for recognition of Ayurveda as an established scientific knowledge system.

The website aims to educate people about parenthood, provides 'best progeny' through prenatal, antenatal and postnatal care, infertil-ity management and educates the medical fraternity about *garbha sanskar*. The profile of the programme's founder, Dr Hitesh Jani, shows a clear allegiance to the RSS and BJP, while its co-founder, Dr Karishma Narwani, has conducted research on scientific insights of ancient antenatal care. It is noteworthy that Dr Jani has also served on the Animal Welfare Board Government of India and has written about cows' milk, nationhood and the divine journey of the womb. This is clearly aligned with the RSS' agenda of worshipping the cow as mother, and foregrounding the agenda of Hindutva nationalism and nation-building through the use of knowledge systems like Ayurveda.

Twitter

#Garbhvigyan Kendra's Twitter page @GarbhVigyan (twitter.com/ GarbhVigyan) has been active since 2015, and had nearly forty-five tweets and about eleven followers at the time the research was conducted. The tweets are a combination of promotional marketing and advertising of the programme through the sale of Ayurvedic products, invoking health, diet, exercise, a positive mindset and paying particular attention to specific Vedic chants, certain 'spiritual books' and the valorisation of motherhood in nation-building. There are tweets marketing the programme's Ayurvedic products, such as *Suvarnaprashan* (processed gold) (23 January, 2019) and *Ved Sutika* kits for prenatal and postnatal care (1 June, 2020),[8] suggestions about listening to Vedic chants (6 March, 2019) and following a particular healthy diet (11 March, 12 September, 2019) during pregnancy to have beautiful and intelligent babies. They also promote reading spiritual books such as *Ramayan* and the *Bhagvad Gita*, arguing that these will lead the child to believe religious thoughts and ethics (27 December, 2018).

Some other tweets liken biological motherhood to divinity, drawing upon the mother-as-god and mother-as-nation metaphors valorising biological motherhood that are so prevalent in Hindutva rhetoric. They liken motherhood to 'a very precious gift from God' (5 February, 2020). The page creators send greetings on *Durga Puja* and *Navratri* – both festivals associated with larger Hindutva projects of nation-building through deifying motherhood by worshipping goddesses embodying *shakti* (power). This is done through images of a healthy mother and child, cuddling newborns and infants with tweets invoking ancient texts such as the Vedas that suggested treating mothers on a par with Gods/Goddesses.

Ironically, while on the one hand, the tweets liken motherhood to divinity and nation-building, one tweet sends greetings to the followers on Women's Day. The celebration of International Women's Day throughout the world acknowledges, commends and reveres the social, economic, cultural and political achievements of women, not specifically or necessarily defined by their roles as mothers. The programme, however, deploys a different kind of marketing strategy to revere women with regard to their role as bearers of children.

The tweets suggest making family of the nation and 'making families *for* the nation (Heng and Devan, 1992; Jolly, 1994). Through metaphors of the nation, men and women are invited into the nation through heterosexual reproduction through being part of the "family of the nation" and through making families *for* the nation' (Jolly and Ram, 2001: 6). This process of the naturalisation of nations is often through 'more subtle processes of persuasion, of soliciting sentiments of attachment on the part of emotions associated with blood and kinship and the melding of the model and familial metaphors of nation – "motherlands" or "fatherlands" and leaders as "fathers" or "mothers of the nation" (Heng and Devan, 1992; Jolly, 1994)' (Jolly and Ram, 2001: 6).

Facebook

The Facebook page of Ved Garbha Vihar (www.facebook.com/vedgarbhavihar) had twenty-seven posts at the time of research, with the last one in August 2019. There were 618 likes, 533 people following the page, and about 80 people who had checked into the programme. The page provides a link to the of the programme's website and is replete with photographs and images of the centre, rites and rituals conducted with the parents-to-be and parents of newborns, infants and toddlers, signifying a well-curated reproductive futurity. The page promotes and markets the programme through the use of visual images of some of the practices, rites and rituals at the centre, I argue, in a bid to legitimise its engagement with traditional knowledge.

In recent times, with the right-wing government in power heavily influenced by extremist groups such as the RSS, there has been a growing emphasis on worshipping the cow as mother, popularly known as *gau mata*. This, in addition to other aspects as previously mentioned, of worshipping the motherland (*Dharti mata*) and the feminised mother image of the nation itself (*Bharat mata*) are trends mobilised on the website through sharing and reposting an article from a health and wellness website which establishes that cuddling animals, especially cows, is a new wellness trend. The Facebook page of Ved Garbh Vihar reiterates the typical RSS strategy of 'We knew it long ago'. Several posts before (May, 2017), a nervous, seemingly clueless toddler is brought in close contact with a cow sitting on the ground as part of *Karn ved sanskar* (the ear piercing ceremony). The conflation of bovinity with divinity further reinforces the programme's recourse to Mother Nature by staging inter-special proximity that brings nourishment to the human race.

In January 2019 one of the posts in Gujarati also had hashtags #vedic motherhood, #garbhsanskar, #vedicchild and #designerbaby, revealing the nature and language register of creating a socio-culturally desirable child, whom the programme claims is intelligent, fair and tall.

The Facebook posts reflect a narrative metaphorical imagination to validate Ayurveda as science, claiming the inherent eugenic ideals within Ayurveda.

Electronic media

Electronic English print media discourses have critiqued the Garbh Vigyan programme, with a few exceptions. A large number of English print media articles online reveal the eugenic agenda of the Hindutva nationalist project of the RSS to portray Hindus (who are a majority in India) as a race who wish to outnumber other groups such as the Muslims and the Christians through Ayurvedic techniques such as *garbh sanskar*. The spread of the programme from Gujarat to other states like West Bengal, wherein it received criticism, is well documented in electronic media.

Textual analysis of online newspaper and website articles has revealed a consistent critique of the state's attempt to produce 'customised babies' as *uttam santati* (ideal babies) for a *samarth bharat* (strong India) with a goal of having 'thousands of such babies by 2020' (Bhardwaj, 2017). The programme's office bearers claimed that the programme had been inspired by Germany, which had 'resurrected itself' by having such such signature children through Ayurvedic practices within two decades after World War II (Bhardwaj, 2017; Outlook Web Bureau, 2017). The National Convenor of *Arogya Bharti* (the health wing of the RSS) even claimed that if proper procedures were followed by dark-skinned parents with lesser height, they could have children with fairer complexions who could grow taller. A veteran RSS activist and Swayamsevak added that having customised babies through such procedures is also mentioned in the (Hindu) *shastras* (scriptures). The office bearers claim that the procedures 'repair genes' by ensuring that 'genetic defects' are not passed on to babies. An RSS *pracharak* (worker) and national organising secretary of Arogya Bharti, Dr Ashok Varshney, said that a university in Jamnagar and two other institutions – Children's University in Gandhinangar and Atal Bihari Vajpayee Hindi University in Bhopal – have incorporated Garbh Vigyan Sanskar in their curriculum. The project was inspired by a senior RSS ideologue who received advice from a woman in Germany called 'Mother of Germany' forty years ago who told him about this resurrection citing the story of Abhimanyu from the Mahabharata, who learnt the art of breaking the *chakravyuh* (blockage) in the womb when his father narrated the method. The procedure prescribes a particular time for sexual intercourse, based on a couple's 'horoscopes and planetary configurations' (Bhardwaj, 2017; see also Daniyal, 2017).

Garbh Vigyan Anusandhan Kendra in Jamnagar 'claims that its programme is based on the advice of ancient Indian seers. The project claims to 'be able to repair genes to prevent defects from being passed on, and claims to have produced 450 perfect babies so far' (Chaudhuri, 2017). The project 'spotlights a certain section of Indians' obsession with the west, its economic muscle and beauty standards. Prejudice against dark skin is deeply ingrained in Indian society' (Outlook Web Bureau, 2017).

Sayantani Sur (2018: 20) calls garbh sanskar 'a set of medico-cultural and religious practices, which when adopted during conception and pregnancy claims to produce *su-santan* or *uttam santan* (a superior child or perfect child). Rakhi Ghoshal (2018) writes about Garbh Vigyan Sanskar as the process of 'sanitising the womb' aimed at purifying otherwise 'impure' wombs. Subramaniam's (2019) concept of 'archaic modernity' looks at Ayurveda as well as the RSS' attempt to modernise and nationalise Ayurvedic tradition to make it appear as credible as western biomedicine. The appeal of a knowledge system like Ayurveda has gained national and global prominence with Ramdev who has 'done a disservice to Ayurveda'

(Banerjee, 2020). Banerjee further argues that it is unreasonable for two varied systems and knowledge traditions to compete with each other.

Conclusion

This chapter gives a brief overview of neo-eugenics in the larger context of 'repronationalism' (Franklin, 2016) in India. Broadly conceptualising reproductive nationalism, I argue that eugenic agendas have been perpetuated through male and female bureaucrats in India since the postcolonial period. With earlier aims at a 'bourgeois nationalism' (Ahluwalia, 2008) and 'maternalist eugenics' (Nadkarni, 2014) through the control and surveillance of subaltern bodies, and the continual demographic paranoia through coercive sterilisation during the Emergency, more recent Hindutva nationalistic agendas towards a 'saffron demography' (Rao, 2007) are deeply problematic. The xenophobic sentiment displayed by the current government through violent pogroms, aggressive campaigns and othering of marginalised bodies (Muslims, Christians) manifests its aim in building a Hindu Rashtra.

VGV is not just a programme, it is a repronational neo-eugenic project aimed at creating a Hindu Rashtra, with prodigious children, especially men. The aggressive marketing of the programme, the likening to the procedures involved as 'scientific', and the marketing of Ayurveda as inherently 'eugenic' reproduce the early Hindutva leaders' ideals.

The neo-eugenic agenda as part of the RSS' Hindutva nationalist project to further a perfect ideal Aryan 'race' is demonstrated through visual imagery, language and symbolism in the social media platforms of the Ved Garbh Vigyan also known as Garbh Vigyan Sanskar programme. The deployment of Ayurvedic practices for eugenic means that are not coercive appeals to the market economy primarily paid for by the socio-economically privileged, in fear of a dying race and Hindu emasculation. This operates in the larger apparatus of the state making certain groups of people, including Muslims and Christians, stateless and turning them into second-class citizens.

With the recent expansion of the programme to other centres in Gujarat, the growing number of websites, webinars, training programmes, and the increasing digital footprint of the programme's mobile applications, it is important to critique and understand the neo-eugenic agenda of Hindutva nation-building and possible growing concerns around 'reproductive surveillance' through digital apps.

Notes

1 I have consistently used the term Hindutva to indicate the RSS', the VHP's and the BJP's militant Hindutva nationalist and 'saffron demography' project. Hindutva and Hinduism are not synonymous in that the former is a militant nationalist ideology and the latter a syncretic religion.

2 The Rashtriya Swayamsevak Sangh (RSS) is a militant Hindutva nationalist organisation and the Vishwa Hindu Parishad (VHP) is an offshoot of the RSS. Both organisations work together closely and BJP is a part of their political wing, and the political party strongly advocates for Hindutva and 'Hindu Rashtra'. The BJP was in power in Gujarat in 1995 and has been in power in the state of Gujarat since 1998.

3 The CAA and NRC are two pieces of legislation which govern the granting of citizenship to particular groups of illegal immigrants (framed as persecuted minorities from Muslim-dominated countries); and a national register of Indian citizens respectively. When read together, many protesters are arguing that they encourage discrimination based on religious grounds and promote the idea that Muslims cannot be Indian citizens (Deka, 2019).

4 For details on the role of each of the Indian male birth advocates, see Ahluwalia (2008). On the role of masculinity during colonial times, see Sinha (1995).

5 Charles Darwin's cousin, Francis Galton, a famous geographer and statistician, coined the term eugenics in the year 1883. Galton defined eugenics as 'the science which deals with all influences that improve the inborn qualities of a race; also with those that develop them to the utmost advantage' (Galton, 1909: 35). The term eugenics implied good genes or heredity, whereby Galton proposed that 'the goodness or badness of character is not absolute, but relative to the current form of civilisation' (Galton, 1909: 35).

6 Marie Stopes was a British author who campaigned for eugenics and women's rights and was responsible for setting up birth control initiatives.

7 The apps, much like the programme and its aspects, have titles with some mythico-historic characters and a continual attempt to call the programme scientific. The programme's expansion to other states through a digital presence is significant in that it deploys technology to further

the Hindutva nationalistic agenda and, possibly, include it as a part of the government's agenda of 'reproductive surveillance' through digital apps.

8 *Suvarnaprashan* is an Ayurvedic immunity booster for 0–16-year-olds that contains processed gold, while *Ved Sutika* kits contain postnatal care for women including massage oils, micronutrients, and fumigation for the surroundings.

References

Ahluwalia, S. (2008). *Reproductive Restraints: Birth Control in India, 1877–1947*. Illinois: University of Illinois Press.

Anand, D. (2007). Anxious sexualities: masculinity, nationalism and violence, *The British Journal of Politics and International Relations* 9:2, 257–69.

Andersen, W. (1972). The Rashtriya Swayamsevak Sangh I: early concerns, *Economic & Political Weekly*, 11 March, 7:11, 589–97.

Banerjee, M. (2020). When one manufacturer pushes an untested product in an unethical manner, why does it vilify Ayurveda as a whole? *Indian Express*, 2 July. https://indianexpress.com/article/opinion/columns/ayurveda-culture-in-india-coronavirus-healthcare-patanjali-baba-ramdev-6485710/. Accessed 3 September 2020.

Banerjee, P. (1998). *In the Belly of the Beast: An Insider's Story*. Delhi: Ajanta Books.

Basu, T., Datta, P., Sarkar, S., Sarkar, T. and Sen, S. (1993). *Khaki Shorts, Saffron Flags*. New Delhi: Orient Longman.

Bhardwaj, A. (2017). RSS wing has prescription for fair, tall 'customised' babies. *Indian Express*, 7 May. https://indianexpress.com/article/india/rss-wing-has-prescription-for-fair-tall-customised-babies-4644280/. Accessed 3 September 2020.

Bhuyan, A. (2018). Chattisgarh's sterilisation deaths have changed nothing for family planning burden on women, *The Wire*, January. https://thewire.in/health/sterilization-family-planning-women-burden. Accessed 3 September 2020.

Biswas, S. (2014). India's dark history of sterilisation. *BBC News*. www.bbc.com/news/world-asia-india-30040790?OCID=fbindia&fbclid=IwAR0krMGUqiDp8uw9fzvI9b-EhQG25Of1rrRn6jRAtJxGGDbAyDnLoVXZLA. Accessed 3 September 2020.

Bunsha, D. (2006). *Scarred: Experiments with Violence in Gujarat*. New Delhi, New York: Penguin Books.

Carney, S. (2010). Inside India's rent-a-womb business. *Mother Jones*. www.motherjones.com/politics/2010/04/surrogacy-tourism-india-nayna-patel/. Accessed 10 August 2021.

Chaudhuri, P. (2017). Still born. *The Telegraph Online*. www.telegraphindia. com/science-tech/still-born/cid/1377755. Accessed 30 November 2021.

Daniyal, S. (2017). RSS' grand plan to help Indians bear fair, bespoke babies exposes Hindutva's obsession with race. *Scroll.in*, 8 May. https://scroll.in/ article/836880/rss-grand-plan-to-help-couples-bear-fair-tall-bespoke-babies-exposes-hindutvas-problem-with-race. Accessed 3 September 2020.

Das, U. (2017). RSS customised baby plan 'Garbh Vigyan Sanskar': 'Get intimate' as per Sevaks' instructions, to have a stronger, taller, fairer and smarter child. *India.com*, 7 May. www.india.com/news/india/rss-customised-baby-plan-get-intimate-as-per-sevaks-instructions-to-have-a-stronger-taller-fairer-and-smarter-child-2106298/. Accessed 3 September 2020.

Datta, P. K. (1993). Dying Hindus: production of Hindu communal common sense in early twentieth-century Bengal, *Economic & Political Weekly*, 19 June, 1305–19.

Dayal, J. (2015). What drove Sanjay Gandhi and his coterie during the Emergency? *Scroll.in*, 26 June. https://scroll.in/article/735576/what-drove-sanjay-gandhi-and-his-coterie-during-the-emergency. Accessed 3 September 2020.

Dayal, J. (2019). Castration and the constitution. *Indian Currents*, May. www.indiancurrents.org/article-castration-and-the-constitution-255.php. Accessed 3 September 2020.

Deka, K. (2019). Everything you wanted to know about the CAA and NRC. *India Today*, 23 December. www.indiatoday.in/india-today-insight/ story/everything-you-wanted-to-know-about-the-caa-and-nrc-1630771-2019-12-23. Accessed 14 September 2020.

Franklin, S. (2016). Changing global fertilities: a third demographic transition? https://static1.squarespace.com/static/578f761446c3c42341a25de5/ t/5eb94731f37be845ff8aed3d/1589200690014/Changing+Global+ Fertilities.pdf. Accessed January 2021.

Ghoshal, R. (2018). A few shades fairer, please. *Indian Journal of Medical Ethics*, 3:3, July–September, 230–4.

Gowen, A. (2017. 'Straight out of the Nazi playbook': Hindu nationalists try to engineer 'genius' babies in India. *The Washington Post*. 8 May.

Green, H. H. (2018). The legacy of India's quest to sterilise millions of men, *Quartz India*, 6 October. https://qz.com/india/1414774/the-legacy-of-indias-quest-to-sterilise-millions-of-men/. Accessed 3 September 2020.

Heng, G., and Devan, J. (1992). State fatherhood: the politics of nationalism, sexuality, and race in Singapore. In A. Parker et al. (eds), *Nationalisms and Sexualities*, 343–64. New York and London: Routledge.

Hodges, S. (2006). Indian eugenics in an age of reform. In S. Hodges (ed.), *Reproductive Health in India: History, Politics, Controversies*, 115–38. Vol. 13. New Delhi: Orient Longman.

Hodges, S. (2010). South Asia's eugenic past. In A. Bashford and P. Levine (eds), *The Oxford Handbook of The History of Eugenics*, 228–42. Oxford. Oxford University Press.

HT Correspondent (2002). Gujarat experiment to be repeated in Delhi: Togadia, Hindustan Times. www.hindustantimes.com/india/gujarat-experiment-to-be-repeated-in-delhi-togadia/story-KKIkXFDOLZMKA3Gm1JnaWM.html. Accessed 10 August 2021.

Jaffrelot, C. (2007). *Hindu Nationalism: A Reader*. Princeton, NJ: Princeton University Press.

Jolly, M. (1994). Motherlands? Some notes on women and nationalism in India and Africa. *The Australian Journal of Anthropology* 5:3, 41–59.

Jolly, M. and Ram, K. (eds) (2001). *Borders of Being: Citizenship, Fertility and Sexuality in Asia and the Pacific.* Ann Arbor: The University of Michigan Press.

Nadkarni, A. (2014). *Eugenic Feminism: Reproductive Nationalism in the United States and India.* Minneapolis, MN: University of Minnesota Press.

Nadimpally, S., Marwah, V. and Shenoi, A. (2011). Globalisation of birth markets: a case study of assisted reproductive technologies in India, *Globalization and Health* 7:27, 1–9.

Nanda, M. (2003). *Prophets Facing Backward: Postmodern Critiques of Science and Hindu Nationalism in India.* New Brunswick, NJ: Rutgers University Press.

Outlook Web Bureau (2017). RSS wing knows how to get dark, short low IQ parents to deliver tall, fair bright kids, *Outlook India.* 7 May.

Pande, A. (2010). Commercial surrogacy in India: manufacturing a perfect mother-worker, *Signs: Journal of Women in Culture and Society* 35:4, 969–92.

Pande, A. (2015). 'Global reproductive inequalities, neo-eugenics and commercial surrogacy in India', *Current Sociology* 64:2, 244–58.

PRS India (2020). The Surrogacy (Regulation) Bill, 2019. https://prsindia.org/billtrack/the-surrogacy-regulation-bill-2019. Accessed 10 August 2021.

Rao, M. (2007). India's saffron demography: so dangerous, yet so appealing. *Different Takes.* A Publication of the Population and Development Program at Hampshire College, No. 48.

Rao, M. and Sexton, S. (2010). *Markets and Malthus: Population, Gender, and Health in Neo-liberal Times.* New Delhi: Sage Publications India.

Sarkar, Tanika (2002). Semiotics of terror: Muslim children and women in Hindu Rashtra, *Economic & Political Weekly*, 13–19 July, 37:28, 2872–6.

Savarkar, V. D. (1923). *Essentials of Hindutva.* Himani Savarkar, Savarkar Bhavan, Raja Thakur Path, Shanivar Peth, Pune. https://savarkarsmarak.com/activityimages/Essentials%20of%20Hindutva.pdf. Accessed 30 November 2021.

Sharma, A. (2002). On Hindu, Hindustān, Hinduism and Hindutva. *Numen* 49:1, 1–36.

Sinha, M. (1995). *Colonial Masculinity: The 'Manly Englishman' and the 'Effeminate Bengali' in the Late Nineteenth Century.* Manchester: Manchester University Press.

Spodek, H. (March 2010). In the Hindutva laboratory: progroms and politics in Gujarat, 2002, *Modern Asian Studies* 44:2, 349–99. www.jstor.org/stable/27764659?read-now=1&seq=1#page_scan_tab_contents. Accessed 10 August 2021.

Subramaniam, B. (2019). *Holy science: the biopolitics of Hindu nationalism.* Seattle, WA: University of Washington Press.

Sur, S. (2018). Garbha Sanskar and the Politics of Masculinity in West Bengal, *Economic and Political Weekly* LIII:5, 20–22.

Tarlo, E. (2003). *Unsettling Memories: Narratives of India's Emergency.* New Delhi: Orient Blackswan.

Thapar, R. (1996). The theory of Aryan Race and India: history and politics, *Social Scientist* 24:1/3, 3–29.

Thapar, R. (2014). Can genetics help us understand Indian social history? *Cold Spring Harbor Perspectives in Biology* 1–9.

Thapar, R., Noorani, A. G. and Sadanand, M. (2016). *On Nationalism.* New Delhi: Aleph Book Company.

Wilson, R. A. (2018). Eugenics never went away. *Aeon.* https://aeon.co/essays/eugenics-today-where-eugenic-sterilisation-continues-now. Accessed 3 September 2020.

Websites

Garbhvigyan Anusandhan Kendra. https://garbhsanskar.org.in/index.php. Accessed 10 May 2021.

Twitter @GarbhVigyan. https://twitter.com/GarbhVigyan. Accessed 8 March 2022.

Facebook Ved Garbha Vihar @vedgarbhavihar. www.facebook.com/vedgarbhavihar. Accessed 8 March 2022.

4

Racialising ancient skeletons: how haplogroups are mobilised in the re-writing of origin stories in the Indian media

Devika Prakash

In 2015, four skeletons were unearthed in Rakhigarhi, well-preserved enough by the sandy soil of the area to excite the possibility of extracting DNA that could answer questions about who the occupants of the ancient city were. The site lies in the north-west of India and is thought to be one of the biggest remnants of the Indus Valley Civilisation, a sophisticated, urban civilisation that existed between 3300 BCE and 1300 BCE (Deswal, 2015). The Indus Valley Civilisation is a key node in the story of Indian history because it is the earliest known 'Indian' civilisation.[1] One of the points of contention among political factions is whether the Indus Valley Civilisation is Vedic or whether the Vedas and their associated culture and language were brought into the subcontinent by migrants from outside of India (Thapar, 1996). The discovery of the Rakhigarhi skeletons and the subsequent analysis of the ancient DNA extracted from them resulted in a flurry of activity in Indian media. The narrative of genetics holding the key to the human past is an exciting idea sold by books that tell us that, through contemporary technologies of gene sequencing, we can unveil our pasts with high accuracy (Joseph, 2018; Reich, 2018). Of course, casual scientific curiosity is not the only thing that interests people about their genetic past. Questions of ancient history are important tools for nation state building: creating a narrative that binds together certain people and not others within modern day national borders are politically charged discussions, and potentially dangerous ones. The symbiosis of race and nationalism is evident most famously in Germany's history of National Socialism and the idea of an 'Aryan race'. This symbiosis is again made visible in the problem of the 'non-white' immigrants to European countries and the US, which reinforces the idea of a white nation (El-Haj, 2007; Schinagl, 2019). More recently, the focus of citizenship and belonging has been reframed within the language of genomics, as observed by scholars looking at Taiwan (Tsai and Lee, 2020), India (Subramaniam, 2019), South Africa (Erasmus, 2017), and Korea (Gottweis and Kim, 2009) within the framework of what is largely referred to in these publications as 'bionationalism'.[2]

The following discussion contributes to a history of Hindu nationalism and its dialogue with biology, blood and population, and more recently with the unit of reproduction that revolutionised twentieth-century biology: DNA. The chapter extends the biomedicalisation of reproduction (Pande, Chapter 1, this volume) to the biomedicalisation of national belonging. In India, questions of belonging, rooted in right-wing Hindu fundamentalism, often revolve around the idea of an unbroken lineage of Hindus versus invaders and colonisers. The current government in power is led by a political party called the Bharatiya Janata Party (BJP) whose ideological parent organisation is a Hindu Nationalist outfit called the Rashtriya Swayamsevak Sangh (RSS) (Krishnan, 2018). The RSS espouses the idea that India's Hindu past is what gives the country its integrity, as opposed to the narrative of a nation bound together by the colonising forces of the British Empire.[3] The RSS was founded by K. B. Hedgewar based on the ideas of V. D. Savarkar's book *Hindutva* (Curran Jr., 1950). Savarkar spoke of the common cultural identity of Hindus, where 'Hindus' were followers of religions that originated within India – such as Vedic Hinduism, Buddhism, Jainism and Sikhism. This imagination of India translating to official policy can, arguably, already be seen through the example of the Citizenship Amendment Act (CAA). The act expedites the granting of Indian citizenship to undocumented migrants and refugees of Hindu, Sikh, Buddhist, Jain, Parsi or Christian extraction, thus excluding Muslim refugees.[4] Those who oppose the CAA 2019 claim that it sets a precedent for classifying citizens as Muslim and non-Muslim, and defining India as the 'rightful home' of Hindus, and that the ethos of Hindutva goes against the constitutionally enshrined values of India as a secular nation and advocates for India as a Hindu nation or *Hindu Rashtra* (Hasan, 2020).

Another hotly contested issue in this vein is the origin of Indian peoples. Hindutva followers lobbied for a history of India where the origins of Vedic religion (or Hinduism) are indigenous to India, going so far as to persuade the State of California to change its school history textbooks (Bose, 2008). This is at odds with the 'Aryan Migration Theory' that posits that Indo-European language speakers following an early version of Vedic religion migrated to India from the steppes of Central Asia. These opposing points of view have been contested both in scholarly publications and outside of them, most noticeably through mass media (Thapar, 1996). With the prevalence of genetic analysis, these discussions have taking a new turn, where genetic evidence in the form of ancient DNA has become a highly politicised object in which opposing groups have high stakes (Subramaniam, 2019).

This chapter situates the media discussion around the Rakhigarhi DNA within the framework of sociotechnical studies, focusing on the importance of genetic evidence in the twenty-first century and the intertwining of race and genes (El-Haj, 2007; Fujimura et al., 2008; Fullwiley, 2007), using Amade M'charek's (2014) concept of the topological object, where race is framed as a 'spatio-temporal' object. As M'charek et al. (2014a: 460) note, race becomes a matter of concern through 'specific historical and political trajectories' because 'science is never isolated from the "prevailing culture value-system of its time" (Latour 2004)'. In the process it finds that the dissection of ancient DNA within a scientific network that extends across continents has important implications for existing typologies of humans in Indian society and for narratives of nation-building. My objective is not to determine whether the media portrays the science behind the controversy accurately or not, but to observe how the media is involved in the intertwining of social, political and scientific ideas. I also hope to bring to light how the tricky concept of race continues to rear its head in modern discussions, often changing its form in different manifestations but continuing to carry with it the inherent idea that humans are fundamentally members of some typological category, manifesting as races or castes – among many others, that carry certain predispositions inherited from debunked theories on race.

A disclaimer

I have tried to ensure that I refrain from making the claim of impartiality when I certainly do have a personal political opinion – that Hindutva ideologues do not get to decide who belongs to India. Science and Technology Studies (STS) as a field arose from the idea that scientific knowledge and truths are socially constructed; Maria Puig de la Bellacasa (2011) discusses the role of the STS researcher in deconstructing science – the researcher too is a part of the topic of research, and not outside of it. She reminds us to be accountable to the stories that we tell and to not position ourselves outside of them. I have a stake in telling this story that may affect how I approach my sources and interpret then. That being said, I try not to argue strongly for one version of the story versus another, keeping in mind that there is no presumption of a socially and politically 'untainted' science. I say this because empirical material from both sides of the political spectrum contributes to essentialising social typologies into biological artefacts, such as DNA, while discussing the Rakhigarhi case.

In the debate surrounding the question of 'who really belongs to India', different groups have different things at stake. When I say, 'we Indians', who is the 'we'? This is the discussion that the authors of the newspaper articles surrounding the Rakhigarhi DNA samples do not dissect. As a Hindu (at least by birth), I would automatically be enfolded into the majority 'we' of the Hindus of India. Using Hindutva logic, I am then able to trace my roots back through hundreds of generations to a Vedic past that supposedly sprung out of Indian soil. On the other hand, being south Indian and lower caste, my claim to the sacred Vedas is made more distant despite the various social justice movements that have ensured that lower castes have also been included in the umbrella of Hinduism where previously they would be barred from entering Hindu temples due to ritual pollution (Galanter, 1955).[5] Furthermore, there is the Aryan-Dravidian divide between north and south India, very much a part of everyday discussion, identity formation and politicisation (Annamalai, 2010; Subramaniam, 2019). In this case whether the Aryans 'invaded' or 'evolved naturally' is not a question that should shake any self-professed Dravidian's sense of self.[6] While drawing attention to the ambiguities and the making and unmaking of different kinds of social groups associated with terms such as 'Aryan', 'Dravidian', 'Hindu', 'Indian', etc. one must begin to ask how DNA evidence is interpreted within a social context, for example through public discourse as constructed by popularly read media outlets. These bubbles of identity descriptors with their various value-laden associations (indigeneity, supremacy, invasion) are influential in interpretations of scientific results – especially at the public discourse level.

Race, caste and bionationalism

The analytical direction in this chapter comes from writings in STS and allied fields concerning the effect of modern genetics on the concept of race (El-Haj, 2007; Fullwiley, 2007; Fujimura et al., 2008; Tallbear, 2013). Modern genetic sciences allow for a 'genetics of difference' (Fujimura et al., 2008); while race is dismissed by many scholars as scientifically invalid, existing notions of racial difference continue to permeate genetic science. Duana Fullwiley (2007) writes about the 'molecularisation of race' where DNA is classified racially through self-declarations of people it is extracted from, and 'pure' DNA is sought after from 'unmixed populations'. Through this 'molecular vision of life', the scientific concept of race makes a transition from a phenotypic phenomenon to a genotypic one (El-Haj, 2007). Kim Tallbear (2013) writes about how genetic science takes centre stage in defining indigeneity and belonging – the privileging of the 'genomic articulation of indigeneity' over traditional practices of adjudicating belonging. El-Haj (2007) further investigates the concept of race within new genetics versus the older form of race science. Even while genomic categories moved away from typological classifications of 'race', she argues that probabilistic distinctions are enough to propagate racism, and that through 'genealogical origins ... the practices of race science continue to haunt population genetics even now' (El Haj, 2007: 287).

M'charek et al. (2014a: 461) note that most critical discussions about race and genetics have been North America centric. They raise the point that, 'the historical, political, and representational baggage that race carries is not the same everywhere'. They propose a 'topological approach' to 'show how race gets assembled in specific historical contexts by associating different kinds of entities ... biological and religious differences' (2014: 461). The 'folded object' is introduced by Amade M'charek (2014) in her discussion on HeLa cells:[7] it takes into consideration the effects of both time and space in the making of objects, where historical practices are folded into the object. She shows in his article how 'race becomes an irreducible, spacio-temporal thing, one that moves and changes shape depending on the times and places that are drawn together' (2014: 48). Erasmus (2017: 128) shows that population genetics 'mobilises already existing forms of social identification premised on race, tribe, nation, first people, indigeneity, and diversity'. The literature reviewed in this section shows that race is a product of a particular time and space. Even though race does not mean much as an identity marker in India, the global mobility of the concept of race forces a reckoning with it, particularly when it comes encapsulated into globally mobile objects such as DNA. In order to allow comparison, I extend the idea of race to the 'identity-bubble' which is multiple and contradictory but offers a heuristic when discussing DNA and bionationalism on a transnational level. While the word 'race' itself makes very little sense in Indian society to label its members in current parlance, it has been discussed at several points in history.

Another important move in literature on the field of genomic science and biopolitics is the turn to 'bionationalism' where previous frameworks to define the thread holding together a population within a national boundary shifts from being one based on 'blood' to one based on 'genes' (Gottweis and Kim, 2009; Simpson, 2000). Gottweis and Kim (2009: 519), studying scientific fraud in human embryonic cloning explains that 'bionationalism in Korea went beyond traditional ethnic nationalism insofar as the traditional ethnicity marker of "blood" became increasingly displaced by biologically and scientifically grounded concepts such as stem cell or the oocyte that were defined as "Korean"'. Wade et al. (2015: 775) have shown how 'genomic knowledge can unsettle and reinforce ideas of nation and race' in various Latin American countries and become part of political debate. Subramaniam (2019: 165) discusses how the 'Indian genome' is created through practices such as the Indian Genome Variation Project, which takes as its representative samples existing divisions based on caste, region and community in India. Similarly, Erasmus (2017) shows how groups such as 'Malay' and

'Khoi-San' in South Africa are given genetic basis, collapsing a history of inter-mingling, religion and migration into biologically essentialised population groups. In Taiwan, Tsai and Lee (2020) elaborate on how the co-production of a Taiwanese biobank and the Taiwanese genome are rooted in bionationalism. In many of these cases, the genomic focus arises out of state-sponsored 'genome variation' projects serving a global competition of biocapital (Rajan, 2006). However, Ayo Wahlberg (2009: 248) speaks of bionationalism as something 'not unique to ... global bioeconomy' but as something invoking healthcare for the 'collective vitality' of the national population in the case of Vietnam. In India, nationalism arose as an opposition to imperial rule and colonisation as it did in other colonised nations (Gottweis and Kim, 2009). One of the ways in which the linguistically, ethnically and culturally diverse population within the national boundaries of India is brought together is through a population united in their fight against a colonial power; the other, not strictly distinct notion, is that of the Hindu nation or Hindu *Rashtra*.

A significant publication from which modern questions surrounding race, nationalism and religion in India have arisen is V. D. Savarkar's (1969) book *Hindutva*, an important ideological basis for modern Hindu Nationalism. Savarkar makes a case for a Hindu 'race', and Indians being united by 'the bonds of common blood. They are not only a nation but also a race-*jati*' (Savarkar, 1969: 84). Savarkar minimises the division of society by caste, saying that castes have often mixed to create new castes and ultimately all Indians have the same bloodlines. Savarkar's definition of the word 'Hindu' includes all religions that have their roots in India – Buddhism, Jainism, Sikhism and Vedic Hinduism. Categorically excluded are the religions of Christianity and Islam. He argues that followers of religions where the 'holy land' lies outside the 'land of birth' causes such groups to be conflicted about where their loyalties lie. Subsequently, one of the key arguments of Hindutva ideologues is that India is the holy land of Hinduism. This is one of the main reasons that the Vedas originating outside India are such an intense point of contention. One of the articles I analyse, a piece by Shukla and Venkataraman (2018) from *Swarajya*, particularly emphasised this point. Incidentally, the authors are members of the American Hindu Foundation, one of the groups that lobbied against the story of Aryan migration into India being included in school textbooks in California.

The questions of race and caste were addressed by several scholars of India from the nineteenth and twentieth centuries and race-thinking has permeated ideas about caste for years, shaping the modern construct of caste in India (Thapar, 1996). Romila Thapar (1996) brings out the race-caste debates that have existed in scholarship on India and its links with the Indus Valley debate. Banu Subramaniam (2019) charts out comprehensively more recent attempts at bringing together race and caste, including the embracing of reading caste as race by anti-caste activists to bring more global attention to caste-discrimination and forge solidarity with anti-racist activists. In another form of religion-based racialisation, Zaheer Baber (2004) has written about the racialisation of communal identity in India, pointing out similarities between racial conflicts elsewhere and communal conflict in India.

The ghosts of earlier scholarship continue to haunt modern scholarship and, possibly, everyday understandings of caste and race; in other words the topological approach (M'charek, 2014) is imperative in seeing how historical ways of social differentiation do not disappear but remain enfolded within objects or become folded objects. Even while modern scholarship would not explicitly equate caste and race, the effects of nineteenth- and twentieth-century understandings of the caste-race relationship continue to exist in narratives of Hindu Nationalism today (Egorova, 2010: 35) and even within scientific work. Yulia Egorova (2009, 2010) has written about the effect of genetic studies on the essentialisation of caste and how scholarship on genetics and caste in India pre-supposes caste as a genetic category, looking for heritability of 'phenotypes' such as skin pigmentation and genetic markers in blood groups between castes (Arya et al., 2020; Chavhan, 2011; Jonnalagadda et al. 2016; Lanchbury et al., 1996).[8] Subsequently, one could assume that new genetic evidence is interpreted again in the light of existing literary and archaeological evidence. Egorova (2010) has analysed the paper published by Reich et al. (2009), which, along with DNA from the Rakhigarhi skeletons, set-in motion the debates in the news articles I analysed. She also interviewed scientists working on the project and analysed media articles discussing the Reich paper findings around the time period of 2009 and 2010. Egorova notes that the Reich paper provides a basis to biologise and pathologise castes. While it positions the importance of finding disease risks in population groups as a future use of the research, the implication that certain population groups (castes, tribes, races) are genetically prone to disease reifies racialised ideas of human difference. There are also striking similarities between public discourse surrounding the issue, which are almost a decade apart, notably encouraging Indians to inter-marry between castes for 'genetic diversity' (Pai, 2018). My work speaks closely to Egorova's (2009) analysis of the landscape of caste and Hindu nationalism tied to genetic studies but is now situated within a political landscape dominated by a Hindu Nationalist political party since 2014 along with a shift in the media landscape with considerably more right-wing representation (Bhat and Chadha, 2020).

Methods

Since my main aim was to investigate how genetic evidence is discussed at the level of national public discourse, I chose to study newspaper articles that discussed and argued the topic of the Rakhigarhi skeletons using a discourse analysis framework recommended by Schneider (2013). My choice of newspaper articles was limited by language – I chose only English-language articles – and by their availability online. This already limits the 'public' who are involved in reading, writing and commenting on these articles. They are a small selection of English-speaking, almost always digitally literate, individuals who are not representative of the entire population of India but are still a relevant and possibly powerful group in Indian society. My total sample size was thirty-one articles across seven sources dated between 2017 and 2019, most of which are in conversation with each other and in response to the news report that the Rakhigarhi skeltons lacked the R1a haplogroup, choosing my sample size using what Schneider (2013) citing Jäger (2004: 171) calls a synchronous analysis. Three of the sources were magazines – *The Caravan, Swarajya* and *India Today*, of which *India Today* had featured the Rakhigarhi discovery and discussions around it as a cover story. Two are online news websites – *Scroll.in* and *The Print*. Two are print newspapers with national circulation – *The Hindu* (the second most widely read English-language newspaper in India) and *The Economic Times* (a subsidiary of the Times Group – the most widely read

English-language newspaper in India) (Audit Bureau of Circulations, 2020). Most articles are opinion pieces, while a minority are reports.

Following the thread of news articles referencing each other, there seems to be a consistent group talking about this issue, often critiquing or arguing with other articles in this list. Despite my attempt to incorporate multiple political leanings, I could only find one credible right of centre source (*Swarajya*) that discussed this issue. I tried to find descriptions on the websites of these publications in which they categorised themselves as left or right leaning. *Swarajya* magazine declares itself as 'a big tent for liberal *right of centre discourse* that reaches out, engages and caters to the new India' (Swarajya, n.d., emphasis added). The other sources were categorised according to the 'Media Bias Fact Check' website.

In the articles, I identified: (1) words that reinforce the conclusiveness of genetic evidence – such as 'conclusive', 'undeniable', 'cannot be refuted'; (2) the references to population groups with words such as – 'Aryans', 'Dravidians', 'south Indians' etc.; (3) the emphasis on scientific language (haplogroups, mitochondrial DNA, 'DNA markers' and others that indicated that the author was doing the work of translating scientific terms); and (4) scientific actors (scientists, names of institutes). The idea behind these codes was that authors translating scientific findings for a lay audience would activate scientific actors and language to back up the use of genetics as evidence. Further, in the process of discussing ancient DNA as genetic evidence, authors would reinforce or question groups such as 'Aryans' and 'Dravidians' – sometimes using them normatively and otherwise questioning them as language groups that are being conflated with population groups bound together by common genes.

I also read abstracts of scientific papers referred to in these articles in order to get a sense of what the 'non-translated' version of the genetic evidence was saying. But this was not the focus of my research.

Understanding the Rakhigarhi case

The setting behind the politically charged nature of the Rakhigarhi discussions is the historical question of where Indo-European language speakers originated from.[9] There are two schools of thought – the Aryan Migration Theory and the Indigenous Aryans Theory. After the Indus Valley Civilisation was discovered in 1920, the Aryan Invasion Theory was put forward by archaeologist Mortimer Wheeler. This idea of a hostile 'invasion' that destroyed the Indus Valley Civilisation was later replaced by an Aryan *Migration* Theory where Indo-European language speakers with oral tradition of the Vedas mixed in waves with the existing population (Possehl, 2002). On the other hand, the Indigenous Aryan Theory posits that the Indo-European language speakers are indigenous to India. Another strain of this theory elaborates that the Indo-European languages spread from India to the rest of Central Asia and Europe (Bryant, 2001). Despite the fact that the Aryan Invasion Theory no longer has credence in history and other disciplines, the term continued to be used in the news articles – almost always in ones that espoused a Hindu Nationalist point of view.

A brief history of the Rakhigarhi findings is easiest understood from a piece in the magazine *The Caravan* by Hartosh Singh Bal. In March 2018 a paper titled *The Genomic Formation of South and Central Asia* was published from the Lab for Ancient DNA at Harvard Medical School headed by David Reich, which posited two migrations into South Asia:

> The first, by Iranian farmers less than 9000 years ago, and the second, by the steppe pastoralists less than 5000 years ago. The first migration mingled with the pre-existing hunter gatherer population of South Asia and gave rise to what the authors term as Indus Periphery people – the latest study clarifies that this represents the population of the Indus Valley Civilization, and not another distinct population. The second migration of steppe people, which coincided with the decline of the Indus Valley Civilization, around 4000 years ago, mixed with the Indus Periphery People to give rise to the ANI[10] population. Simultaneously, the Indus Periphery People also migrated southward and further mixed with the indigenous hunter-gatherers who lived in the area to give rise to the ASI population. (Bal, 2018)

The Rakhigarhi findings would provide DNA from within an Indus Valley site instead of the stand-in population used in the above-mentioned scientific study. Indian newspapers have been abuzz with news about Rakhigarhi since the discovery of two mounds in 2014 made it the largest Indus Valley settlement to be discovered to date (Subramanian, 2014). The star object in these stories is the R1a haplogroup passed on through male lineage from father to son. The

R1a haplogroup is supposed to be found in higher frequencies in north Indian, upper castes (Friese, 2018). The presence of the R1a gene is supposed to indicate a continuity between the Indus Valley Civilisation and the Hindu, upper-caste north Indian people in modern day India. This haplogroup is contested because in the Migrant Aryans narrative, a group of people from the steppes of Central Asia carrying the haplogroup entered India at some point along with some preliminary version of Vedic culture. There are multiple contestations here. The mainstream perspective is of the R1a originating 'outside India' and being carried into the country by a group of migrants ('the Aryans') who arrived after the Indus Valley Civilisation. This narrative means that the Vedic culture (associated with the Aryans) was brought in by people not indigenous to the modern idea of what is territorially India. The Hindu Nationalist narrative also proposes that the R1a haplogroup is indigenous to India and could have spread outwards from India. The haplogroup being associated with 'north Indian, upper castes', already raises several questions on the objective of unifying all of India as a single homogenous entity with unbroken lineage. It also reinforces the assumption that north Indian, upper castes are a discernible population group. The intertwining of nationalist aspirations, ideas of race and differences between populations, religion and belonging with genetics becomes difficult to separate.

Findings

Genetics as evidence

The imaginaries associated with genetics are visible in the language used to describe the Rakhigarhi DNA and new technologies of analysing ancient DNA. Genetics is described as 'the key to', 'unlocking', 'settling the debate', 'an open door', 'unambiguous evidence'. For example, one newspaper editorial declared that 'population genetics coupled with ancient DNA extraction and analysis will tell us true tales about the human past' (Joseph, 2019: 9). The internationality of science is an important contributor to the plausibility of genetic evidence (Joseph, 2019). The role of reputed institutions, such as Harvard, and international teams of scientists are used to drive home the fact that this new genetic evidence is rooted in hard science that displays all the characteristics of Mertonian science (Merton, 1979). Current genetic evidence is spoken of (in opposition to older genetic evidence) in metaphors such as an 'open door' as opposed to 'peeking through the keyhole'. In this way, earlier genetic evidence is minimised as 'fuzzy' while new genetic evidence is revelatory. While scientific discoveries often take this linear path of replacement or improving upon earlier theories, this clashes with reinforcements that the current evidence is 'indisputable', as scientists are quoted as saying in several articles.

Other forms of evidence (linguistic, archaeological) are not explicitly diminished but used together with genetic evidence to support the argument. Thus new evidence continues to be interpreted in the light of existing evidence, repeating the reading of archaeological evidence through literary interpretations of Vedic text since these were 'used in reconstructing the past, prior to the availability of archaeological evidence' (Thapar, 1996: 11). In an opinion piece in *The Hindu*, Tony Joseph (2017) quotes Shinde (one of the archaeologists of the Rakhigarhi dig) as saying 'we may have excavated a lot of pottery ... but what is new in that?' emphasising the new angle that genetics will give to archaeological findings.

The magnitude of genetic evidence is enlarged or diminished based on which theory it supports or destabilises. Those opposing the Aryan Migration Theory are more critical when it comes to looking at the genetic evidence. Sanjeev Sanyal, an economist who writes popular books on revisionist Hindutva history, is quoted in *Swarajya* articles saying that R1a is an Indian haplogroup that spread to Central Asia. This is an example of how scientific terms are important tools in the hands of interpreters who make differing claims often backed by niche groups of scientists.

'Hard evidence', different interpretations

One news article from the *Economic Times* (Vishnoi, 2018), published the results of the DNA study with the conclusion that the Indus Valley Civilisation had been confirmed as 'indigenous' and therefore the Vedas too were indigenous. It quotes the archaeologist responsible for the dig, Dr Shinde, seemingly to reinforce the idea that the claim was coming directly from the expert. This is, of course, a counter narrative to the one in which the lack of R1a haplogroup indicated that the Indus Valley Civilisation preceded a 'Vedic civilisation'. The article claims that the lack of R1a haplogroup 'rubbishes' the 'Aryan Invasion Theory'. This claim was questioned almost immediately by a *Scroll.in* article (Venkataramakrishnan, 2018) published two days later. This article points out that the Aryan Migration Theory posits that 'migrants from the steppes, who were earlier referred to as Aryans' (Venkataramakrishnan, 2018) entered the sub-continent towards the decline of the Indus Valley Civilisation, meaning that the lack of R1a indicates a conformance of this discovery to the Theory. The Vishnoi (2018) article is the only instance of an extrapolation of results that went explicitly against the grain and interpreted a Vedic Indus Valley without questioning the genetic evidence found. At the time this chapter was written, the *Economic Times* article was still online without any corrections. An article in *The Print* (Khan, 2018) again quotes Shinde, its headlines stating that 'Archeologist who found 4,500-yr-old skeletons in Haryana doesn't buy Aryan invasion theory'.

The *Swarajya* articles did not take the DNA as conclusive evidence of the Indus Valley Civilisation not being Vedic. They were more likely to dilute the implications of such evidence. They note that in the March 2018 paper, 'no actual IVC or South Asian DNA' was used and so 'we are left with a major assumption that the Swat Valley of northern Pakistan is a reasonable placeholder for IVC' (Shukla and Venkataraman, 2018). Moreover, they emphasise that Brahmin DNA from north India may show admixture from the steppes but are 'seven times closer to the Indian mix of the IVC than to the Steppe where they may have originated' (Shukla and Venkataraman, 2018). It also diminishes the importance of the DNA from the Rakhigarhi skeletons – another article states that the 'Rakhigarhi skeletons are just a few from a single site', and 'it's too early to say if they belonged to South Indians or North Indians or … to the Indus Valley people at all' (Suri, 2018). It reinforces the diversity of the Indus Valley Civilisation, which was spread over a large area and states that the 'DNA obtained from the available skeletons will not be representative of the entire Bronze Age Indus population' (Suri, 2018). Despite diminishing the evidence that the Rakhigarhi skeletons provided, the article does not wipe away the importance of genetic evidence in its entirety, saying that, 'obviously such questions will be definitively answered only when we have *adequate* ancient DNA from Neolithic sites in the Indus Valley region and the Ganga plain' (Suri, 2018; emphasis added.). Meaning, it is merely a question of adequate sample size and not a problem with the DNA evidence itself: hard evidence is coming, but always in the future. Another article repeats that the 'DNA sample itself is meagre' (Swarajya, 2018) and goes on to reinforce the view of geneticist Dr Gyaneshwar Chaube that the R1a haplogroup is most likely of Indian origin – a controversial counter to the mainstream argument that supports an 'out-of-India' emergence of the 'Aryans'. In this, the authors make an additional move of disputing whether the so-called steppe DNA could be of Indian origin, meaning that the movement of migration was from India to the steppes.[11] The right-wing articles were keener to make the observations that genetic evidence was not proof of language or culture.

Population groups and indigeneity

The term 'Aryan' is used normatively in most news articles. A few do recognise that the term is not to be taken normatively – sometimes putting it in quotes – but then the same article would use it in another paragraph as a normative classification (Suri, 2017). The *India Today* magazine piece puts forth a summary of the results including: 'Q[uestion]. Were they closer to popular perceptions of 'Aryans' or 'Dravidians'? A[nswer]: Dravidians. Q: Were they more akin to the South Indians or North Indians of today? A: South Indians' (Friese, 2018). The article then goes on to say that steppe ancestry marks 'many North Indian high castes' (Friese, 2018). Most articles quote researchers as saying that the DNA found indicates that the Rakhigarhi man was genetically most similar to the *Irula* tribe of South India. One article in *The Print* goes on to use genetic evidence based on David Reich's work to advise Indians to marry outside of caste because 'intermixing is good for our genes' (Pai, 2018).

The genetic findings speak to the possibility of unveiling what the 'Harappans looked like' (Kumar, 2019). One news article asks if the Harappans might look like the popular Bollywood actor Hrithik Roshan who is from Punjab (ET Bureau, 2019). While this is amusing, it also demonstrates that there seems to be a presumption that figuring out how the Harappans look would help us place them geographically into some part of India, and DNA analysis held the key to unravel how we could visualise (and categorise) these people. Through all these practices, the bond between genetics and population groups is reified in India. Two outcomes arise out of this – one, saying that there are genes linked with north Indian upper castes, implies that there is a genetic basis for castes and for tribes. The second is the angle of indigeneity.

A fundamental question in this debate is who is indigenous and who is not. Although most of the left-leaning articles end with statements about all humans being migrants, the question of indigeneity is still positioned as important. Ancient Ancestral South Indians, for example, are 'native to the subcontinent' (*India Today* Web Desk, 2018), while in the *Economic Times* article (Vishnoi, 2018), the Indus Valley Civilisation is 'indigenous with only a few minor strains of Iranian DNA'. Indigeneity is prized in this interpretation of DNA because in this narrative, indigenous people have the strongest claim to national belonging in discussions about who 'real Indians' are. In modern India, indigenous groups – called *adivasis* (first inhabitants) – are often displaced for dam building projects (Biswas, 2019) and form one of the most marginalised groups in the country. Thus, while indigeneity may be prized in discursive constructions of nationalism, in practice, 'being indigenous', in the sense that this group is constructed within Indian society, has little social power.

Discussion

Chatterjee, Roy and Subramaniam (in Chapter 2 of this volume) urge a rethinking of biological politics in South Asia, where the 'hauntings of colonisation', which Deboleena Roy talks about being visible in this entanglement of biology and politics in India, need to be considered seriously when deploying theoretical terms such as biopolitics. The Hindu Nationalist narrative in India seems to mobilise anti-racist and decolonialist discourse to argue against the Aryan Migration Theory saying that it presumes that an advanced civilisation of fair-skinned people came in and oppressed the dark-skinned group of natives.[12]

Another argument is that western science and especially colonialist science during the 1920s influenced the telling of the Indus Valley story. The use of colonial science and racism as means to discredit mainstream scholarship on Indian history that does not agree with the Hindu Nationalist narrative of the 'Aryan Past' is elaborated upon by Lars Martin Fosse (2005). These details show the need to intricately examine questions of race and genetics in different national settings (M'charek et al., 2014b) and to problematise the idea that science is apolitical.

Tallbear's (2013) example of genetic science taking precedence in defining tribal belonging over traditional practices of adjudicating belonging shows how genetic evidence can undermine traditionally embedded ways of seeing kinship. The centring of genes and DNA thus has the capability to collapse histories of human relationships into narrow genomic rationalities of knowing, in ways that are not innocent but explicitly seeking to otherise. The star objects in this discussion – the R1a haplogroup and its absence in the Rakhigarhi DNA is what sets off a heated debate in Indian media. As noted earlier, these bubbles of identity descriptors of Aryan/Dravidian, south Indian/north Indian, upper caste/lower caste, Hindu/non-Hindu have value-laden associations In this case, the R1a haplogroup, with its presence in north Indian, upper castes and absence in the Rakhigarhi skeletons, unravels the stakeholders of a Hindu nation in which the Vedic-Hindu tradition provides the framework for how we should exist as a nation and what people are privileged within its boundaries. Erasmus (2017: 106) reminds us that attempts by scientists to tell us 'who we are' is more accurately a question of 'how we should be ruled'.

Gottweis and Kim (2009) refer to bionationalism as means by which the population within the boundaries of the nation state is seen as a 'biological unit' and Wahlberg (2009) emphasises the focus on 'collective vitality'. In this case study, there seems to be more of an activity of fragmentation or differentiation of the imagined 'national population' and in the process removing certain populations from this framework. In India, as in previously colonised countries, nationalism was invoked to oppose an occupying imperialist power (Gottweis and Kim, 2009). Various attempts to forge linguistically, ethnically and culturally diverse groups of people in the country include the 'Hindu nation' narrative among others. The 'bonds of blood' that Savarkar speaks about now has the possibility to be extended to bonds of DNA. In this discussion surrounding the R1a haplogroup, what is revealed is that the biological population is not one monolith but is composed of sub-populations, some more important than others. As Stinson and Lunstrum (2021: 5) note in their literature review of national populations and biopolitics, this bionationalistic imagination can also result in the necropolitics of removing undesirable populations and 'outsiders'.

Vailly (2017) talks about how human genome sequencing has led to far reaching effects outside the lab in the sphere of race in societies where racial differences and discrimination exists. Genomes relating to specific population groups may carry with them essentialised understandings of how populations can be grouped and named – i.e. the population group is created in the process of the study. It is not something that exists in the wild or 'out there to be found'. In her case, the use of DNA profiling of suspects in criminal investigation shows how DNA analysis of population groups is based on essentialised understandings of population groups – in this case based on a continent of origin. Vailly, quoting Duster (2011), explains how in order to have an indication of whether a person was 'probably' of African origin, the creators of the DNA tests would first need a reference group that is 100% African. What would this 100% African group consist of? The academic articles, on which several of these reports are based (Basu et al., 2016; Metspalu et al., 2011; Moorjani et al., 2013), themselves contain problematic groupings of populations.[13] The articles talk about samples taken from ethnic groups from around India. Here we see socially defined typologies of humans based on conventional practice getting inscribed into genetic categories that are then accepted as 'hard science' and 'hard evidence' to adjudicate questions of national belonging and so on. Despite this, genetic evidence vis-a-vis other forms of evidence (archaeological, linguistic) is taken as the (almost) final word on the topic in public discourse.

Betsy Hartmann (in the Foreword to this volume) reminds us against the uncritical acceptance of biomedical research. In the Rakhigarhi case, we see that even when the controversies surrounding a scientific finding are publicly discussed in mass media, all factions seem to believe in the existence of untainted genetic evidence. They create a distinction between a science untainted by ideology and politicised science even as the articles themselves perform the work of piecing together and interpreting various scientific papers to translate a coherent story to the reader, bolstered by quotes from scientists involved in the projects or email correspondences of authors with the scientists. By underlining the 'science' involved in the story, the media contributes to an essentialised understanding of population groups becoming part of the conversation of national belonging.

Conclusion

This chapter frames DNA and its surrounding discourse as socio-technical object, showing that genetic evidence being publicly contested is especially visible in highly politicised matters and can result in the discursive creation of population groups outside of the lab, in this case through media discourse. The validity of genetic evidence can be questioned, or further investigation sought, when it does not support one narrative; articles from the Hindu right seemed to dissect the evidence with greater nuance.[14] Despite this, the idea of the scientific and the social being separate spheres and that of science being somehow not 'tainted' by societal/political ideas remains in these articles. There is little to no discussion about scientists having ideological biases or the enfolding of social groups with their inherent political biases into the creation of scientific objects such as genetic markers. The translation activity practised by news article writers surfaces when opposing narratives meet one another, but is otherwise hidden.

The media discussions surrounding genetic analysis of ancient DNA also seemed to reinforce a genetic basis of population groups along caste-, language- and region-based lines. This corroborates the findings of Yulia Egorova (2010), with some media articles – a decade apart between Egorova's study and mine – interpreting the scientific journal results in strikingly similar ways, including raising questions about whether 'inter-caste marriage' was good for genetic diversity (Pai, 2018). Indigeneity is a prized commodity to identify the 'real Indian' in this discourse, where the claim to nationality is rooted in having an unbroken lineage that can be traced through genetic analysis. Thus, the media discursively creates biologically essentialised population group centred around sometimes coherent and sometimes blurry and overlapping population groups – Dravidian/ Aryan, south Indian/north Indian, upper caste/lower caste, tribal/ indigenous. These discourses reinforce the idea of populations, which from their 'inception has been a focus of both political economy (Malthus) and biology (Darwin) and continues to be so' as noted by Hinterberger (2012: 88), who draws attention to the continued presence of population thinking in the sciences. Malthusian and Darwinian focuses on populations have, in turn, reinforced notions of population limits and selection of superior populations, as discussed in the Introduction to this book. This form of bionationalism is especially problematic when read alongside the developments of a right-wing Hindu nationalist government that continues to other populations that do not fit within its preferred ambit, more tangibly through its policy decisions such as the Citizen Amendment Act 2019 and the proposed Population Control Bill 2019.[15] This idealised population could be 'religions that originate within India' – Sikhism, Buddhism, Jainism (Savarkar, 1969); it could be also be limited to Hindus or more specifically Hindu upper-castes.[16] The discursive creation of biologised population groups through media discussion of ancient DNA shows how the ideal progeny is co-constructed parallel to neo-eugenic practices, such as those exemplified in the Ved Garbh Vihar project (see Chapter 3, this volume).

In the prevailing atmosphere of political Hinduism and the fashioning of India as a Hindu nation, the creation of DNA-based population groups have potentially dangerous consequences for India. Population groups are important tools for the Government to create policy and for parties to gather votes. In this context, the role of ancient DNA in determining whether a civilisation that existed thousands of years in the past aligns with modern religious groupings is not just a question of lay interest but is used to make arguments against those who 'do not belong'. The story of the nation, stretching from the Indus Valley Civilisation to the present day, is now mediated through DNA within the framework of bionationalism, setting the scene to remove those who do not genetically belong to this national population. The possibility of ancient DNA revealing the secrets to our path can set a dangerous precedent to the creation of groupings along caste, linguistic and perhaps religious lines that are reinforced with a hard 'genetic' basis.

Notes

1 The Indus Valley Civilisation (IVC) straddles two countries, one Muslim and the other constitutionally secular, but majority Hindu. Both countries attempt to create a narrative for their existence in which the imagined religion of the inhabitants of the IVC is intertwined with, or at least does not contradict, stories of their nations. The first sites discovered of the IVC are in modern-day Pakistan. While India attempts to reinforce the 'Hinduness' of the Civilisation, it is the lack of a clear 'Hindu' link that ensures that the Pakistani Government embraces rather than rejects the IVC in its version of national history (Khalid, 2018). The question of whether the IVC was Hindu is, in this story, answerable through the R1a haplogroup, as though the haplogroup has Hinduness within it.

2 Wahlberg (2017) uses the word 'bionationalism' outside of the genomic focus and to refer to a nationalistic focus on the health of the 'national population as a whole', while Erasmus (2017) does not use the term 'bionationalism' but nevertheless refers to the genome being centred in creating 'South African' populations.

3 Gottweis and Kim (2009) draw attention to how nationalism in colonised nations was often a response to imperialism and therefore has very different connotations than in the west.

4 While Parsis and Christians are outliers in the list, it should be noted that the BJP Manifesto 2019 includes only Hindus, Sikhs, Jains and Buddhists.

5 Ritual purity among the caste Hindus prevents inter-dining and worship at Hindu temples (see Galanter (1964) for more information). The barring of lower caste people into Hindu temples was opposed by various social justice movements, resulting in the 1936 Temple Entry Proclamation in the Princely State of Travancore. The Madras Temple Entry Proclamation in 1947 later granted access to Hindu temples for lower castes in the Princely State of Cochin and the Madras Presidency (Sivathambika 1991).

6 E. Annamalai (2010: 232) notes that it was with the rise of the Dravidian political movement in 1916 that the term Dravidian became used to refer to a political group where previously it had 'historically been used to refer either to a region in the southern part of India, a language family, or a "racial" group, often conflating the three'.

7 The HeLa cell is a widely used cell line in biology extracted without consent from a Black woman, Henrietta Lacks, who suffered from a particularly fast-replicating form of cervical cancer.

8 As another example, Banu Subramaniam (2019: 164) points out that the Indian Genome Variation Project, in attempting to create a '"representative database" of India's genome, relies on familiar modes of difference in its sampling techniques – region, religion, caste, subcaste, community, and so on', reproducing, 'old categories of difference as valid biological categories for modern India'.

9 In this case, there also seems to be a conflation between the language group and the assumed 'racial group'.

10 ANI – Ancestral North Indian; ASI – Ancestral South Indian.

11 This theory is called the Out-of-India theory, also espoused by a section of Hindutva ideologues – in this scenario the origin of Indo-European languages itself lies in India.

12 The leftists oppose this argument by pointing out that if the incoming migrants did displace the Indus Valley Civilisation, the incoming group of pastoralists was in no way more 'advanced' than an urban settlement of agriculturalists (Shahane, 2018).

13 Erasmus (2017: 128) says, 'Population genetics both inside and outside the laboratory mobilises already existing forms of social identification premised on race, tribe, nation, first people, indigeneity and diversity'.

14 See Latour (2004) on 'artificially maintained controversies'.

15 The BJP included in its manifesto and proposed in 2019 the Population Control Bill which seeks to incentivise families in India to have not more than two children. News reports note that the Population Control Bill is largely discussed through the narrative of the Muslim population overtaking the Hindus (Purohit, 2019).

16 See Kalpana Wilson's paper on the reproductive politics in BJP led India, and the conflation of caste-based thinking and neo-eugenics (2018). Notably, the population-based focus on reproductive control has included the lower castes and lower classes well before the BJP, particularly in the era of Indira Gandhi and the sterilisation campaign led by her son, Sanjay Gandhi. See also Prashant Jha's book (2017) on the image make-over of the BJP from a party of upper-class, upper-caste north Indian Hindu men to a party representing 'all Hindus' post-2014.

References

Annamalai, E. (2010). The political rise of Tamil in the Dravidian movement in South India. In Joshua A. Fishman and Ofelia García (eds), *Handbook of Language and Ethnic Identity, Volume 2*. Oxford: Oxford University Press.

Arya, R., Duggirala, R., Comuzzie, A., Puppala, S., Modem, S., Busi, B. and Crawford, M. (2002). Heritability of anthropometric phenotypes in caste populations of Visakhapatnam, India, *Human Biology* 74:3, 325–44. www.jstor.org/stable/41466058. Accessed 21 April 2021.

Audit Bureau of Circulations (2020). Highest circulated dailies, weeklies and magazines amongst member publications (across languages). Audit Bureau of Circulations. Accessed 10 January 2020.

Baber, Z. (2004). 'Race', religion and riots: the 'racialization' of communal identity and conflict in India, *Sociology* 38:4, 701–18.

Bal, H. S. (2018). Indus Valley people did not have genetic contribution from the steppes: head of ancient DNA lab testing Rakhigarhi samples. *The Caravan*, 27 April. https://caravanmagazine.in/vantage/indus-valley-genetic-contribution-steppes-rakhigarhi. Accessed 6 September 2020.

Basu, A., Sarkar-Roya, N. and Majumder, P. P. (2016). Genomic reconstruction of the history of extant populations of India reveals five distinct ancestral components and a complex structure, *Proceedings of the National Academy of Sciences of the United States of America* 113:6, 1594–9.

Bhat, P. and Chadha, K. (2020). Anti-media populism: expressions of media distrust by right-wing media in India, *Journal of International and Intercultural Communication* 13:2, 166–82.

Biswas, S. (2019). Why a million Indian tribal families face eviction. *BBC*, 22 February. www.bbc.com/news/world-asia-india-47317361. Accessed 14 September 2020.

Bose, P. (2008). Hindutva abroad: the California textbook controversy, *The Global South* 2:1, 11–34.

Bryant, E. (2001). *The Quest for the Origins of Vedic Culture: The Indo-Aryan Migration Debate*. Oxford: Oxford University Press.

Chavhan, A., Pawar, S. and M. Baig (2011). Allelic frequency of ABO and Rh D blood group among the Banjara Backward Caste of Yavatmal District, Maharashtra, India. *Nature Precedings*. DOI:10.1038/npre.2010.5482.1.

Curran Jr, J. A. (1950). The RSS: militant Hinduism, *Far Eastern Survey* 19:10, 93–8.

de la Bellacasa, M. P. (2011). Matters of care in technoscience: assembling neglected things, *Social Studies of Science* 41:1, 85–106.

Deswal, D. (2015). Four Harappan era skeletons found near Hisar. *Tribune India*. 14 April 2015. www.tribuneindia.com/news/archive/features/four-harappan-era-skeletons-found-near-hisar-67080. Accessed 14 September 2020.

Duster, T. (2011). Ancestry testing and DNA: uses, limits, and caveat emptor. In S. Krimsky and K. Sloan (eds), *Race and the Genetic Revolution:*

Science, Myth, and Culture, 99–115. New York: Columbia University Press.

Egorova, Y. (2009). De/geneticizing caste: population genetic research in South Asia, *Science as Culture* 18:4, 417–34.

Egorova, Y. (2010). Castes of genes? Representing human genetic diversity in India, *Genomics, Society and Policy* 6:3, DOI:10.1186/1746-5354-6-3-32.

El-Haj, N. A. (2007). The genetic reinscription of race, *Annual Review of Anthropology* 36, 283–300.

Erasmus, Z. (2017). *Race Otherwise: Forging a New Humanism for South Africa*. New York: New York University Press.

ET Bureau (2019). What if Rakhigarhians really did look like Hrithik Roshan? *The Economic Times*, 31 January. https://economictimes.indiatimes.com/magazines/panache/what-if-the-rakhigarhians-really-did-look-like-hrithik-roshan/articleshow/67767794.cms. Accessed 6 September 2020.

Fosse, L. M. (2005). The polemics and politics of indigenous Aryanism. In E. Bryant and L. Patton (eds), *The Indo-Aryan Controversy: Evidence and Inference in Indian History*, 434–66. London: Routledge.

Friese, K. (2018). 4500-year-old DNA from Rakhigarhi reveals evidence that will unsettle Hindutva nationalists. *India Today*, 3 September. www.indiatoday.in/magazine/cover-story/story/20180910-rakhigarhi-dna-study-findings-indus-valley-civilisation-1327247-2018-08-31. Accessed 6 September 2020.

Fujimura, J. H., Troy, D. and Ramya R. (2008). Race, genetics, and disease: questions of evidence, matters of consequence, *Social Studies of Science* 38:5, 643–56.

Fullwiley, D. (2007). The molecularization of race: institutionalizing human difference in pharmacogenetics practice, *Science as Culture* 16:1, 1–30.

Galanter, M. (1964). Temple-entry and the Untouchability (Offences) Act, 1955. *Journal of the Indian Law Institute* 6:2/3, 185–95. www.jstor.org/stable/43949802. Accessed 8 November 2021.

Gottweis, H. and Kim, B. (2009). Bionationalism, stem cells, BSE, and Web 2.0 in South Korea: toward the reconfiguration of biopolitics, *New Genetics and Society* 28:3, 223–39.

Hasan, Z. (2020). The anatomy of anti-CAA protests. *The Hindu*, 1 January. www.thehindu.com/opinion/op-ed/an-anatomy-of-anti-caa-protests/article30446145.ece. Accessed 2 March 2021.

Hinterberger, A. (2012). Investing in life, investing in difference: nations, populations and genomes, *Theory, Culture and Society* 29:3, 72–93.

India Today Web Desk (2018). Think the Harappans were the source of Vedic Hinduism? Think again. *India Today*, 1 September. www.indiatoday.in/india/story/think-the-harappans-were-the-source-of-vedic-hinduism-think-again-1329605-2018-09-01. Accessed 7 September 2020.

Jäger, S. (2004). *Kritische Diskursanalyse: Eine Einführung.* (Discourse Analysis: An Introduction). 4th ed. Munster: UNRAST-Verlag.

Jha, P. (2017). *How the BJP Wins: Inside India's Greatest Election Machine.* New Delhi: Juggernaut.

Jonnalagadda, M., Norton, H., Ozarkar, S., Kulkarni, S. and Ashma, R. (2016). Association of genetic variants with skin pigmentation phenotype among populations of west Maharashtra, India, *American Journal of Human Biology* 28:5, 610–18.

Joseph, T. (2017). Who built the Indus Valley civilisation? *The Hindu,* 23 December. www.thehindu.com/news/national/who-built-the-indus-valley-civilisation/article22261315.ece. Accessed 6 September 2020.

Joseph, T. (2018). *Early Indians: The Story of our Ancestors and Where we Came From.* New Delhi: Juggernaut.

Joseph, T. (2019). How genetics is settling the Aryan migration debate. *The Hindu,* 16 June. www.thehindu.com/sci-tech/science/how-genetics-is-settling-the-aryan-migration-debate/article19090301.ece. Accessed 6 September 2020.

Khalid, H. (2018). In Pakistan, appreciation of the Indus Valley civilisation ties in with attempts to erase its Hindu past. *Dawn,* 30 August.

Khan, F. (2018). Archeologist who found 4,500-yr-old skeletons in Haryana doesn't buy Aryan invasion theory. *ThePrint,* 14 September. https://theprint.in/culture/archeologist-who-found-4500-yr-old-skeletons-in-haryana-doesnt-buy-aryan-invasion-theory/113852/. Accessed 6 September 2020.

Krishnan, M. (2018). RSS – India's Hindu nationalists spread their wings far and wide. *DW,* 9 August. www.dw.com/en/rss-indias-hindu-nationalists-spread-their-wings-far-and-wide/a-44588126. Accessed 14 September 2020.

Kumar, A. (2019). Soon you can see how the Harappans looked. *The Hindu,* 27 January. www.thehindu.com/todays-paper/soon-you-can-see-how-the-harappans-looked/article26102844.ece. Accessed 6 September 2020.

Lanchbury, J., Agarwal, S. and Papiha, S. (1996). Genetic differentiation and population structure of some occupational caste groups in Uttar Pradesh, India, *Human Biology* 68:5, 655–78. www.jstor.org/stable/41465513. Accessed 21 April 2021.

Latour, B. (2004). Why has critique run out of steam? From matters of fact to matters of concern, *Critical Inquiry* 30:2, 225–48.

Merton, R. K. (1979). The normative structure of science, *The Sociology of Science: Theoretical and Empirical Investigations,* 267–78.

Metspalu, M., Gallego, R. I., Yunusbayev, B., Chaubey, G., Mallick Chandana, B., Hudjashov, G., Nelis, M., Mägi, R., Metspalu, E., Remm, M., Pitchappan, R., Singh, L., Thangaraj, K., Villems, R. and Kivisild, T.

(2011). Shared and unique components of human population structure and genome-wide signals of positive selection in South Asia, *The American Journal of Human Genetics* 89:6, 731–44.

Moorjani, P., Thangaraj, K., Patterson, N., Lipson, M., Loh, P., Govindaraj, P., Berger, B., Reich, D. and Singh, L. (2013). Genetic evidence for recent population mixture in India, *The American Journal of Human Genetics* 93:3, 422–38.

M'charek, A. (2014). Race, time and folded objects: the HeLa error, *Theory, Culture and Society* 31:6, 29–56.

M'charek, A., Schramm, K. and Skinner, D. (2014a). Technologies of belonging: the absent presence of race in Europe, *Science, Technology, and Human Values* 39:4, 459–67.

M'charek, A., Schramm, K. and Skinner, D. (2014b). Topologies of race: doing territory, population and identity in Europe, *Science, Technology, and Human Values* 39:4, 468–87.

Pai, N. (2018). Inter-caste marriages are good for health of Indians. That's what DNA testing tells us. *ThePrint*, 20 September. https://theprint.in/opinion/inter-caste-marriages-are-good-for-health-of-indians-thats-what-dna-testing-tells-us/121098/. Accessed 6 September 2020.

Possehl, G. L. (2002). *The Indus Civilization: A Contemporary Perspective.* Altamira: Rowman.

Purohit, K. (2019). The Islamophobic roots of population control efforts in India. Al Jazeera. www.aljazeera.com/features/2019/8/9/the-islamophobic-roots-of-population-control-efforts-in-india. Accessed 14 April 2021.

Rajan, K. S. (2006). *Biocapital: The Constitution of Postgenomic Life.* Durham, NC: Duke University Press.

Reich, D. (2018). *Who We Are and How We Got Here: Ancient DNA and the New Science of the Human Past.* Oxford: Oxford University Press.

Reich, D., Thangaraj, K., Patterson, N., Price, A. L. and Singh, L. (2009). Reconstructing Indian population history, *Nature* 461, 489–95.

Savarkar, V. D. (1969). *Hindutva: Who is a Hindu?* Bombay: Veer Savarkar Prakashan. 5th ed.

Schinagl, R. C. (2019). One only needs an island/Alone in a vast sea: 'We refugees' – the waves of refugees of 2015/16, *Stellenbosch Theological Journal* 5:1, 361–81.

Schneider, F. (2013). How to do a discourse analysis. www.politicseastasia.com/studying/how-to-do-a-discourse-analysis. Accessed 29 January 2018.

Shahane, G. (2018). Why Hindutva is out of steppe with new discoveries about the Indus Valley people. *Scroll.in*, 6 September. https://scroll.in/article/893308/why-hindutva-is-out-of-steppe-with-new-discoveries-about-the-indus-valley-people. Accessed 6 September 2020.

Shukla, A. and Venkataraman, S. (2018). Why the latest genetic study does not rewrite India's history. *Swarajya*, 22 April. https://swarajyamag.com/ideas/why-the-latest-genetic-study-does-not-rewrite-indias-history. Accessed 6 September 2020.

Simpson, B. (2000). Imagined genetic communities: ethnicity and essentialism in the twenty-first century, *Anthropology Today* 16:3, 3–6.

Sivathambika, E. L. (1991). *The untouchables and their struggle for temple entry in Kerala, since 1920*. Doctoral Thesis. Union Christian College, Aluva, Mahatma Gandhi University, Kerala. http://hdl.handle.net/10603/317. Accessed 25 November 2021.

Stinson, J., and Lunstrum, E. (2021). Biocultural nation making: biopolitics, cultural-territorial belonging, and national protected area, *Environment and Planning E: Nature and Space*, DOI:2514848621995189.

Subramaniam, B. (2019). *Holy Science: The Biopolitics of Hindu Nationalism*. Seattle, WA: University of Washington Press.

Subramanian, T. S. (2014). Rakhigarhi, the biggest Harappan site. *The Hindu*, 27 March.

Suri, A. K. (2017). So what happened to the 'unambiguous' genetic evidence of Aryan migration? *Swarajya*, 25 December. https://swarajyamag.com/culture/so-what-happened-to-the-unambiguous-genetic-evidence-of-aryan-migration. Accessed 6 September 2020.

Suri, A. K. (2018). Bones of contention: who do the Rakhigarhi skeletons really belong to? *Swarajya*, 2 September. https://swarajyamag.com/politics/bones-of-contention-who-do-the-rakhigarhi-skeletons-really-belong-to. Accessed 6 September 2020.

Swarajya. (n.d.). About Swarajya. https://swarajyamag.com/. Accessed 15 April 2021.

Swarajya Staff (2018). Rakhigarhi DNA: what does it really reveal as of now? *Swarajya*, 14 June. https://swarajyamag.com/insta/rakhigarhi-dna-what-does-it-really-reveal-as-of-now. Accessed 6 September 2020.

Tallbear, K. (2013). Genomic articulations of indigeneity, *Social Studies of Science* 43:4, 509–33.

Thapar, R. (1996). The theory of Aryan race and India: history and politics, *Social Scientist* 24:1, 3–29.

Tsai, Y. Y. and Lee, W. J. (2020). An imagined future community: Taiwan Biobank, Taiwanese genome, and nation-building, *BioSocieties*, 1–28.

Vailly, J. (2017). The politics of suspects' geo-genetic origin in France: the conditions, expression, and effects of problematisation, *BioSocieties* 12, 66–88.

Venkataramakrishnan, R. (2018). Do Rakhigarhi DNA findings debunk the Aryan Invasion Theory or give it more credence? *Scroll.in*, 13 June. https://scroll.in/article/882497/do-rakhigarhi-dna-findings-debunk-the-aryan-invasion-theory-or-give-it-more-credence. Accessed 6 September 2020.

Vishnoi, A. (2018). Rakhigarhi DNA study questions Aryan invasion theory, claims author. *The Economic Times*, 6 September.

Wade, P., López-Beltrán, C., Restrepo, E. and Santos, R. V. (2015). Genomic research, publics and experts in Latin America: Nation, race and body, *Social Studies of Science* 45:6, 775–96.

Wahlberg, A. (2009). Bodies and populations: life optimization in Vietnam, *New Genetics and Society* 28:3, 241–51.

Wilson, K. (2018). For reproductive justice in an era of Gates and Modi: the violence of India's population policies, *Feminist Review* 119:1, 89–105.

5

Bio-power and assisted reproductive technologies in the global south: an ethical response from South Africa informed by vulnerability and justice

Manitza Kotzé

The Universal Declaration on Bioethics and Human Rights (UDBHR), adopted by the General Conference of UNESCO in October 2005, expresses a number of essential principles in bioethics. As indicated by the title, the Declaration 'anchors the principles it endorses in the rules that govern respect for human dignity, human rights and fundamental freedoms (UNESCO, 2006) when faced with ethical questions brought about by medicine and related technological developments. Rheeder refers to the UDBHR as 'one of the most important instruments in the development of human rights and bioethics' (2017: 59), for the reason that is was unanimously accepted in 2005 by the international community of 191 member states (Rheeder, 2017: 59). This chapter is situated in the global south, and written from the South African context. The UDBHR is also explicitly aimed at developing countries such as South Africa, stating:

> The aims of this Declaration are ... to promote equitable access to medical, scientific and technological developments as well as the greatest possible flow and the rapid sharing of knowledge concerning those developments and the sharing of benefits, with particular attention to the needs of developing countries. (UNESCO, 2006)

Two articles in the UDBHR are especially relevant to the issue of assisted reproductive technologies (ARTs) in the global south, and in South Africa in particular. Article 8 mentions respect for human vulnerability, while article 10 calls for equality, justice and equity. In this chapter, these two articles will be brought into conversation with the issue of ARTs in the global south, taking the South African context as the point of departure.

Briefly stated, articles 8 and 10 of the UDBHR underscore the necessity for vulnerable groups and individuals to be protected in the application and advancement of scientific knowledge, medical practice and associated technologies, while also emphasising all human beings should be treated in a just and equitable manner. In the context of South Africa, where the majority of the population are unable to access and afford most forms of ART, the issues of biopower and misuse of power in particular come to the fore. Especially in forms of biotechnology where donor material is utilised, donors are often from vulnerable groups, while those that benefit are in positions of privilege where they can both access and afford these treatments. This also raises the issue of intersectionality in the ethical discussion on ARTs in the South African context. I examine this subject by drawing on an ethos that values vulnerability and justice in its response.

Conversation around ARTs, where third parties and government-controlled policies become involved in the conceiving and birthing of children, invariably also then raises questions of eugenics. In the South African context, questions of nationalism are often raised in the same breath. In the first section of this chapter, the issue of reproductive technology in this regard is discussed, first in general and then more specifically in the South African context, before turning to the two articles of the UDBHR. I will look at vulnerability, article 8 of the UDBHR, and then justice, article 10, as guiding bioethical principles in responding to the issue of biopower, ARTs and the question of belonging in South Africa.

ARTs and possible ethical and social concerns

With the continuing development of ARTs, more and more choices become available to those who wish to make use of it, for a variety of reasons. This includes medication to induce ovulation or improve fertility, or more invasive procedures such as intrauterine insemination (IUI), either with one's own or donor sperm, in vitro fertilisation (IVF) with one's own or donor ova and/or sperm, as well as pre-implantation genetic diagnosis (PGD), where embryos undergo genetic screening, after which a decision is made which to implant based on the genetic information. In most instances of PGD, screening is done to identify genetic disorders (Kotzé, 2019: 248–9).

There are a number of ethical and social concerns when donor material is utilised, particularly around the 'monetization of human reproduction' (Shapiro, 2018: 75). This is especially the case when there exist 'multiple conflicts of interest for every party involved; the fertility centre, the physician, the recipient patient and the donor' (Shapiro, 2018: 75). The risk of financial coercion and the commodification of human body parts, including genetic material, are further issues of concern, as are the health risks involved, including ovarian hyper stimulation syndrome, which could occur in egg donors (Shapiro, 2018: 75–6).

The issue of commodification, and whether donors are reduced to their reproductive capacities, are serious ethical issues that are raised by ARTs, to which I return later in the chapter. Discussions on reproductive technology also often raise issues of eugenics. Daar notes that when first considered, eugenic practices of the past, 'discouraging and disallowing reproduction by institutional segregation and surgical sterilization seem to bear little resemblance to the reproductive enthusiasm embodied by' the ARTs of our present time (2017: 2). The relationship, however, lies in the 'transfer of such a personal and intimate decision into the hands of third parties' (Daar, 2017: 2). From a perspective of biopower, this is also then a pressing issue, in particular surrounding the access to reproductive technology.

As noted by Sarah Franklin (1997: 166) reproductive technology can be viewed as the coming together of 'two of the most powerful Euro-American symbols of future possibility: children and scientific progress'. As such, it follows that biopower should be included in the conversation on ARTs. Mason and Ekman define eugenics as 'the belief and practice of improving the genetic quality of the human population' (2017: 7).[1] While the term 'eugenics' most often bring to mind notions of "the monstrous Nazi race hygiene project or … an American sterilization assault against the disadvantaged and racially "inferior"' (Crook, 2008: 135), the issue of eugenics is not this simple. Various factions existed, including '"leftist and "reform" eugenists as well as "mainline" or reactionary eugenists, with dedicated opposition coming more from liberal and religious quarters' (Crook, 2008: 135).

Within South African society, an important aspect of the discussion of eugenics within the conversation on ARTs is, who has access to these forms of biotechnology? It is estimated that while roughly 10% of the population worldwide are infertile and unable to conceive without medical treatment, including ARTs, in sub-Saharan Africa, the number of subfertile adults grow to between 10% and 25% (Kotzé, 2019: 251). From a eugenics perspective, it is therefore an alarming phenomenon if only certain groups within the broader South African context are able to access biotechnological assistance to reproduce. In the following section, the South African context and ARTs within it are examined further.

Transnational ART utilising donor material in South Africa

There are numerous factors that influence access to reproductive technology – financial access being the most obvious, with the utilisation of reproductive technology in most instances being very expensive. However, many factors also contribute to access or the lack thereof, such as geographic locality or issues of cultural taboos (Kotzé, 2019: 249). In the South African context, all of these factors play a decisive role.

Financially, South Africa and Brazil are the two countries world-wide with the biggest gap between the rich and the poor (Kotzé, 2019: 250). With this ever-widening gap, and extremely high unemployment levels, the vast majority of South Africans cannot afford access to reproductive technology. Statistics South Africa indicated in 2017 that over 70% of the populace are reliant on public healthcare services (2017: 3). There are only two hospitals in South Africa covered by public healthcare where fertility treatments are offered, while two others are able to provide limited treatment through partnerships with the private sector (Kotzé, 2019: 252).

One of the most striking features of the reproductive technology landscape, particularly when donor material is utilised, is the increase in transnational access to treatment (Homanen, 2018: 28). This also affects the South African context, with South Africa being a significant destination for many people from other countries who seek to utilise reproductive technology treatments (Homanen, 2018: 28). There are a variety of reasons for people seeking to engage in the highly challenged term 'fertility tourism'.[2] It could be as simple as treatment not being available to specific groups within their home countries, such as ARTs not being offered or accessibility to single women or same-sex couples. The reasons include the desire to make use of treatments that are banned in certain countries, such as the donation of gametes or technological treatments, like PGD for example, or the belief that better standards and quality of care will be experienced in the country the patient is travelling to (Kotzé, 2020: 245). However, in the majority of instances, affordability is given as one of the most significant reasons, as well as 'a shortage of donor gametes in some countries' (Wilson, 2016: 49). The possible shortages of donors in certain countries, particularly egg donors, are also tied up with financial reasons, as one of the biggest motivations behind egg donation is financial. In the developed world, countries where there are strict regulations in terms of donor compensation are often faced with a limited donor pool, whereas countries that allow generous compensation, such as the US, follow Shapiro's argument that the best way to ensure a steady supply of egg donors is to ensure payment (2018). In the US, while the American Society for Reproductive Medicine has stated that it is 'not appropriate' to compensate egg donors above ten thousand dollars (still just below R140,000.000 based on the exchange rate at the time of writing, which is twenty times the compensation South African donors can expect), advertisements offer much higher amounts for young women graduating from high-ranking universities and matching criteria in terms of height, academic achievements and other benchmarks (Mason and Ekman, 2017: 103).

In the South African context, financial motivation is a genuine reality for many donors. As a student at Stellenbosch University, advertisements from clinics seeking egg donors were found in many of the female restrooms on campus, with the compensation highlighted on most of these posters. One agency who advertised in this manner, included in the FAQ on their website the question 'How many pairs of shoes can I buy with my financial compensation?' and used the term 'ka-ching' in answering regarding the amount donors could expect. This has since been removed from the website, but the implications that donors should be focusing on financial reimbursement was clear to potential donors perusing the website.

While regulations in South Africa indicate that advertising for egg donation should be done in such a manner that the wording avoids statements 'about "earning money" or "financial gain"', it also notes that 'reference to reimbursements or compensation is acceptable' (SASREG, 2020). This further raises question of biopower; it was mentioned earlier that one of the reasons for transnational utilisation of ARTs, and donor eggs in particular, is shortage of available donors in the recipient's home country. It was indicated that this is partially due to the lack of compensation offered to prospective donors. Individuals and couples travelling from the developed world to the developing world, motivated by the availability of donors, would then conceivably have been willing to pay what would be viewed as fair compensation in their own country, but instead pay the much lower price enforced by South African policies. South African donors, often in desperate financial situations, are grateful to receive the R7000.000, which is the maximum compensation allowable under the National Guidelines from the Southern African Society for Reproductive Medicine and Gynaecological Endoscopy as of 2020 (SASREG, 2020).

South African fertility clinics also market themselves in particular to the international market. One well-known clinic located in Cape Town has various packages on their website catering to overseas patients, which include, in addition to the ART treatments, accommodation in the V&A Waterfront (a tourist hotspot), and day trips to tourist attractions such as Robben Island and Table Mountain. In instances such as these, 'fertility tourism' might be an apt description of the services rendered.

In addition, egg donors being motivated by financial compensation also raises a number of other ethical issues, including the reality that the risks involved in the process are rarely discussed with donors and whether the criteria of informed consent are indeed met (Lahl, 2017: 241). Issues concerning the commodification and objectification of human body parts were mentioned earlier, and are worth bringing up again: the fear of commodifying human beings, and making a human person the 'subject of a contract'; that surrogacy is 'considered a breach of human dignity under Article 1 of the Constitution' in Germany; while the French Supreme Court has also banned surrogacy, claiming that it is a violation of a woman's body (Mason and Ekman, 2017: 157).

Regarding the commodification of the human body, Sharp mentions that, historically, numerous forms of slavery emerge as an expression of objectification and 'one party owning or purchasing temporary or permanent rights to another' (2000: 293). A related theme, and one of extreme importance for the South African context, is that of colonisation. Colonised or commodified bodies, she suggests, are often disciplined through the combined effect of, amongst others, colonial power and medical practices (Sharp, 2000: 293). This can also be expressed as the transformation of persons into economic objects and the dehumanising of individuals for profit (Sharp, 2000: 293). Within the context of biotechnology, this raises questions of ownership 'of entire bodies, their processes, their tangible (and, increasingly, microscopic) parts' (Sharp, 200: 299). In turn, issues of justice and equality are highlighted, which will be revisited later in the chapter.

The question of belonging is a central issue in this volume, and also comes strikingly to the fore in terms of the possible psychological issue of identity. SASREG indicates that all egg donations in South Africa should be anonymous, with the exception of instances 'qualifying as a "known donation"' and specifies that 'No contact will be allowed between the donor and the potential child in the future' (2020). This can have profound implications for the notion of belonging: children born from donor material might feel a lack of connection with their siblings, or even their parents and other family members in a way which impacts on their identity and self-worth (Daar, 2017). Daar indicates that the website used most often in the US for connecting 'donors and donor-conceived persons … reports attracting twelve thousand visitors to its website each month' (2017: 252).

Children born using other forms of reproductive technology, such as children with three genetic parents, might also suffer 'both psychological and physical damage' (Mason and Ekman, 2017: 7). When ART is utilised with donor material, which in the majority of instances are anonymous, the 'naturalized definition of genetic lineage … becomes complicated' (Bergmann, 2011: 283). This has further implications for the "legal definitions of kinship" (Bergmann, 2011: 283) and accordingly, in terms of transnational ART, is not only a psychological question of 'fitting in' and identity, but also becomes a biopolitical question of belonging.

The other side of the coin is also that it is for the very reason of 'belonging' that transnational ARTs could be sought. Bergmann relates instances of couples travelling in order to find donors that share their phenotype or would 'look like them' (2011: 286). In these cases, the argument could be made that rather than posing a challenge to the notion of belonging, these parents are ensuring that their future child feels that they fit in and truly belong. How notions of kinship, relatedness and belonging are understood and conceived of in future might very well change as a result of transnational ARTs.

A further issue, and one of extreme importance, that has been implied previously but not yet explicitly referred to, centres on the possible exploitation of donors. In the South African context in particular, where donors are often financially desperate and the recipients are from the developed world, often able to pay greater amounts of compensation than they are charged, the vulnerability of donors is thrust into the spotlight in bioethical reflection. The remainder of this chapter considers two guiding bioethical principles for the reflection on ARTs in South Africa, especially when donor material is used. In the first instance, the principle of vulnerability is discussed in the following section.

Vulnerability as bioethical principle

Morais and Monteiro remark that the concept of vulnerability was introduced into the setting of research involving human beings as an attribute that assigns particular population groups who are viewed as 'more exposed and less able to defend themselves against abuse and ill-treatment by others' (2017: 312). That such protection is necessary is clear from history, as also previously mentioned as part of the history of eugenics.

The *Belmont Report: Ethical Principles and Guidelines for the Protection of Human Subjects of Research* (1979), created by the National Commission for the Protection of Human Subjects of Biomedical and Behavioral Research, was the first to refer to 'vulnerability' (Rheeder, 2017: 62). Vulnerability within the context of bioethics can have both broad and narrow conceptions, and is not a self-evident notion. From a broad perspective, it can be viewed as the foundation that underlies all ethics and one that stresses the most fundamental aspect of bioethics for profoundly conveying the human condition as finite – vulnerability being an intrinsic part of being human (Morais and Monteiro, 2017: 313). From this viewpoint, then, all human beings are vulnerable. According to such such a view view, vulnerability 'has the constitutive element of universality', as a state shared by all human beings and 'complemented by constancy'; it can manifest itself in various manners and cannot be concealed, but is a condition marked by the pervasive possibility of harm (Ippolito, 2019: 545). Vulnerability, however, is also more than this universal condition and certain individuals and communities or groups can be said to be vulnerable in a more narrow conception, and be vulnerable to harm or risk in a way that many other individuals or communities are not.

'From the perspective of autonomy as the normative ideal', Ten Have indicates, 'vulnerability is diminished autonomy' (2016: 1). This is of particular importance in the discussion on ARTs. It was mentioned earlier that part of the ethical challenges are raised by these forms of biotechnology are the fears of commodification or reducing donors to their reproductive capacities. From such a definition of vulnerability as reduced autonomy, then, it is not a stretch to argue that donors in reproductive technology could be seen as vulnerable.

There are a variety of dimensions to differentiate between in terms of vulnerability as a bioethical principle. Vulnerability can relate to individual persons, or a collective of groups, communities or even countries. When used to identify a collective, however, it does not necessarily mean that every individual within that group is vulnerable, or that vulnerability is an unchanging constant. Accordingly, vulnerability is also both a gradual and a relational notion (Ten Have, 2016: 11). It is possible to distinguish different forms of vulnerability; while medical vulnerability often comes to mind first in bioethical discussions, Ten Have also mentions 'physical, psychological, social, economic, and environmental vulnerabilities' (2016: 11). Within the context of egg donation in South Africa, discussed earlier, all donors are then not necessarily vulnerable. In the same way that the South African population could be described as vulnerable, belonging to the global south, but not all individuals living within South Africa are automatically vulnerable according to the narrow conception, the same is true for egg donors.

In the UDBHR, article 8, under the heading 'Respect for human vulnerability and personal integrity', the article states:

> In applying and advancing scientific knowledge, medical practice and associated technologies, human vulnerability should be taken into account. Individuals and groups of special vulnerability should be protected and the personal integrity of such individuals respected. (UNESCO, 2006)

It is noteworthy that the UDBHR does not simply mention vulnerability, which could be construed according to the broad conception and interpreted merely as part of the human condition, as mentioned earlier. By such a definition, all human beings are vulnerable. The wording of the declaration calls for the protection of 'individuals and groups of *special* vulnerability' (italics added), thereby emphasising that it is not this broad conception of being vulnerable that is referred to.

It is, then, also necessary to clarify further who is meant by those who have special vulnerability. As Ten Have indicates, the notion 'that persons are vulnerable simply because they belong to specific groups or populations is inadequate' (2016: 75). When reference is made to vulnerable populations, it does not necessarily mean that within the particular group, all individual persons are affected in the same way (Ten Have, 2016: 131). As mentioned previously, if this bioethical principle of vulnerability is applied to egg donors within the South African context, many donors might have special vulnerability, in particular those who are drawn to donation for the financial compensation and who live in conditions that make it unlikely they will be in a position to utilise the ART treatments themselves, should they need or desire it. Yet they donate so that others can benefit from a biotechnology they are unable to access.

For bioethics, the concept of vulnerability is important because 'vulnerable groups are prone to exploitation in medical research'; in other words, 'they are easily taken unfair advantage of to serve another's interests' (Schroeder and Gefenas, 2009: 113). Within the context of ARTs in South Africa, this has been alluded to earlier. It is very often the vulnerable who take part in systems that they do not benefit from, such as through the donation of genetic material, for example. When young low-income women from vulnerable communities in the developing world are lured to egg donation in order to be financially compensated, and the recipients of that donation are wealthy people from the developed world, this description of vulnerability rings true. Accordingly, it becomes a serious bioethical issue of biopower.

Schroeder and Gefenas, after discussing and defining vulnerability as a bioethical principle, identify as one of the challenges for future work, 'how to address the justice concern within vulnerability discussion, which has for decades focused mostly on autonomy concerns. It is here that the topic of benefit sharing will gain importance' (2009: 120). The following section turns to the concern for justice, addressing justice as a bioethical principle in guiding the response to ARTs in the South African context.

Justice as bioethical principle

In the UDBHR, article 10, under the heading 'Equality, justice and equity', states: 'The fundamental equality of all human beings in dignity and rights is to be respected so that they are treated justly and equitably (UNESCO, 2006). The recognition of the intrinsic worth and dignity of every human being can be viewed as the basis for the recognition of the equality of all human beings. The connection between the notions of human dignity, equality and the rule of law is also stressed by John Rawls in his influential theory of justice (1971). Rawls focuses on 'the least advantaged, respect for all people and the essential role of community in the formation of just individuals and a just society (Wright, 2012: 306). Rawls recognises the reality that there will always be some forms of injustice in any society, and, accordingly, the load of unjust results has to be 'more or less evenly distributed over different groups in society' (1971: 312). While not explicitly referring to the notion of vulnerability, Rawls does acknowledge that the 'duty to comply' is problematic for those who have for many years suffered under the weight of injustice, and that such individuals or communities rather have the 'duty to resist' (Bankovsky, 2012: 76; Rawls, 1971: 312). Bankovsky indicates that by making this argument in the defining of conditions, Rawls 'limits any opposition to only those *clear and obvious* infractions of basic liberties and of a very basic and uncontroversial equal opportunity principle' (2012: 78, italics in original).

Similarly, the relation between dignity and equality is unified in the South African Constitution, where the Bill of Rights sets out to 'enshrine the rights of all people in our country and affirms the democratic values of human dignity, equality and freedom'. Justice is also an important principle when discussing ARTs. 'Reproductive justice' is a concept devised by Black feminist scholars and activists in the US. Reproductive justice activist Loretta Ross defines the term as:

> based on three interconnected sets of human rights: (1) the right to have a child under the conditions of one's choosing; (2) the right not to have a child using birth control, abortion, or abstinence; and (3) the right to parent children in safe and healthy environments free from violence by individuals or the state. (2017: 290)

She further notes that the notion of reproductive justice is embedded in the idea that decision making around having and raising children has always been formed by the realty of systemic inequality, and that this has especially been the case for vulnerable women (Ross, 2017: 291). Within the South African context, for example, it was mentioned previously that the young low-income women who are drawn to egg donation for the financial compensation are unlikely to access or afford the biotechnological treatments they make possible for others. This systemic inequality that Ross mentions are, then, also a feature within the South African landscape in terms of reproductive technology. In addition, the first aspect of reproductive justice that Ross articulates, the 'right to have a child under the conditions of one's choosing', is also not one of the rights that all South African women share. It was previously mentioned that up to 25% of adults in sub-Saharan Africa are subfertile, and it follows that many individuals and couples who greatly desire to have children would need to make use of ARTs to be able to do so. Being unable to access or afford these treatments is not in keeping with this first right of reproductive justice.

At present then, the principle of justice as set out in the UDBHR, where all people are treated justly and equitably, are not met within the South African ART sphere. It is one thing to claim the rights and equality of all people as the Constitution does, but the UDBHR specifically refers to the manner in which people are *treated*.

Returning to the notion of belonging, ARTs should also be guided by the principle of justice in allowing people the space to belong and live out their identity. Robertson notes that reproductive experiences 'are central to personal conceptions of meaning and identity. To deny procreative choice is to deny or impose a crucial self-defining experience, thus denying persons respect and dignity at the most basic level' (in Daar, 2017: 153). If vulnerable individuals within the South African context are used by a system that they are unable to access themselves, and as such, are excluded from this self-defining experience, then the principle of justice as envisioned in the UDBHR is not met. This exclusion can also be categorised as the opposite of belonging.

Conclusion: biopolitics, reproductive technologies and belonging in South Africa

Conversation around ART raises a number of bioethical questions, some of which were examined in this chapter. ART share with eugenics that third parties and government-controlled policies become involved in the conceiving and birthing of children. The chapter used two guiding bioethical principles from the UDBHR to provide a response to some of the issues raised by ART: vulnerability as set out in article 8, and justice as set out in article 10. Issues of biopower and the question of belonging were emphasised, in particular, within the focus of this volume, and situated within the South African context.

Vulnerability is provisional; to refer to an individual or a community as vulnerable implies that they are at risk of being hurt or harmed, but that the hurt has not yet happened. This can and should produce the responsibility to take pre-emptive action, to prevent the possible hurt or harm from occurring. As such, it is possible for vulnerable individuals, also young low-income women who are lured to egg donation in South African for the financial gain, to be freed from the category of vulnerability. If the second guiding principle of justice, and then justice as formulated in the UDBHR is followed, where all human beings are not only viewed as equal, but treated in a manner that embraces equity and equality, fears of commodification, objectification and exploitation need not be an aspect of ARTs in South Africa.

Notes

1 The term 'liberal eugenics' is often used to refer to the improvement of human beings through biotechnology such as genetic engineering, and can be seen in movements such as transhumanism, where the aim is to transcend the current limitations of humanity. This, however, will not be the focus in this chapter.

2 'Fertility tourism' as a term is highly contested, with 'tourism' implying, in most instances, travel for recreation and enjoyment. For this reason, many argue, this it is not an appropriate moniker to use in cases where individuals or couples travel in order to obtain access to, or to make use of reproductive technology. Bergmann prefers to speak of 'transnational economies' or 'the circumvention routes of reproduction' when referring to the intricate and multifaceted collection of travellers, who include 'traveling users, mobile medics, sperm and egg donors, locally and globally operating clinics, international standards, laboratory instruments, pharmaceuticals, biocapital, conferences and journals, IVF internet forums, and differing national laws' (2011: 283). Others prefer to make use of other terminology, such as Matorras, who refers to 'reproductive exile', or Sirpa Soini et al., who use a 'crossborder flow of patients' (in Kotzé, 2020: 245). 'Fertility tourism' can be differentiated from 'medical tourism', where the same controversy exists regarding the term itself, but the debate mostly focuses on aspects of health policies and medical competition on a global scale; transnational travel in terms of ART includes the characteristic of 'promissory capital', in that it remains unpredictable without any guarantee (Bergmann, 2011: 283).

References

Bankovsy, M. (2012). Perfecting Justice in Rawls, Habermas and Honneth: A Deconstructive Perspective. *Continuum Studies in Political Philosophy*. London: Continuum.

Bergmann, S. (2011). Fertility tourism: circumventive routes that enable access to reproductive technologies and substances, *Journal of Women in Culture and Society* 36:2, 280–9.

Crook, P. (2008). The new eugenics? The ethics of bio-technology. *Australian Journal of Politics and History* 54:1, 135–43.

Daar, J. (2017). *The New Eugenics Selective Breeding in an Era of Reproductive Technologies*. New Haven: Yale University Press.

Franklin, S. (1997). *Embodied Progress: A Cultural Account of Assisted Conception*. London: Routledge.

Homanen, R. (2018). Reproducing whiteness and enacting kin in the Nordic context of transnational egg donation: Matching donors with cross-border traveller recipients in Finland. *Social Science Medicine* 203, 28–34.

Ippolito, F. (2019). Vulnerability as a normative argument for accommodating 'justice' within the AFSJ. *European Law Journal* 25, 544–60.

Kotzé, M. (2019). Whose reproductive health matters? A Christian ethical reflection on reproductive technology and exclusion. In M. Kotzé, N. Marais and N. Müller van Velden (eds), *Reconceiving Reproductive Health: Theological and Christian Ethical Reflections.* Reformed Theology in Africa Series volume 1, 247–63, Cape Town: AOSIS.

Kotzé, M. (2020). A Christian ethical reflection on transnational assisted reproductive technology. In M. Kotzé and R. Rheeder (eds), *Life in Transit: Theological and Ethical Contributions on Migration.* Reformed Theology in Africa Series Volume 2, 239–56. Cape Town: AOSIS.

Lahl, J. (2017). Surrogacy, *The Handmaid's Tale,* and reproductive ethics: egg donation, sperm donation and surrogacy, *Issues in Law and Medicine* 32:2, 241–4.

Mason, M. A. and Ekman, T. (2017). *Babies of Technology: Assisted Reproduction and the Rights of the Child.* New Haven: Yale University Press.

Morais, T. C. A. and Monteiro, P. S. (2017). Concepts of human vulnerability and individual integrity in bioethics, *Revista Bioetica* 25:2, 311–19.

Rawls, J. (1971). *A Theory of Justice.* Cambridge, MA: Harvard University Press.

Rheeder, R. (2017). An ethos of vulnerability: a kingdom perspective on the principle of respect for vulnerability within the UNESCO Declaration on Bioethics and Human Rights, *Asia Journal of Theology* 31:1, 58–81.

Ross, L. J. (2017). Reproductive justice as intersectional feminist activism, *Souls: A Critical Journal of Black Politics, Culture, and Society* 19:3, 286–314.

SASREG (Southern African Society for Reproductive Medicine and Gynaecological Endoscopy). (2020). SASREG guidelines for egg donation agencies. Online: www.sasreg.co.za. Accessed 9 May 2021.

Schroeder, D. and Gefenas, E. (2009). Vulnerability: too vague and too broad? *Cambridge Quarterly of Healthcare Ethics* 18, 113–21.

Shapiro, D. B. (2018). Payment to egg donors is the best way to ensure supply meets demand, *Best Practice and Research Clinical Obstetrics and Gynaecology* 5, 73–84.

Sharp, L. A. (2000). The commodification of the body and its parts, *Annual Review of Anthropology* 29, 287–328.

Statistics South Africa (2017). Mid-year population estimates P0302. South African Government, Department of Statistics.

Ten Have, H. (2016). *Vulnerability: Challenging Bioethics.* New York: Routledge.

UNESCO (2006). *Universal Declaration on Bioethics and Human Rights.* Paris: UNESCO Publishing.

Wilson, T. L. (2016). Unravelling orders in a borderless Europe? Cross-border reproductive care and the paradoxes of assisted reproductive technology policy in Germany and Poland, *Reproductive Biomedicine & Society Online* 3, 48–59.

Wright, J. A. (2012). Justice between fairness and love? Christian ethics in dialogue with Rawls and Niebuhr, *International Journal of Public Theology* 6, 306–28.

Part II

Birth violated

6

Injectable contraceptives: technologies of power and language of rights

C. Sathyamala

Birth control is not a modern concept and individuals, couples, families, and societies have prevented conception and births through means available to them at different points in history. However, it is in the second half of the nineeenth century, that birth control methods began to be deployed by emerging nation states to regulate populations. In *The History of Sexuality, Volume I*, Foucault argues that one of the juridical powers of the sovereign was the right to decide life and death which 'was in reality the right to take life or let live' (Foucault, 1978: 136). Later on, this sovereign power was, 'complemented by a new right which does not erase the old right but which does penetrate it, permeate it. This is the right, or rather precisely the opposite right. It is the power to "make live" and "let die"' (Foucault, 2003: 241).

Incorporating the earlier disciplinary power on individual bodies which he termed 'anatomo politics of the human body' (Foucault, 1978: 139), this new form of 'non-disciplinary' 'biopower', 'is applied not to [hu]man-as-a-body but to … [hu]man-as-species' (Foucault, 2003: 242). The right of death is now manifested as 'the right of the social body to ensure, maintain or develop its life', exerting 'a positive influence on life … endeavor[ing] to administer, optimize, and multiply it, subjecting it to precise controls and comprehensive regulations' (Foucault, 1978: 136–7). With this transformation, life and biological processes are taken control of and all vital events such as birth rates, death rates, morbidity rates, and life expectancy of *populations* become objects for study/knowledge and intervention in order to 'achieve overall states of equilibration and regularity' (Foucault, 2003: 246). Control of sexuality and fertility, then, becomes critical in regulating the size of a nation's population and one of the critical biopolitical projects of the state.

With the technological revolution of the late nineteenth century and the rise of the pharmaceutical industry, nation states were in a better position to fine-tune their biomass to suit their bio-needs. However, given that not all bodies were deemed of equal importance in achieving specified bio-objectives, natalist policies were opera-tionalised differentially by the enhancement of some by 'making them live' while others were negated by 'letting them die'. In liberal democratic states, the project of elimination of bodies deemed superfluous and irrelevant to the economy had to subscribe, at least overtly, to 'letting die' rather than 'making die'. It was in this context that contraceptive technologies such as the long-term hormonal injectables that did not require compliance were developed and marketed. Initially these technologies were promoted as health products but when serious adverse life-threatening effects began to manifest, they were positioned as technologies of empowerment. It was argued that such technologies enabled women, particularly those who were subjugated under patriarchy, to exercise their individual freedom and choice.

This chapter examines the three-decade-long resistance against the introduction of the injectable contraceptives into the Indian family planning programme (FPP), a struggle that I have been closely associated with. It argues that by positioning them as products that avert death, their inherent hazardous, anti-life nature is camouflaged, as are the underlying eugenic intents in deploying them. Further, that by promoting them as tools of empowerment, women are invited to participate in their subjugation through self-discipline and self-surveillance. Finally, by promoting anti-life contraceptive technologies at the national and global level, nation states are reverting back to the biopolitical project of a sovereign state by shifting from a passive 'letting die' to actively 'making die'.

The chapter begins with a brief description of family planning policy in India from the time of Independence in 1947 up to the 1970s. By the mid-1970s, however, by evoking a state of emergency, India deployed a sovereign's right to 'make die' as the biopolitical strategy, turning it into what Giorgio Agamben (2005) terms a 'state of exception'. When overt coercion threatened political stability, the Indian state introduced the life-negating injectable contraceptive in its population control programme under the guise of 'making live'.

The chapter goes on to describe the struggle, spearheaded by the autonomous women's and health movement in the country, against its inclusion into the Indian FPP. It analyses the context within which this struggle gained currency and the context within which it lost out. It ends by concluding that, notwithstanding the rhetoric of reproductive choice and women's empowerment, promotion of life-threatening contraceptives, aided by transnational capital, demonstrates the class, gender, caste, and racist dimensions of the eugenic biopolitical project of 'making die'. By continuing to operate within a legal framework, the state of exception has now become the enduring paradigm of government as certain populations are rendered into 'bare lives' stripped of their rights, who can then be killed with impunity as *Homines sacri*, as argued by Agamben (1995).

Population control programme in post-independent India

As India gained freedom from colonial subjugation in 1947, in the initial period of state formation, reducing fertility was one of the first projects of the Indian state. This was not surprising because the need to control population had been articulated by several Indian elites prior to Independence. The Indian elites, even as they were participating in the struggle for freedom from colonial rule, subscribed to the Malthusian logic of 'too many people' as a cause of poverty in India, reflecting their class background and westernised leanings. In 1952, a state-led population control programme was included as an integral part of the planned economy and a key to developing the nation.[1] However, when, contrary to expectations, the 1961 census showed a higher birth rate, for the first-time incentives and disincentives began to find a place in policy recommendations (Government of India, 1962).[2] Through intense propaganda, attempts were made to normalise the concept of 'small' families. Restrain of fecundity was equated with patriotism and service to the nation, and citizens were urged to embrace the small family norm subscribing to the Foucauldian concept of governmentality and self-care.

By the 1970s, rising unemployment, inflation and scarcity of food began to manifest as civil unrest. It was thus that in 1975, when Indira Gandhi, the then Prime Minister, declared an internal 'Emergency' and suspended all civil liberties, the individual citizen's right to procreate was also appropriated by the state. With that, men and women were forcibly sterilised with a brutality and violence which is difficult to grasp today.[3] The slogan coined by Indira Gandhi, *garibhi hatao* (remove poverty) in reality became, *garib hatao* (remove the poor) demonstrating that it was turning into a state of exception and reverting to a sovereign's rule of actively 'making die'. By specifically targeting the poor, lower-caste, and Muslim populations, the upper-class, upper-caste, Hindu ethos of the power-elite became apparent, as did the genocidal proclivity of the postcolonial Indian state. As Foucault observed, 'If genocide is indeed the dream of modern powers, this is not because of a recent return of the ancient right to kill; it is because power is situated and exercised at the level of life, the species, the race, and the large-scale phenomena of population' (Foucault, 1978: 137). But 'Where there is power, there is resistance' (Foucault, 1978: 95), and the subsequent fall of Indira Gandhi's party from power in 1977 was ascribed to the exercise of power by these marginalised sections of the population through the electoral ballot. This effectively demonstrated that overt power of 'making die' could be anathema in a democratic state which allowed a certain agency to its polity, however tenuous. It was in this context that the availability in the international market of a provider-controlled long-term, hormonal injectable contraceptive (from now on Injectable) for women appeared to provide a solution for controlling their fertility without needing their compliance. However, resistance came from unexpected quarters. The state's attempt to introduce the Injectable into the FPP saw the engagement of a sub-set of middle-class, educated professional women, who, though not necessarily its target, but as informed subjects, raising questions on its safety. The following section begins with a brief history of the introduction of the Injectables into the Indian FPP and the subsequent long-drawn struggle against it that extended from the mid-1980s over the next three decades.

Contesting the Injectables

DMPA (Depot medroxy progesterone acetate, brand name Depo-Provera, parent company, the American Upjohn) and NET-EN (Norethisterone enanthate, brand name Noristerat, parent company, the German Schering AG) are the two injectable contraceptives that were synthesised in the early 1950s and, till the 1960s when they were ready to be marketed, their development proceeded almost neck to neck (Sathyamala, 1998). In 1971, Schering AG on its own withdrew NET-EN from the market because of the development of pituitary and liver nodules in animal studies. Trials with Depo-Provera continued mostly on women from developing countries. In India, the Indian Council for Medical Research (ICMR) carried out a Phase III clinical trial but discontinued it in 1975 because of serious adverse effects.

In early 1978, Upjohn was denied approval by the US Food and Drug Administration (USFDA) citing, among several concerns, its carcinogenic and teratogenic potential (Multinational Monitor, 1985).[4] Given this ruling, the Depo-Provera contraceptive could not be marketed in India because the Indian Drugs and Cosmetics Act forbids the use of a drug banned in the country of its origin. In 1985, members of an autonomous women's organisation,[5] *Stree Shakti Sangatana*, in the Indian state of Andhra Pradesh became aware, through newspaper advertisements, of a special camp to be inaugurated by the district Collector for administering a new Injectable at the government Primary Health Centre in Patancheru. What the advertisement did not reveal was that the camp was meant to recruit women for a Phase IV clinical trial with NET-EN. When the members of the collective arrived, they found that the women, who were mostly poor and illiterate, had been told only that the injection would prevent pregnancies. When the women learnt from the *Sangatana* members that NET-EN was still in an experimental stage, the women left without accepting the Injectable and the camp had to be called off.[6] *Stree Shakti Sangatana* then wrote to the Union Ministry of Health and Family Welfare and the Drugs Controller of India calling attention to the unethical nature of such clinical trials, which recruited women without their knowledge or consent.[7] When the authorities did not respond, the collective decided to take recourse to legal action. The following section describes the legal case against NET-EN that was filed in the Supreme Court of India.[8]

Litigating against the Injectable

There were two reasons for opting for a legal strategy: First, in democracies, law can be a powerful instrument to hold states accountable, resulting in individual or collective redress for rights violations (Ezer et al., 2015). Secondly, in India, the existence of 'Public Interest Litigation' (PIL)[9] law enables any member of the public to file a suit directly in the Supreme Court on behalf of an aggrieved party, provided it can be shown that public interest is at stake. In the case of the Patancheru incident, participation without informed consent was a clear violation of the fundamental rights guaranteed by the Indian constitution. However, the socio-economic background of the potential victims meant that they were not in a position to approach the courts on their own. Thus, in the court case, the victims and the petitioners belonged to two different worlds, so to speak, with the petitioners, as expert witnesses, assuming the right to speak on behalf of the victims. This they did by building a scientific argument against the use of the Injectable, using their particular expertise and voice. In 1986, a PIL was filed in the Supreme Court of India.[10] The original concerns that the clinical trials were unethical, and the potential for abuse in a state-controlled FPP, were broadened to include questions of safety and hazard.[11] The Supreme Court refused to pass an interim stay order restraining the state from proceeding with the unlawful trials till the matter was heard and decided. The Indian government could therefore go on to complete the trials and in the absence of legal bindings, the Drugs Controller granted approval for the marketing of NET-EN in the private sector. Yet the company German Remedies abstained from marketing NET-EN in India.

In 1993, the situation altered as the USFDA granted approval to Depo-Provera, and the Drugs Controller of India followed suit and granted approval for its use in India. The following period saw a series of protests from women's groups (Saheli, 2001), and another round of PIL incorporating Depo-Provera,[12] and the publication of a scientific critique of Depo-Provera (Sathyamala, 2000). During this time, although the Injectables were available in the private sector, they were not distributed through the public sector national FPP.

To summarise, though no direct legal relief was provided through the Indian Supreme Court, a combination of legal, scientific, and popular protest strategies led by a vibrant women and health movement had prevented the distribution of the Injectables through the national FPP in India. The struggle was spearheaded by women from a class that was not the target of the FPP or the Injectables but who, along with other democratic forces, could organise collectively to generate a counter epistemic discourse, challenging truth claims of power elites. The following section analyses the context within which the struggle against the Injectable gained currency and the context within which it lost out.

Objective and subjective conditions of a struggle

Kuumba (2001: 5) notes, 'Mobilization [in social movements] is dependent on a delicate balance between the existence of objective conditions that stimulate the emergence of protest movements and, on a more individual level, the subjective awareness and interpretation of these conditions.' In India, the core of the struggle against the Injectables was founded on a stream of political consciousness that arose as a consequence of extreme levels of oppression experienced during the period of 'Emergency' in 1975 when civil liberties were suspended. This period marked the rise of many democratic movements, notably the civil liberties movement. The autonomous women's organisations that emerged during this time drew their inspiration from a broad left ideology even as they had become disenchanted with the patriarchal values that held sway among the organised left parties. Within the loosely knit movement were women who had experienced the brutal arms of state repression during the period of Emergency, women who as professionals had faced sexism both within their workplace and within the confines of their homes, as well as women from democratic movements who had experienced sexist discrimination by their male comrades (Sathyamala, 2005). Given the voluntary nature of participation, they were self-funded, shunning international donors' funding, viewing it as furthering an imperialist agenda. Comprising educated professional women, issues taken up were diverse, responding to the local situation as well as national ones.

It was thus that in the struggle against the Injectables, *Stree Shakti Sangatna* could respond to the advertisement in the newspaper but later broad based it in collaboration with other similar women's groups and individuals to file the PIL. They could draw upon the medical technical expertise of the *Medico Friend Circle*, an organisation of health professionals that had also emerged in the ferment of the post Emergency period, again, self-funded, and functioning as a collective with no salaried employees. In an environment of heightened sensitivity around population control policies particularly because of the stark violation of human rights witnessed during the Emergency, the Injectable as a technology of power and control acted as a red flag. The NET-EN case, well-constructed from both a scientific and legal point of view, went a long way in establishing the credentials of the autonomous women's groups, not only with the medical establishment but also among other organisations such as the women's wing of political parties and non-governmental organisations (NGOs).[13] What was central to the struggle was that it subscribed to the understanding of women's oppression in the context of population control as emanating from both patriarchy and class subjugation.

The state countered by trying to co-opt individuals and women's organisations, primarily through patronage. For instance, in 1991, the ICMR organised a meeting in New Delhi for those they termed 'health advocates', with the objective of evolving a common perspective on contraception. The meeting excluded vocal opponents of the Injectables, such as *Saheli* but included representatives from the Ford Foundation and United Nations Population Fund, both proponents of the Injectables (Medico Friend Circle Bulletin, 1992). Such selective inclusion and exclusion was not to overtly subvert opposition to the Injectables. It was a part of an overall strategy to test the solidarity among women's groups as well as to contain dissent by identifying and bringing into their fold, individuals and organisations that would subscribe to the biopolitical objectives of the state. During the meeting, it became apparent that the ICMR's primary objective was to evolve a compromise regarding the Injectables and the hormonal sub-dermal implants that were in the pipeline. Since serious adverse health effects with these contraceptives could no longer be denied, the ICMR argued that it should be safe to distribute these Injectables (and implants) through healthcare facilities at the tertiary level, such as hospitals attached to medical colleges, where proper screening and monitoring possibilities existed. This side-stepped one of the important arguments against the Injectables: being a depot injection, irrespective of the level of healthcare available, were life-threatening adverse reactions to take place when the drug was in a woman's body, there was no way the drug could be taken out to limit the threat.

The other strategy of the pro-injectable lobby was to discredit individuals and groups that opposed the Injectables by branding them as 'anti-technology' and playing the 'class' card by positioning them as frivolous upper-class women working against the interests of women from the marginalised sections. For instance, in 1994, R.P. Soonawala, an eminent private gynaecologist from Mumbai, and the principal investigator in the post-marketing surveillance study of Depo-Provera had this to say about the women protesting against the Injectables:

> I am saying let it (Depo-Provera) be available ... Who are these women protesting against it? Ill-informed, so-called feminists, who are just a bunch of college girls with nothing better to do. Without going into the issue they are making a noise about it. Barging into meetings, carrying placards, shouting slogans. (Soonawala as quoted in Sathyamala, 2000: 129)

Most importantly, the argument put forward was that the withholding of the Injectables was tantamount to interfering with an individual woman's right to choose. These strategies had their impact as could be seen in the final handling of the NET-EN case. In August 2000, the NET-EN case was voluntarily withdrawn from the Supreme Court by the petitioners, which spoke of a dilution in the understanding of the merits of the case. The petitioners agreed to 'settle' the case with a written assurance (not a court order) from the Union of India that the Injectables would not be used in the mass FPP and that it would be made available only 'where adequate facilities for follow-up and counselling [were] available' (Saheli, n.d.). This commitment made by the Indian government was nothing remarkable because, as mentioned earlier, the ICMR had already proposed this compromise in their 1991 meeting with the 'health advocates which *Saheli* had then rejected.

Moreover, the assurance was restricted to the inclusion and distribution of the Injectables in the public sector. The issue of the unethical trials, particularly the lack of informed consent, that the PIL had raised were not addressed. Hence the case was 'settled' without holding the Indian state responsible for the violation of the rights of the women participants. Thus, by accepting to withdraw the PIL without legal ruling or legal remedy on these critical issues, the opportunity that the case presented to raise issues pertinent to the conduct of clinical trials in the country was missed.

Though in the early period following the 'settlement' of NET-EN case, women's organisations continued to demand a ban of the Injectables from the FPP (Karat et al., 2005), they soon began to subscribe to a demand of restricted use in medical institutions with adequate facilities for care and follow-up. However, now that the obstacle posed by the legal case was removed – the only deterrent in the previous twenty-five years for the mass use of the Injectables – the Indian state was free to include them in the FPP. In November 2016, under the new 'Mission Parivar Vikas' (Mission Family Development), the state rolled out Depo-Provera 'at one go till Sub-centre level' (Panda, 2016, Annexure I:3). This policy decision made a mockery of the assurance given by the Union of India before the Supreme Court, that the Injectables would be made available only at tertiary care centres; instead, they were to be distributed at the lowest level of healthcare facility, which could provide only a bare minimum of care and by the least trained health provider.

Among the several reasons for the dilution of the earlier uncom-promising position demanding a ban on the Injectables in the FPP as advocated in the PIL, three stand out: one is the power of the truth claims offered by the medical establishment; the second is the discourse around reproductive choice and freedom; and the third is the NGO-isation and the conflation of diverse ideologies under the rubric of 'women's' groups. The following section examines these arguments.

1. Scientific bodies and their questionable authority

A major reason why the NET-EN case was not dismissed outright by the Supreme Court and why the scientific bodies such as the ICMR lobbied with the women's organisations, was the arguments presented in the PIL, which used the language of 'science' to demystify medical knowledge. This process of creating powerful evidence-based counter narratives to dominant truth discourses was an important part of protest strategies. However, this was always somewhat tenuous because, while the Indian state was transparent about its biopolitical objective of curtailing its population, what was not so obvious was the role of scientific bodies such as the ICMR and the World Health Organization (WHO) in furthering these aims at national and global levels. If the studies on Depo-Provera published in peer-reviewed journals had been taken seriously, the conclusion reached would have been as stated in Sathyamala (2000):

> Depo-Provera appears to be hazardous to the health of women and her progeny. The contraceptive appears to be not suitable for nulliparous women, adolescents, breast feeding women, women who have not completed their family and women who are in the reproductive age group. In short, there does not seem to be a single group of women for whom Depo-Provera can be safely recommended as a contraceptive method of choice. (Sathyamala, 2000: 128)

Why then did these scientific bodies deny and minimise the findings from their own studies and those of other scholars? To understand their role in contraceptive development and promotion, one has to go back to the early 1960s when, following the Thalidomide tragedy, strict regulations on drug testing, particularly those to be used by women in the reproductive period were formulated by the USFDA.[14] This meant that the cost of developing contraceptives became prohibitive, and duration of testing lengthened, leading to decrease in the average effective patent life of a contraceptive drug. In addition, product liability issues, increasing litigation, and high compensatory awards made pharmaceutical companies withdraw from developing and marketing contraceptive drugs.[15] This was when allegedly 'neutral' scientific bodies such as the WHO stepped in to bail out the contraceptive research and development sector in the pharmaceutical industry. This led to the virtual camouflaging of vested interests in contraceptive development and population control programmes. Providing an ethical-scientific veneer to the anti-poor, anti-women population policies became the assumed role of these bodies at national and global levels. It was thus that the link between the Injectables and increased HIV transmission, a life-threatening adverse drug reaction flagged in the late 1990s (Sathyamala, 2000), was researched not by Pfizer (current manufacturer of Depo-Provera) but by a consortium, the Evidence for Contraceptive Options and HIV outcomes (ECHO), comprising scientific bodies such as the WHO and donors such as the Bill and Melinda Gates Foundation (Hofmeyr et al., 2018).

The recently concluded ECHO trial subjected women and girl trial participants from four countries in Sub-Saharan Africa to a risk of increased HIV transmission without adequately informing them of the potential risks. Reviewing the trial protocols, Sathyamala (2019a: 12) concluded that the 'ECHO trial is unique in subjecting a group of healthy girls/women knowingly to a contraceptive drug with an intention not of finding out whether it is efficacious as a contraceptive, but to find out how risky or life-threatening its use could be' in violation of the Helsinki Declaration. Moreover, even though the results from the ECHO trial pointed to an increased risk (Sathyamala 2019b, 2020), the WHO downgraded the risk, declaring the Injectable to be safe for unrestricted use even in populations with high rates of HIV (World Health Organization, 2019).

2. The language of rights

It is argued that women desire and choose Injectables because their use can be 'hidden' from their husband/partner. In a state of patriarchal un-freedom, some women could perceive the 'discretion' that such a contraceptive provides as empowering. The 'benefit' of the secrecy-of-use is often pitted against medical risks. For instance, the 1982 issue of *Spare Rib* carried an article entitled, 'Depo-Provera, control of fertility – Two feminist views'. The first feminist viewpoint was that of Hari John, a medical doctor from Tamil Nadu, India, and an advocate of Depo-Provera:

> I am an acceptor of DP [Depo-Provera] and use it myself ... DP is the most popular choice that women in South India make. Women in South India choose DP because they are totally deprived and have no say in any aspect of their lives; they are subject to constant sexual abuse ... Most forms of contraception are very difficult to hide, and DP is the only one their husband won't know about ... Western feminists call for a ban on DP without hearing Third World women's point of view. (John and Hadley, 1982: 51)[16]

The second feminist viewpoint was that of Janet Hadley, member of the *Campaign against Depo-Provera*, London:

> I am wary of claims that Depo-Provera tops the popularity stakes among women at a particular clinic or hospital. Research shows that the most popular contraceptive 'chosen' by women attending a particular doctor reflects the doctor's favoured method … The doctor's prejudices govern the explanations … Upjohn has admitted paying millions of dollars' worth of bribes to government officials, hospital employees and others. (John and Hadley, 1982: 52)

If the two women who were both described as 'feminists' held such diametrically opposite viewpoints, whose voice was to be the representative one? The question really is how to weigh 'empowerment' allegedly afforded by use of the Injectable against its hazardous nature. Do the Injectables really increase possibilities of 'choice'? Countering this viewpoint, Sathyamala and D'Mello (2003) write:

> Market society celebrates the individual's 'freedom to choose'. This is the case also with contraceptives as commodities and products. In this context, in any critical analysis of the claims of 'freedom of choice', it is worth considering that choice also implies the lack of choice. The set of alternatives from which a racially oppressed, gender subordinated, working class woman has to choose are usually those that are presented to her by a patriarchal, racist and class-biased medical-industrial complex. It is most likely that her choice may be distinguished by the lack of choice. … Indeed, given her conditions of life, mired in poverty, misery and degradation, she may 'freely' choose the injectable contraceptive Depo-Provera as a lesser evil, a choice that she would have deemed unwise were she wealthy. (Sathyamala and D'Mello, 2003)

If user rates are any indication of exercising 'choice', in India, though the Injectables have been available in the private sector since the late 1990s and were distributed by several NGOs, often at a subsidised price, the use rate in 2005–6 was a mere 0.1% (India and Family Planning: an overview, n.d.), which rose to 0.7% in 2009 (e-FP, 2012); and in 2018, it was found that 50% of users dropped out after the first use (*Times of India*, 2018). Given the hazardous nature of the Injectables, and the fact that the discontinuation rates are high, Sathyamala and D'Mello (2003) ask: why then do the neo-Malthusian power elite promote Depo-Provera and subsidise its use for the low-income women of the world?

> Our answer has been that this category of women and their families are essentially a growing portion of the labor force in the third world and in the developed market societies that are deemed … to be almost totally superfluous … This 'marginal mass' is deemed irrelevant in market society as it is *presently structured* … The social roots of the misery, degradation and exploitation of millions of poor human beings are then apparently justifiably brushed aside. What mainstream medical and social science and the medical-industrial complex, the UN agencies, the large foundations and the large foundation-financed NGOs then identify is a thing (Depo-Provera) to help poor women avoid an 'unwanted' pregnancy. Overpopulation … is after all supposed to be the main explanation for hunger, indeed, to explain all ecological problems. (Sathyamala and D'Mello, 2003: 23; italics as in original)

3. The women's movement and its NGO-isation

In 2015, when the Indian Drug Technical Advisory Board recommended that Depo-Provera be included in the FPP, a memorandum opposing the move was submitted by over twenty organisations and networks working on public health and women's issues (*Jan Swasthya Abhiyan* et al., 2015). At the same time, a coalition of thirty-two NGOs under the banner of *Advocating Reproductive Choices* welcomed the government's decision, offering their help with introducing the Injectables into the FPP (Dey, 2015). Reflecting on such dissonance, Sarojini et al. (2006) observe:

> Even women's groups cannot be perceived as a homogenous entity with a similar stand on issues related to contraception. One strand of thought within the movement defends the use of such contraceptives like Depo. They believe that using such contraceptives like injectables and implants is the only way poor and powerless women can have control over their lives … So, where does the movement head for and how does it arrive at a consensus? Contrary to the above view, the widespread availability of Depo can dilute efforts to challenge the basic social and economic conditions that produce women's powerlessness. (Sarojini et al., 2006: 61)

The issue is not so much about the homogeneity of the entity called 'women's groups' and its stand on contraception; it is about the politics of population control and how the different organisations within this loose network engage with the state. Roy (2015: 99) remarks that 'the watershed decade of the 1990s – the decade of globalization, privatization and the opening up of the Indian economy – … fundamentally transformed the terrain upon which feminists wage their struggles as well as the nature and form of such struggles.' This period witnessed the NGO-isation of the movement. New forms of women's organisations emerged, with the earlier principles of collective functioning giving way to organisations that were heavily funded, with formalised hierarchies and clear employer–employee relationships. The state moved in by launching its own state-sponsored women's organisations, which co-opted the language and idiom of women's movement sans the ideology. The cracks began to appear quite early. For instance, in the late 1980s, the top-level functionaries of the government-sponsored Women's Development Programme (WDP) in Rajasthan with its large network of grassroots women workers (*sathin*), refused to oppose the linking of population control targets with the government-run famine relief programme. The reason cited was that it would put the survival of the WDP into jeopardy (Sawhny, 1995). The report by a fact-finding effort of members of autonomous women's groups concluded on this note:[17]

> Collaborating with the government to advance the movement has been one clear option for some organizations and activists. While no movement can flourish in isolation, no movement is likely to flourish without an ideology clearly spelt out. At present the movement is in its nascent stage and has to contend with a very sophisticated opposition. Clearly, we don't face suppression – we face cooption. We also have a movement which is extremely amorphous and has obfuscated certain differences among women in the name of universal sisterhood. We are continuing to form alliances within the movement with individuals and organizations of all sorts '*aurat honey ke natey*' (on grounds of their simply 'being women'). This may have been the only way out in the beginning. (*Saheli* et al., 1991: 30)

The fact-finding team highlighted an important issue: 'Why has the movement not systematically questioned the government and its intentions vis-à-vis women? This needs to be analysed in the context of the women's movement's visible critique and suspicion of the established left' (*Saheli* et al., 1991: 30). Fast-forwarding to 2007, by the time of the 7th National Conference on Women's Movement in India in Kolkata, the leadership of the movement was in the hands of NGOs, leading to what Sinha (2007) observed as 'state-sponsored feminism', now with a new legitimacy as part of the 'autonomous' women's movement. Importantly, as Sinha remarked, it was illusionary to view funded NGOs as not being 'carriers of politics'. External funding was one clear reason for their heightened visibility, which had allowed them to occupy centre-stage in less than two decades. As Bernal and Grewal (2014) argued, it was the similarity of such organisation with the state that made them attractive to the funders, since NGOs appeared less threatening than mass movements and though they seemed separate from the state, their appeal was that they are a site of governmentality.

Coming from diverse ideologies, although not explicitly stated, there was no one voice and the issue of who should speak on behalf of the women who formed the target of the Injectables began to assume central importance. International donors funded studies to hear the voices of these 'real' women, and while these were important to access woman users' experiences, what was troubling was that the 'user' perspective was being counterposed to the technical hazard of the contraceptive. However, what was interesting was that often the same donor would fund NGOs who were involved in social marketing of the Injectables, as well as those who were opposing their use, in effect painting them all the same colour.

Hartman and Rao (2015: 12) remark, 'in recent years, on both national and international levels, the strength and independence of such movements have weakened'. According to them, '[i]n the case of India, [it is because] women's groups have had to take on such a host of serious challenges – from sex selection, to gender violence, to new reproductive technologies, to unethical drug trials – that the focus on *population policy* has diminished' (emphasis added). Here, Hartman and Rao define 'population policy' as distinct from all the other specific issues they mention. I would argue that they are not disparate issues but are all very much part of the same *population* policy. It is the lack of coherent theory that has led to the fragmentation of both understanding and response within the women's movement.

Injectable contraceptive and technologies of power

Population reduction and the use of reproductive technologies for birthing subscribe to eugenic ideals and form the two sides of the same biopolitical coin of regulating populations. Taking off from Hartmann's concept of 'revised eugenics script' – the sterilisation of the minorities and assisted reproduction of the upper-class (Hartmann, 2006 as cited in Pande, 2016), Pande (2016: 250) argues that 'Neo-eugenics then becomes the new subtle form of eugenics whereby the neoliberal notion of consumer choice justifies promotion of assisted reproductive services for the rich, and at the same time, by portraying poor people (often in the global south) as strains on the world's economy and environment, justifies aggressive anti-natal policies'. This, Pande remarks, is a 'fundamental paradox' whereby the production of humans is dependent on the maintenance of a global hierarchy which privileges some and denies others (Pande, 2016: 245). I would argue that, rather than a paradox, viewed through the Foucauldian lens, one can see how it eminently fits the biopolitics of 'making live' of some population and of 'letting die' of others, with the stage now broadened from nation states to the global market, all in the interests of capital. Considering the number of 'eligible' women targeted, the worldwide market is indeed huge for both natalist and anti-natalist technologies.

The development and the deployment of long-acting provider-controlled contraceptives as technologies of power in the regulation of a recalcitrant population exhibit the three elements in the exercise of biopower as identified by Rabinow and Rose (2006): an array of authorities considered competent to speak a truth discourse; strategies for intervention upon collective existence in the name of life and health; and modes of subjectification. The notion of women's empowerment through such contraceptive usage fits well with the rhetoric of reproductive rights bringing the neo-Malthusian profes-sional elite and liberal feminists onto a common platform. In the 1990s, finding 'common ground' was the theme of meetings organised for such purposes by the international population lobby. Further, by normalising the life-threatening potential of these hazardous Injectables, women are invited to subjugate themselves through self-discipline and self-surveillance, devaluing their health and lives as part of governmentality. Finally, because past experience has shown that years of social marketing has not had the desired effect of making women 'choose' the Injectables, the current attempt is to further break down resistance by employing community-based workers who will, as 'trusted' members of their community, act as 'an interface between the community and the public health system' (National Health Mission, n.d.), in effect, deployed as the agents of the state.

In *Society Must be Defended*, Foucault (2003) asks: if the basic function of biopower is to nurture life, how is it possible 'for a political power to kill ... to expose not only its enemies but its own citizens to death?' and he points to state racism as an essential part of biopower. Racism, he says,

> is a way of separating out the groups that exists within a population ... That is the first function of racism ... Racism also has a second function ... 'if you want to live, the other must die' ... in a way that is completely new and quite compatible with the exercise of biopower ... [This] is not a military or war like relationship of confrontation, but a biological-type relationship ... the death of the bad race, of the inferior race (or the degenerate, the abnormal) is something that will make life in general ... healthier and purer. (Foucault, 2003: 254–5)

Concluding remarks

The mass distribution of the Injectables through the state-controlled FPP is a clear instance of using technology for eliminating an unwanted section of the population which is redundant to the economy because of its socio-political location in terms of its class, caste, religion, and race. In his analysis of the Holocaust and Third Reich, Agamben (2005: 2) points out that in 'a state of exception, ... a legal civil war ... allows for the physical elimination not only of political adversaries but of entire categories of citizens who for some reason cannot be integrated into the political system'. The

Indian state learnt its lesson that to enforce 'Emergency' and make overt the biopolitics of 'making die' was to make obvious the paradox of modern totalitarian states in the context of their professed democracy. By promoting the Injectables the paradox could be camouflaged because contraceptives are positioned as technologies that save lives by preventing pregnancies, when in reality they pose life-threatening risks.[18] However, as this chapter has shown, where Injectables are concerned, it was possible to raise a counter narrative on the anti-life nature of such technologies.[19] The fact that irrespective of the political party in power at the centre, Injectables have been promoted, goes to show that the nature of the postcolonial Indian state has essentially remained unaltered in its racist intentions since Independence. While the 1975 Emergency was a blatant and transparent use of force to realise the genocidal objective of 'making die', the mass use of the hazardous injectable contraceptive through the state-sponsored FPP is a clear form of state control with equal genocidal intents. The population that Agamben (1995) terms 'Homo Sacer', of lives that are deemed redundant and 'bare', are stripped of all legal rights and can be eliminated even while remaining within the framework of legality.

The long-drawn struggle against the Injectable has shown that the state has a much longer staying power in pursuing its biopolitical objectives than social movements, however powerful they may be at a particular point in history. It has also shown that to counter the genocidal intentions of the state, engagement with the state is not enough. There is a need to spell out what the politics of this engagement ought to be. The analysis and conclusions presented in this chapter are relevant not only to India but to all countries and populations that the current global economy deems redundant and therefore targets with such anti-life technologies to make them cease to exist.

Notes

1 That India was the first country in the world to make population control a national policy is upheld as a matter of pride even today (Ministry of Health and Family Welfare, n.d.). For an extensive discussion on the history of the Indian Family Planning programme, see Rao (2004).

2 Tax penalties, withdrawal of maternity benefits, and limitation of welfare provisions were some of the measures suggested (Government of India, 1962).

3 For instance, men were rounded up by the police and taken to clinics for sterilisation (Morse and Mosher, 2014). Peaceful protesters against such forcible sterilisations were shot at by police. In just one year, 6.2 million men were sterilised, a number fifteen times higher than those sterilised by the Nazis (Biswas, 2014). For a graphic description of the forcible sterilisation of Muslim men from a village in Haryana, see Shah Commission (1978).

4 For a chronology of events, see Multinational Monitor (1985).

5 The autonomous women's groups in India are non-party affiliated, non-funded, women's organisations that emerged in the post-Emergency period.

6 This trial was part of a multi-national, multi-centre study, carried out by ICMR under the aegis of the WHO.

7 Letter dated 18 October 1985, signed by Dr Suzie Tharu, Convenor, *Stree Shakti Sangatana*, Hyderabad, Andhra Pradesh.

8 This was when I became involved with the case. Being Delhi-based at that time, I was requested to help with the filing of the petition, and it was decided to involve *Saheli*, an autonomous women's group in Delhi, with whom I was volunteering.

9 Public Interest litigation is a rule of law devised by the Supreme Court of India following the Emergency period to reach out to people to address their grievances.

10 Writ Petition (Civil) No. 680 of 1986: *Stree Shakti Sangatana*, and 8 others vs. Union of India and Others. Respondents were Union of India, The Drugs Controller, the ICMR, Ministry of Health and Family Welfare, and the state of Andhra Pradesh. The drug company German Remedies (the Indian subsidiary) was not added as a respondent because the PIL is a grievance against the state. Though the Indian trials were part of the WHO multicentric trials, the WHO could not be made a party because of its immunity as an International Organisation. The technical case had to be built from scratch as nothing much was known about NET-EN since the campaign by women's group in the west had focused on Depo-Provera. The research was carried out primarily by Sathyamala and Nalini Bhanot, on behalf of *Saheli*. Members of *Stree Shakti Sangatna* and the Medico Friend Circle contributed to the formulation of the technical arguments.

11 For a detailed discussion on the Supreme Court case see Sathyamala (1998).

12 This was because the PIL against NET-EN did not cover Depo-Provera and, therefore, Depo was treated as a 'new' drug by the Drugs Controller of India.
13 The NET-EN case became a legal prototype for opposing other similar tendencies in the country; for instance, the PIL against quinacrine sterilisation (Viswanathan and Rao, 1997).
14 In the late 1950s Thalidomide was prescribed as a sedative and for morning sickness in pregnancy. In 1961, it was withdrawn as it caused serious birth defects such as shortened, absent, or flipper-like limbs in children born to mothers who took the drug when pregnant.
15 Recall of Dalkon Shield, an intrauterine contraceptive device, by A. J. Robins Company in the 1980s is a case in point. More than 300,000 lawsuits were filed against the company. In 1985 the company filed for bankruptcy. The payout has been estimated to be as large as US$2.4 billion.
16 Later on, the health facility discontinued distribution as some women acceptors including Hari John developed benign breast nodules (P. C. John, 13 March 2019, personal communication).
17 I was a member of the fact-finding team on behalf of *Saheli*.
18 However, even this is debatable at a population level. As far back as the 1980s, it was shown that in India, pregnancy-related causes formed only a small proportion among the causes of death in the reproductive age group; major causes of death in women in this age group were infectious diseases, and 'accidents' (Sathyamala et al., 1986).
19 These arguments would apply to other hazardous contraceptives such as the sub-dermal implants and anti-fertility vaccines as well.

References

Agamben, G. (1995). *Homo Sacer: Sovereign Power and Bare Life*, trans. Daniel Heller-Roazen. Palo Alto, CA: Stanford University Press.
Agamben, G. (2005). *State of Exception*, trans. Kevin Attell. Chicago: University of Chicago Press.
Bernal, V. and Grewal, I. (2014). Introduction: the NGO form: feminist struggles, states and neoliberalism. In V. Bernal and I. Grewal (eds), *Theorizing NGOs: States, Feminisms, and Neoliberalism*, 1–18. Durham, NC: Duke University Press.
Biswas, S. (2014). India's dark history of sterilisation. *BBC News*. www.bbc.com/news/world-asia-india-30040790. Accessed 1 July 2018.

152   *Injectable contraceptives and technologies of power*

Dey, S. (2015). Government to allow injectable contraceptive for women? *Times of India*. https://timesofindia.indiatimes.com/home/science/Government-to-allow-injectable-contraceptive-for-women/articleshow/48979064.cms. Accessed 4 February 2019.

e-FP (2012). Injectable contraception in India: what does the future hold? India e-FP Synthesis Brief #2.

Ezer, T., Mckenna, R. and Schaaf, M. (2015). Accountability and legal empowerment: allied approaches in the struggle for health rights. Working Paper, Open Society Foundation.

Foucault, M. (1978). *The History of Sexuality, Volume I: An Introduction*, trans. Robert Hurley. New York: Pantheon Books.

Foucault, M. (2003). *Society Must be Defended: Lectures at the College De France 1975–76*, ed. M. Bertani and A. Fontana. New York: Picador.

Government of India (1962). *Report of the Health Survey and Planning Committee August 1959–October 1961*. Volume I. www.nhp.gov.in/sites/default/files/pdf/Mudalier_Vol.pdf. Accessed 15 November 2021.

Hartman, B. and Rao, M. (2015). India's population programme: obstacles and opportunities, *Economic & Political Weekly* 50:44, 10–13.

Hofmeyr, G. J., Morrison, C. S., Baeten, J. M., Chipato, T., Donnell, D., Gichangi, P., Mugo, N., Nanda, K. Ree, H., Steyn, P., and Taylor, D. (2018). Rationale and design of a multi-center, open-label, randomized clinical trial comparing HIV incidence and contraceptive benefits in women using three commonly-used contraceptive methods (the ECHO study). *Gates Open Research* 1, 17.

India and Family Planning: an overview (n.d.) www.searo.who.int/entity/maternal_reproductive_health/documents/india-fp.pdf?ua=1. Accessed 20 July 2018.

Jan Swasthya Abhiyan et al. (2015). A Statement Protesting Approval to Introduce Injectable Contraceptives in the National Family Planning Programme. 23 September. www.facebook.com/permalink.php?story_fbid=528260140662635&id=456131594542157&__tn__=-R. Accessed 24 May 2021.

John, H. and Hadley, J. (1982). Depo-Provera, control of fertility – two feminist views, *Spare Rib* 116, 49–53.

Karat, B., Sundararaman, S., and Sarojini, N. B. (2005). *Letter to Shri S. P. Hota, Secretary, Ministry of Health and Family Welfare, New Delhi*. Dated 26 April.

Kuumba, B. M. (2001). *Gender and Social Movements*. New York: Alta Mira Press.

Medico Friend Circle Bulletin (1992). *The Debate: Report of the Meeting Held on the 6th and 7th of December 1991 by the Indian Council of*

Medical Research, at the ICMR headquarters, New Delhi for what they termed 'Health Advocates' 180–1, pp. 5–8.

Ministry of Health and Family Welfare (n.d.). *National Family Planning Programme*. https://humdo.nhp.gov.in/about/national-fp-programme/. Accessed 24 May 2021.

Morse, A. and Mosher, S. (2014). *A Once and Future Tragedy: India's Sterilization Campaign 39 Years Later*. Population Research Institute. www.pop.org/a-once-and-future-tragedy-indias-sterilization-campaign-39-years-later/. Accessed 7 May 2017.

Multinational Monitor (1985). The case against Depo-Provera. 6 (2 and 3). www.multinationalmonitor.org/hyper/issues/1985/02/problems-us.html. Accessed 13 July 2018.

National Health Mission (n.d.). About Accredited Social Health Activist (ASHA). http://nhm.gov.in/communitisation/asha/about-asha.html. Accessed 22 July 2018.

Panda, A. K. (2016). *'Mission Parivar Vikas' for improved access to contraceptives and family planning services in 145 High Fertility Districts in 7 states*. D.O. No. N. 11023/2/2016-FP; 10 November. Additional Secretary, Ministry of Health and Family Welfare, Government of India.

Pande, A. (2016). Global reproductive inequalities, neo-eugenics and commercial surrogacy in India, *Current Sociology Monograph* 64:2, 244–58.

Rabinow, P. and Rose, N. (2006). Biopower today, *Biosocieties* 1:2, 195–217.

Rao, M. (2004). *From Population Control to Reproductive Health: Malthusian Arithmetic*. New Delhi: Sage Publications India.

Roy, S. (2015). The Indian women's movement: within and beyond NGOization, *Journal of South Asian Development* 10:1, 96–117.

Saheli (2001). *NET-EN: Another Chapter in the Saga of Injectable Contraceptives*. https://sites.google.com/site/saheliorgsite/health/hazardous-hormonal-contraceptives/net-en. Accessed 15 August 2018.

Saheli (n.d.). *Report of a Historic Event: NET-EN Case Comes to a Close on 24 August 2000*. https://sites.google.com/site/saheliorgsite/health/hazardous-hormonal-contraceptives/report-of-a-historic-event. Accessed 11 May 2017.

Saheli, Sabla Sangh, Action India, Disha, Women's Centre, FAOW, and Awaz-e-Niswan (1991). *Development For Whom? A Critique of Women's Development Programme*. New Delhi: Saheli.

Sarojini, N. B., Chakraborty, S., Venkatachalam, D., Bhattacharya, S., Kapilashrami, A., and De, R. (2006). *Women's Right to Health*. New Delhi: National Human Rights Commission.

Sathyamala, C. (1998). Hazardous contraceptives and the right to life, *Journal of the Indian Law Institute* 40:1–4, 174–99.

Sathyamala, C. (2000). *An Epidemiological Review of the Injectable Contraceptive, Depo-Provera.* Pune: Medico Friend Circle; Mumbai: Forum for Women's Health, pp 164. Reprint 2001.

Sathyamala, C. (2005). Women's health movement in independent India. In A. K. Bagchi and K. Soman (eds), *Maladies, Preventives and Curatives – Debates in Public Health in India*, 96–108. New Delhi: Tulika Books.

Sathyamala, C. (2019a). In the Name of Science: Ethical Violations in the ECHO Randomised Trial. *Global Public Health.* https://doi.org/10.1080/174 41692.2019.163 4118.

Sathyamala, C. (2019b). Depot contraception and HIV: an exercise in obfuscation, *British Medical Journal* 367:l5768. www.bmj.com/content/367/bmj.l5768. Accessed 15 November 2021.

Sathyamala, C. (2020). Depo-Provera and HIV transmission: Who to trust? *Differentakes* 95.

Sathyamala, C. and D'Mello, B. (2003). *Depo-Provera Contraceptive in India: Towards a Guiding Light in 'The Great (International) Debate'.* Paper presented at the 10th Annual International conference 'Ethics: The Guiding Light', sponsored by the Vincentian Universities, 22–24 October, New York.

Sathyamala, C., Sundharam, N. and Bhanot, N. (1986). *Taking Sides: The Choices Before the Health Worker.* Madras: Anitra Trust.

Sawhny, A. (1995). Women's empowerment and health experiences in a state sponsored programme. *Medico Friend Circle Bulletin*, 221–2, pp. 1–6 and 9.

Shah Commission (1978). *Shah Commission of Inquiry: Third and Final Report.* 6 August. New Delhi: Government of India. https://ia600401.us.archive.org/3/items/ShahCommissionOfInquiry3rdFinalReport/Shah%20Commission%20of%20Inquiry%203rd-Final-Report.pdf. Accessed 12 July 2018.

Sinha, A. (2007). Whither autonomous women's movement, *Counter Currents.* www.countercurrents.org/anjali130407.htm. Accessed 7 May 2017.

Times of India (2018). 50% Antara contraceptive users drop out after first dose. 12 July. https://timesofindia.indiatimes.com/city/jaipur/50-antara-contraceptive-users-drop-out-after-1st-dose/articleshow/64953103.cms. Accessed 1 February 2019.

Viswanathan, N. and Rao, M. (1997). Women at risk: quinacrine sterilization, a practice that defies accepted international norms, continues in India,

Frontline 14:19. www.frontline.in/static/html/fl1419/14190940.htm. Accessed 16 July 2018.

World Health Organization (2019). Contraceptive Eligibility for Women at High Risk of HIV. www.who.int/reproductivehealth/publications/contraceptive-eligibility-women-at-high-risk-of-HIV/en/. Accessed 15 November 2021.

7

Stratified and violent: young women's experiences of access to reproductive health in southern Africa

Kezia Batisai

Introduction: policies governing gender, sexuality and reproductive health

This chapter analyses young women's reproductive health issues in the context of limited (to no) access to contraception and termination of pregnancy, and limited (if any) comprehensive sexuality education in southern Africa. The chapter frames the cumulative effects of not having access to these intersecting services as core to our understanding of the 'what, why, where, how and when questions' of young women's reproductive health in different countries in the region. Thus, young women's reproductive health experiences in southern Africa cannot be understood independent of the international policies and discourses that govern access to contraceptives and termination of pregnancy services in the region. The chapter draws insight from the reproductive and sexual rights discourses that emerged in the policy sphere subsequent to the Cairo Programme of Action, 1994, and the Beijing Platform of Action, 1995 – platforms where diverse aspects of women's sexuality took centre stage (Gruskin, 2000). The policy discourses in the Cairo Programme of Action and the Beijing document lay the foundation on which scholars dedicated to the politics of gender and sexuality entrench their theorisations (Tamale, 2008). These discourses are in discussion with feminist interests in reforming the shape of the state to achieve gender equality. For instance, feminist chapters on reproductive health and sexual rights that were published post Cairo and Beijing seek to provide 'missing theoretical and practical sparks to ignite the commitment required from both the state and non-state actors to implement them' (Tamale, 2011: 3), to ensure that ideas about the sexual body are integrated into policy.

The extent to which countries in southern Africa and the continent at large commit to ensuring access to reproductive health against a backdrop of numerous international and regional policy documents they have ratified has been the subject of analysis (Amnesty International, 2017). South Africa and Zimbabwe, for instance, ratified the Convention on the Elimination of All forms of Discrimination Against Women (CEDAW), the African Charter on Human and Peoples' Rights, and the Maputo Protocol to the African Charter on Human and Peoples' Rights on the Rights of Women in Africa (Maputo Protocol). Although the principles governing these committees are deeply enshrined in the need to advance and promote human rights discourse (Amnesty International, 2017), literature on policy, including reproductive health and sexual rights policies, points at implementation challenges in southern Africa.

Empirical evidence from Lesotho and Zimbabwe reveals the challenges of a universalistic approach to and application of international or regional treaties and policies (Batisai, 2014, 2015a, 2015b; Batisai et al., 2010; International Organisation for Migration, 2009). Lesotho and Zimbabwe do not merely inherit and make these treaties and policies part of their national policy structures. Instead, the two countries, through their constitutions, call for the domestication of international policies before applying or integrating any guidelines and frameworks at national level. Domestication means that the government has the liberty to adapt the international policies and treaties to ensure that they align with the laws of the land, especially when they contradict customary law. A dualistic approach to international instruments means that whenever a country fails to domesticate such treaties, they 'only play a persuasive role in the legal system' (Batisai et al., 2010: 14). Policy documents such as the 1994 Cairo Programme of Action emerge as 'soft law', which is not binding on governments but rather serves as a tool for lobbying and advocating women's reproductive rights and health (Nair et al., 2004), and 'a tool that strives to hold governments accountable under international human rights law' (Amnesty International, 2017: 7).

This chapter argues that southern African countries domesticate international policies that govern reproductive health in a way that perpetuates reproductive violence, defined here as the institutional or structural, physical and emotional violence that women suffer in their effort to access termination of pregnancy services. The liberty to domesticate international policies and treaties, in the context of reproductive violence and injustice, somewhat explains why countries in sub-Saharan Africa – a region which includes southern Africa – are among those that have been reported by Loi et al. (2015) as having restrictive termination of pregnancy laws. The observation above does not in any way undermine the positive efforts by African countries (excluding Botswana) that have ratified the protocol, which at least authorises women in Africa to terminate pregnancy in cases of maternal health and pregnancy that is a result of any sexual intercourse considered unlawful, including rape and incest (Chiweshe et al., 2017; Johnson et al., 2002; Sekele, 2014). These include: Zimbabwe's Termination of Pregnancy Act No. 29 (1977); Zambia's Termination of Pregnancy Act No. 13 (1994); and the Abortion and Sterilisation Act of South Africa (1975), which Namibia inherited in March 1990 after it became independent from South Africa.

Furthermore, the chapter is particularly alert to the progressive Constitution of the Republic of South Africa (1996) which gives women the right to safe and legal termination of pregnancy guided by the timeline for pregnancy and conditions for termination stipulated in the Choice on Termination of Pregnancy Act (CTOPA) No. 92 (1996). The CTOPA, which has been credited for advancing women's health and their rights, specifies that women and girls have the right to request termination up until the twelfth week and with certain conditions before the twentieth week of pregnancy (Amnesty International, 2017: 3). In addition, South Africa's commitments to human rights 'place clear obligations on the government to safeguard women and girls' access to safe abortion care' (Amnesty International, 2017: 4). Despite the legal status, literature points at the alarming rate of illegal termination of pregnancy and the high rates of maternal deaths in South Africa (Amnesty International 2017; Saving Mothers 2011–2013) dating back to the late 1990s (Guttmacher et al., 1998). The deaths resonate with evidence from Zimbabwe where 'high maternal mortality rate of 280 per 100,000 live births in the country' at the turn of the twenty-first century was attributed to illegal termination practices (World Bank, 2000: 243). Parallels can be drawn from Argentina in South America where various circumstances force young women and girls to suffer unnecessarily because of their reproductive capacity, yet pregnancy is not even a debilitating condi-tion (Human Rights Watch, 2010).

The realities above expose the reproductive violence inherent in the barriers and implementation challenges stemming largely from unequal access and lack of access (Bennett, 2011; Harries et al., 2015; World Health Organization, 2012). Limited access to termination of pregnancy is indeed stratified and violent because the lives of young women in southern Africa, like South America, are put at risk by prevailing structural circumstances that perpetuate reproductive violence and injustice. Considering the policy gaps above, this chapter draws on the work of Rosalind Pollack Petchesky (2003) who, through an intersectional lens, questions the extent to which a woman could enjoy reproductive health and sexual rights when she occupies spaces in which ideological and material realities are gendered (Nair et al., 2004). Underlying Petchesky's analysis is a centuries-long interplay between sexuality and the political economy which frames 'sexual life as a contested territory where meaning and power intersect as part of on-going social and political processes' (Parker, 2010: 59). Hence the need to consider the various socio-political dynamics that influence the national policy priorities that have a huge bearing on reproductive health. Overall, the chapter analyses the various intersecting contextual socio-legal, cultural, political and economic structures that young women navigate and negotiate in their effort to either access reproductive health services or assign meaning/s to the realities of being a woman within specific countries in southern Africa. These structural factors include, but are not limited to: the healthcare systems; financial and human resources allocation; and the socio-cultural belief systems that limit and stigmatise access to reproductive health. These often translate into the broad racial-ised, classed, age-based and gendered dynamics that either limit or facilitate access to sexual and reproductive healthcare in these countries.

Emerging out of the structural forces above is the first section of this chapter, which explores the interplay between healthcare and body politics in southern Africa to provide the broader context in which young women experience the stratified and violent reproductive injustice. Thereafter, the chapter unpacks the theoretical and meth-odological choices that informed the empirical engagements with young women's experiences of reproductive violence in Hillbrow. The subsequent section presents and analyses young women's empirical voices, which articulate the politics of the reproductive body. The politics section paves the way for the conclusion of the chapter, which reflects on the violence the gendered body suffers, and critically discusses how to redress institutionalised reproductive injustice in southern Africa.

Contextual realities: the intersection of healthcare and body politics in southern Africa

Towards the end of the twentieth century, Pretorius (1991: 12) broadly framed 'the African medical care blanket [as] too small to cover the health care needs of all its inhabitants'. Pretorius' (1991) observation supports preceding and subsequent scholars who point out that healthcare systems in many African countries have historically failed to meet demands of the public irrespective of the attempts at reforming these structures (Chiwire, 2016; Good et al., 1979; Kautzky and Tollman, 2008). Some of the key obstacles that continue to hinder the provision of healthcare in southern Africa include: HIV and AIDS; tuberculosis; malaria; poverty; malnutrition; shortages of health workers and medical equipment; unequal distribution of resources; mismanagement of healthcare funds; bureaucracy; corruption; poor political, public sector and medical/health leadership; and a complex and lengthy health transition (Kautzky and Tollman 2008; Rispel, 2016).

   Although there is reference to inequalities in the list above, the question of social stratification and access to healthcare in southern Africa needs further interrogation. Inequalities in the South African context, where the wide gap between the rich and the poor is attributed to the high unemployment rate (Chiwire, 2016), have produced a healthcare system that is stratified along class, gender and racial lines (Cockerham, 2013; Shisana et al., 2012). As the rich of South Africa exclusively access private healthcare, the poor, who often bear the brunt of mass unemployment estimated at 26.7% by the end of June 2016 (Statistics South Africa, 2016), not only rely on a failing healthcare system, but resort to parallel or alternative systems (Batisai, 2020; Trueman and Magwentshu, 2013). This reality is not peculiar to South Africa. Rather, it characterises the health and therapy-seeking behaviour of many poor Black Africans in Botswana, Lesotho, Zambia and Zimbabwe among other countries in the region (Batisai, 2016a, 2020; Bene and Darkoh, 2014; O'Brien and Broom, 2014; Shewamene et al., 2017). The same has been observed in countries from other regions on the continent (Gyasi et al., 2016; Mahomoodally, 2013; Umar et al., 2011; World Health Organization, 2013) as well as other developing contexts in the world such as India (Das et al., 2018).

Gendered stratification, over and above classed and racialised inequalities, produces hierarchised differences that are central to the marked disparities toward health services (Batisai 2016a; Courtenay, 2000). These disparities become more pronounced when one analyses the realities of access to reproductive health in southern Africa. In addition to the challenge of limited access to general healthcare, women have reproductive health issues which stem from several intersecting realities. As wives, women are exposed to the risk of HIV infection because of the longstanding gendered traditional beliefs and cultural values which make it difficult for them to negotiate safe sex (Jaiantilal et al., 2015). Their role as traditional caregivers of the sick, which intensified in the context of HIV/AIDS, and the subsequent home-based care programme aimed at reducing the pressure on healthcare facilities, puts them at further risk of infection (Jackson, 2002; Siliwa, 2007).

Empirical evidence from South Africa, Zimbabwe, Lesotho and other countries from east, west and north Africa also shows that about 80% of African women utilise herbs during pregnancy and for general reproductive health (Gudhlanga and Makaudze, 2012; Shewamene et al., 2017). Though the reasons vary from context to context, women often utilise herbs in settings where men make decisions about the 'what, why, where, how, and when' women may seek healthcare, and in settings where women have faith in the knowledge and intervention of traditional birth attendants compared to that of midwives in hospitals and clinics or where access to biomedical maternity care is limited or non-existent (Shewamene et al., 2017). The reality of limited access to biomedical reproductive care or its non-existence, due to either poor service delivery or prohibitive legal frameworks, adds an age-based layer to the classed, racialised and gendered stratification hierarchy.

The hierarchy alluded to above is evidenced by how adolescent and young low-income Black African women in Botswana and Zimbabwe, countries with legal frameworks that prohibit termination of pregnancy, risk their lives and resort to illegal reproductive health services (Batisai, 2013, 2014, 2015a; Raphuti, 2014; Seleke, 2014). The way young low-income migrant and South African women are lured by illegal adverts to explore an avenue that puts them at risk of either maternal death or longstanding reproductive health complications (Amnesty International, 2017; Trueman and Magwentshu, 2013) – in a country that is celebrated for its progressive constitutional position on pregnancy termination (Mutua, 2011) – opens space for conceptual and empirical interrogations. The chapter argues that illegal pregnancy termination illuminates the realities of reproductive violence that stem from the limited and inaccessible service in South Africa's public healthcare system (Bennett 2011; Harries et al., 2015). It further exposes what Moyo (2021) refers to as transnational care which, in this context, is evident in the huge influx of regional migrants to South Africa in search of reproductive justice. Hence the inference that access to reproductive healthcare in southern Africa is not only stratified along class, race gender and age lines but is violent too.

This chapter, against the backdrop of limited (if any) access to reproductive health, high risk of maternal death (Amnesty International, 2017), and very little research that documents the experiences of women who are denied access to legal abortion services (Harries et al., 2015), seeks to capture and analyse the reproductive violence that young and low-income Black women in southern Africa constantly grapple with. The chapter complements the notion of 'obstetric violence', defined by Chadwick in Chapter 5 of this volume as violation that potentially occurs during labour or birth. This is achieved through an analysis of the reproductive violence that takes the form of institutional or structural, physical and emotional violence that women suffer in their effort to access termination of pregnancy services. This echoes Rucell (2017), who singles out direct physical violence as one of the forms of obstetric violence that manifest within gendered reproductive healthcare services. Overall, this section is not a mere overview of reproductive violence in southern African contexts but, rather, it is a way into critical analyses of the struggles and injustice that young migrant women escape in their home countries and ironically continue to suffer in South Africa despite the progressive constitution.

Theoretical and methodological choices

This chapter builds on theoretical and political standpoints that often emerge as feminist scholars interrogate and engage with the body. Fairly recent feminist efforts include a focus on questions of gender, bodies and justice located in the contemporary medico-legal terrain. The terrain is framed by the scholars as key to producing reproductive injustice because women's bodies are entangled in the interaction between law and medicine in very complex ways (Steele et al., 2016). Scholars in southern Africa have engaged with these theorisations by exploring the power dynamics inherent in women's narratives of their reproductive decision (Chiweshe et al., 2017) and the relationship that exists between the state and its citizens (Batisai, 2013, 2014, 2015a, 2015b; Trueman and Magwentshu, 2013). The chapter works with the theorisation that when juxtaposed with the reality of a failing hierarchised healthcare system, young women's experiences of averting birth tell an interesting narrative about reproductive violence and stratified access to reproductive health in the region. The experiences emerged as young migrant women, who escaped from reproductive injustice in their home countries responded to questions about access to termination of pregnancy services in southern Africa. The empirical gaze was on South Africa because of its liberal legal framework governing termination of pregnancy (Trueman and Magwentshu, 2013), yet women in the same context resort to illegal means, which violates the right to reproductive and general healthcare deeply enshrined in Section 27(1) of the Constitution (1996). The illegal termination of pregnancy adverts pasted on almost every wall, freeway bridge and street light pole across the City of Johannesburg speak volumes about the tensions between the progressive legal framework and the realities of reproductive violence.

Similar to organisations such as Amnesty International (2017) and scholars who are alert and sensitive to questions about, and the realities of body politics, I immediately read the adverts or posters as theoretical and methodological avenues for accessing women's narratives of reproductive health in South Africa. The posters for me raised questions such as: 'why is backyard termination of pregnancy widely advertised when safe and legal services are offered by healthcare centres in the country? Is this because the backyard service providers are capitalising on the legal status of pregnancy termination or is this an insight into the realities of limited and inaccessible services in South Africa's public healthcare centres? Or are they exposing the influx of migrants to South Africa from countries in the region in search of reproductive health among other services? The questions opened space for conceptual and empirical interrogations of the institutionalised/structural, physical and emotional injustice that undermines access to termination of pregnancy services by young low-income migrant and South African women.

Research methods: exploring 'the field'

The unanswered questions above provoked me to explore reproductive health realities with a particular focus on the termination of pregnancy in Hillbrow, a high-density suburb located one kilometre from the central business district in Johannesburg, South Africa. Guided by snowball sampling, which allowed initial participants to refer me to more people, I negotiated access to Hillbrow and young women through fellow Zimbabwean women who were part of my previous study on shifting gender and sexual realities in South Africa (Batisai, 2016b). It was through these Zimbabwean women that I first got insight into the realities of termination of pregnancy in Hillbrow and eventually negotiated access to more young women residing in the suburb. Upon receiving ethical clearance from the university, I conducted qualitative in-depth interviews between January and May 2017 with twelve[1] young women, mainly from Botswana, South Africa and Zimbabwe. Despite the sensitive nature of the topic, I managed to establish a rapport with the young women who were eager to share their experiences to ensure that their narratives expose the reproductive violence that women suffer in the region. I conducted the interviews confidentially at the young women's places of residence, without other people present. Thereafter, I anonymised all interview transcripts and stored them in a password-protected laptop. The stories of the young women are profiled and analysed in this chapter under the shield of randomly selected pseudonyms[2] to avoid violating the principles of anonymity that require researchers to conform to the ethical standards of privacy and confidentiality.

Although the United Nations (2001) defines the category of 'youth' as those aged 15–24, who are still transitioning to adulthood, focus during data collection was on women who were 20 years and above who could consent to participate in the study independent of their guardians. This methodological choice does not disregard the reproductive health challenges that those aged 15–19 battle with (Chareka et al., 2021), given that girls constituting this category account for 25% of all unsafe pregnancy terminations in sub-Saharan Africa (Sawyer et al., 2012). Over and above their relatively young age, the selected women were either South African citizens from less privileged backgrounds with limited access to opportunities and resources, or migrants from Botswana, Lesotho, Namibia and Zimbabwe – countries where termination of pregnancy is restricted (Batisai, 2015a; Chareka et al., 2021; Harries, 2015; Raphuti, 2014; Seleke, 2014).

The contextual binaries, along with the age, class, race and gender-based divides, also used by Chareka et al. (2021), produced situated and intersecting meanings and experiences of reproductive violence stemming from the interplay between structural factors and these identifying categories. To complement the empirical findings presented below, the chapter uses secondary data responses to the thought-provoking questions about the 'what, how and when' of young women's reproductive health in different countries in the region. The chapter carefully draws on literature that has profiled the complex realities and dynamics of access to reproductive health in southern Africa (Amnesty International, 2017; Appasamy, 2016; Chareka et al., 2021; Chiweshe et al., 2017; Harries et al., 2015; Loi et al., 2015; Trueman and Magwentshu, 2013).

Empirical findings: politics of the reproductive body – young women's experiences

To adequately explore notions of reproductive violence and stratified access to reproductive health in the region, this section focuses on young women's lived experiences. The interview narratives reveal the reproductive violence that young women grapple with in their attempt to access and enjoy their reproductive health rights, including the right to contraception, and legal and safe state-sponsored termination of pregnancy services in public healthcare centres in South Africa. For instance, the reproductive violence or injustice is articulated by young women who, in their previous attempts to access legal termination services, had to move from pillar to post due to the complexity of the process, especially in cases where women needed surgical abortion. Such experience confirms the observation that South Africa's primary care service is not only over-bureaucratised but rigid as well (Kautzky and Tollman, 2008). The young women also raise the challenge of a long queueing system at public healthcare centres. Aya, a 25-year-old woman, relays: 'The service at these public healthcare centres is poor, I tell you. If you are pregnant, you can even give birth I promise you; and if you are seriously ill, you can even die before a practitioner attends to your needs. The idea of queueing the whole day for a service is very problematic.'

The combination of poor service delivery in the form of queuing, and the ultimate lack of access to the service, emerge as tools for institutionalised reproductive injustice that perpetuates the reproductive violence that women suffer in southern Africa. It is against this backdrop that Dean (2016) finds unattended queues at public healthcare facilities very challenging in a context where someone needs medical attention. Generally, the young women end up not accessing the service at the public facilities, as observed in a Cape Town study where 45% of the women were turned away for various reasons ranging from advanced gestational age, no clinic staff available to perform the procedure on that specific day, and lack of funds to pay for the procedure (Gerdts et al., 2015; Harries et al., 2015). Young women who do not have enough resources consider locally available illegal and unsafe pregnancy termination services a better option than travelling to and from respective healthcare centres with no guarantee of being served. Sithembile, a 24-year-old woman, for that reason uses the shortcomings of the healthcare system to justify illegal backyard procedures:

> I would rather visit a local illegal service provider than waste limited resources going to these government healthcare centres. There is poor service delivery for the poor ... yes ... you do not see a rich black or

white person at these centres ... they are only meant for us. I do not see the difference between my 'practitioners' here in Hillbrow and those in government healthcare centres ... besides that one is categorised as illegal and the other is legal. Their services are all poor ... hence I take the risk and go the illegal route knowing that I will surely get the procedure done ... cheap and quickly.

Young women, from this standpoint, infer that the illegal backyard pregnancy termination service is not only an indication of how the poor resort to parallel medical systems but a reflection of the way in which a failing public healthcare system institutionalises reproductive violence. Indeed, the narrative [captured below] that 'when you are poor, your options are very limited' speaks volumes about the structural reproductive healthcare realities the poor in South Africa confront daily. The narrative also illuminates the realities of transnational care, which in this context is a direct manifestation of the effects of the restrictive laws experienced in Namibia, Botswana and Zimbabwe that force women to travel beyond their national borders (Batisai, 2014; Harries et al., 2015; Seleke, 2014; Smith, 2012) in search of reproductive justice. Thus, distress, frustration and emotional violence with the healthcare system is even worse for those who travel several kilometres from Namibia, for instance, to access the service in South Africa (Harries et al., 2015). Anele, a 26-year-old woman, reiterates the stratified effect of class on access to reproductive health:

The rich do not go through what we go through I tell you ... they have the luxury to know that they are pregnant very early ... they have access to disposable income to go private whenever the need arises. For some of us, poor women, we have to rely on the public service, and this is what I do not like at all such that I simply opt for the illegal route ... very risky business ... dicing with death ... I tell you. What can you do? When you are poor, your options are very limited.

The narrative above also concurs with findings from Cape Town where women knowingly resorted to illegal providers of pregnancy termination services because of previous disappointment with the public sector facilities (Harries et al., 2015). Hence the need to improve public sector service delivery in the best interest of 83% of the South African population that relies on the public healthcare system (National Health Care Facilities Baseline Audit National Summary Report, 2013). The reliance happens in the absence of money for transport costs to and from healthcare centres (Kautzky and Tollman, 2008), as observed in Botswana and Zimbabwe (Bene and Darkoh, 2014; O'Brien and Broom, 2014), let alone costs for private termination (Chareka et al., 2021; Harries et al., 2015).

The intersection of gender and class illuminates the reproductive violence that stems from the mismatch between the legal right to termination of pregnancy and the lived experiences of young low-income women. Contrary to women in previous studies, who were aware of the legal status of termination of pregnancy in South Africa (Harries et al., 2015), the young women argue that their socio-economic class locates them in Hillbrow, where access to information about such rights, let alone services, borders between being limited and completely absent. Their narratives of reproductive violence that takes the form of lack of information validate the observation that gaps in the knowledge of one's legal sexual and reproductive rights and risks, particularly those relating to the how and where of accessing legal and safe pregnancy termination services, is one of the key barriers to progress or justice in the field of sexual and reproductive health (Amnesty International, 2017; National Department of Social Development, South Africa, 2015). Why? Because women, in the absence of information, make ill-informed decisions (Waldman and Stevens, 2015). Zinzi, a 27-year-old woman, mentions the absence of information in geographical spaces like Hillbrow: 'I have stayed in Hillbrow for all my adult life, and I have no idea where to get information about these rights. I am actually hearing it from you that there are such rights and services in this country. No one tells you about these things.'

It is clearly discernible from Zinzi's narrative that the habitus determines the social and economic capital(s) that one can access to deconstruct the stratified healthcare realities and escape the reproductive violence inherent in these structures. Two other participants, both 28-year-old women, have experiences that suggest access to reproductive health knowledge is not only power but life: 'When I got pregnant in 2010, I was referred to a backyard facility in Hillbrow by a colleague and the procedure was quick ... but very painful ... it was hell ... I bled severely ... it was bad ... let me spare you the details ... and just say, I almost died'. The emotional and physical reproductive violence deconstructs the widely advertised 'cheap, quick and pain free' termination process.

Likewise, Thuli relates the emotional and physical reproductive violence she suffered, putting her at risk of maternal death:

> I got pregnant in 2008 and I only became aware of that reality very late ... I desperately wanted to get rid of it because I was not ready for the baby. I consulted this guy in Hillbrow, and he claimed that he was able to assist ... he was keen to do it ... and he terminated the pregnancy ... but the procedure was not successful and none of us knew that. I went home and I bled heavily, and the pain was not going away. After three ... four days, the pain was excruciating ... that was when I decided to seek medical advice and I was referred to a hospital for women and children, West of Johannesburg. I was examined ... it was concluded after a sonar that the termination had failed, and the opening of my uterus had closed. I was admitted immediately, and I was sent to the theatre for a surgical procedure. That is how I survived. To this day, if I think of the pain, I get goose bumps all over my body because of the near-death experience.

The young women's narratives further reveal that reproductive violence or injustice is also experienced in the form of very limited access to contraceptives, which should help them prevent unplanned pregnancies and the subsequent need to terminate. The young women, in the absence of either contraceptive or termination services, end up pregnant and become young mothers who are constantly shamed by not only healthcare workers, but also teachers in the case of teenagers (Appasamy, 2016). These are the same healthcare workers who have been negatively framed in scholarship for denying young women access to reproductive health services in sub-Saharan Africa (Amnesty International, 2017; Harries et al., 2015; Maternowska et al., 2014; Trueman and Magwentshu, 2013) and South-East Asia as well (Loi et al., 2015). The denial is a form of reproductive injustice deeply rooted in the cultural belief system governing termination of pregnancy (Chiweshe et al., 2017), which often frames it 'as killing and inevitably destructive of cultural values and traditions' (Macleod et al., 2011: 237). These cultural sentiments further manifest as unregulated conscientious objection to termination of pregnancy, where healthcare practitioners abuse their right to freedom of conscience often guided by their morals and beliefs (Amnesty International 2017; Harries et al., 2015). Consequently, young women constantly deal with the injustice stemming from the moral discourse and the stigma attached to termination of pregnancy as well as the use of contraceptives by 'young people' even though they are not teenagers anymore. Anna, a 24-year-old woman, says:

> I have tried to get contraceptives from both a Government hospital and clinic, but I was told that I am too young to use contraceptives. The nurses at these centres yelled at me and noted that it is against our culture to indulge in sexual activities at my age, but I am an adult not a teenager. The approach that these nurses adopt is very prohibitive. At the end of the day, I decided not to worry about getting free contraceptives and I told myself that I will either buy whenever I have money, or I will terminate if I conceive.

Anna's narrative takes us to parallel evidence from Zimbabwe where the politics of gender and sexuality among Zimbabwe's youth point at how contested the terrain of reproductive health education is. The law clearly prescribes who should have unrestricted access to reproductive health services. For instance, young people below the age of 16 can only be supplied with family planning legally when 'parental consent is given or [when] they are married' (Mashamba and Robson, 2002: 274–5). The legal waiver draws on the argument that when a minor is sexually active, the risk of sexual infection increases indisputably. However, research findings expose that reproductive justice is denied as some service providers deny sexually active teenagers access to contraceptives (Maternowska et al., 2014) despite the legal waiver (CEDAW/Zimbabwe, 1998). In South Africa, it was reported that 72,000 girls under the age of 18 delivered babies in 2015 alone (Appasamy, 2016). While Appasamy's analysis does not show a correlation between the statistics and lack of access to contraceptives and pregnancy termination services, the chapter is written in the context of lack of support from rude healthcare staff – a trend that has been observed by other scholars (Harries et al., 2015; Ramiyad and Patel, 2016). Strong-minded 21-year-old Welma Mukuba from Soweto, who became a mother in her teens when she was still in grade eleven, describes the healthcare workers as 'the worst for teenage mothers' (Appasamy, 2016) based on how she was violently treated when she first visited the clinic at eight months.

Beyond the legal restrictions, women's access to pregnancy termination services in South Africa, among other countries that have liberalised their legal framework, is often hindered by religious concerns around the ethics of termination (Bennett, 2011). As such, the narratives point at the stigma that characterises both legal and illegal termination of pregnancy. Stigma-related violence in South Africa, where the service is legal, is experienced by South African women who ensure privacy and anonymity by opting to do the procedure in a town kilometres away from the prying eyes of familiar people in their neighbourhood (Harries et al., 2015). This has been observed in Botswana where termination of pregnancy is not only illegal but is literally defined as 'spoiling or destroying the stomach' (Smith, 2013a: 172). Similarly, women of the older generation in Zimbabwe are distressed by the way young women leave the country and go to foreign countries where they 'destroy the tummy, leaving it empty [hysterectomy]' (Batisai, 2013: 162). The intergenerational stigmatisation not only points at the pro-choice and pro-life dynamics which often leave countries polarised, but also hints at a transnational care system which has led, over the years, to women in the region migrating to South Africa in search of reproductive services and justice.

When classed access to termination of services is juxtaposed with the notion of migrancy, an interesting dynamic to transnational care, reproductive violence and stratified access to reproductive health services emerges. While the choice of young low-income women in the context of restrictive laws in Botswana is limited to very risky illegal and sometimes self-administered practices, those who have disposable income travel beyond the national borders to South Africa – whether accessing the service legally or paying medical practitioners to perform it safely outside the confines of the law (Seleke, 2014; Smith, 2012). Likewise, Zimbabwean migrant women in South Africa resist violent structures of gender hierarchy from home by exploring new ways of engaging with their gendered and sexualised bodies through termination of pregnancy (Batisai, 2016a). As Nyasha, a 35-year-old reveals, Zimbabwean women gain control and reclaim power over their bodies by renegotiating and exploring new gender and sexual identities in the diaspora.

In the context of transnational care, the young migrant women acknowledge that they are aware of the legal status of pregnancy termination in South Africa but because of their illegal immigration status, and the subsequent fear of deportation, they hardly bother to access the service legally. As such, illegal backyard services are quite convenient for them as they serve as tools for circumventing the double effects of institutionalised reproductive violence stemming from illegal immigration status and medical xenophobia. This is substantiated by the reality that the backyard service providers come not only from South Africa but from different countries on the continent, predominantly Zimbabwe and Malawi, which helps the young migrant women escape the widely profiled medial xenophobia and its effects on undocumented migrants. Medical xenophobia manifests as unfriendliness of service providers, insensitivity and inferior care, insults, delays and denial of treatment, and non-recognition of foreign identity cards (Pollock et al., 2012; Zihindula et al., 2015). Medical xenophobia on the one hand unravels the subliminal institutionalisation of reproductive violence in the context of transnational care, and at the other end of the continuum illuminates that increased migration aggravates the challenges to the public healthcare system, which is already failing to meet the overwhelming medical demands of a rapidly increasing population (Chiwire, 2016; Yeld, 2013) in ways that violate South Africans' constitutional right to reproductive and general healthcare.

Conclusion: discussing the way forward

The young women's experiences of access to contraception and pregnancy termination have served as a lens through which the chapter revealed how stratified and violent reproductive and general healthcare is in southern Africa. Their narratives have exposed the classed, racialised, age-based and gendered healthcare structures that violate women's access to reproductive health in southern Africa. These narratives indicate the need to pay attention to contextual healthcare specificities if these violent structural realities are to be confronted and addressed. For instance, lack of access to pregnancy termination services in South Africa is perpetuated by the National Department of Health's (2016) estimates that only 264 of the 505 health facilities that are designed to provide this service are doing so in the first and second trimesters (Amnesty International, 2017). The figures validate earlier observations that about half of these facilities offer the services (Trueman and Magwentshu, 2013), and that less than 40% were operational in 2014 (Stevens, n.d.). Limited access to reproductive healthcare in South Africa takes one back to the violence and injustices of the apartheid era where low-income women, who could not afford medical fees, resorted to illegal services offered by less skilled midwives, lay practitioners or non-registered doctors who had not completed their training (Guttmacher et al., 1998).

Similarly, limited access to information and contraceptives that are supposed to reduce the number of unplanned pregnancies and sexual infections locates sexually active young women across southern Africa in an awkward position. The situation is worse in Zimbabwe, where state regulations still resemble the colonial order through which authorities expelled pregnant teenagers from school (Seidman, 1984). To date, pregnant teenagers in Zimbabwe can neither proceed with their studies nor easily access conditional termination of pregnancy. Adolescents' experiences of 'being nationalised' through the legal structure leave the young women themselves, as well as reproductive rights and health activists, questioning the meaning of citizenship for Zimbabwean women. What then is new about these independent southern African countries when the effects of their legal structures resemble those from the colonial and apartheid systems? Hence the need for further legal reform to ensure that the failures of the public healthcare system in South Africa, for example – currently attributed to the colonial legacy and apartheid past (Amnesty International, 2017; Coovadia et al., 2009) – are decolonised and that they speak to contextual healthcare necessities and realities. Further reform will ensure that the healthcare systems provide services, including reproductive care, that are accessible, affordable, effective and efficient (Batisai, 2016a). As such, effort should shift towards 'incorporating innovative health system designs that reorient today's over-bureaucratised and often rigid primary care system' (Kautzky and Tollman, 2008: 17) to make access to reproductive health easy for young women and redress institutionalised and violent reproductive injustice.

Furthermore, those involved in public health initiatives should bear in mind that there is no need to deny sexually active young women and adolescents access to reproductive care because they are at the stage of their life where 'adult health behaviours are set' (Ramiyad and Patel, 2016: 105). Young womanhood and/or adolescence is a foundation that influences the health of future generations because these are the same women who will grow into adulthood with existing and established patterns of reproductive health challenges (Sawyer et al., 2012), which require the attention of all key stakeholders. It is worth reiterating that restricted access to reproductive care often happens in a context of lack of knowledge about (contraception and termination of pregnancy) rights one is entitled to, such that in the absence of these rights, progress (justice) in the field of sexual and reproductive health is hindered (Ramiyad and Patel, 2016; National Department of Social Development, South Africa; 2015). Thus, Harries (2016: 1) leaves us with the thought-provoking observation that questions around 'how women learn about and seek illegal abortions in South Africa' remain unanswered. Assessments of (young) women's knowledge level of their rights and the legislation that specifically focuses on adolescents are few and far between, for example the work of Harries et al. (2015) in Cape Town; Ramiyad and Patel's (2016) in one of Durban's low socio-economic suburbs; and that of Macleod et al. (2014) in the Eastern Cape Province exposing the cracks in reproductive health rights through Buffalo City grade eleven learners' knowledge of the legislation governing termination of pregnancy. Therefore, there is a need not only for more research into the area but to broaden the scope of the research so that young women aged 20 years and above are also included in a comprehensive approach to sexuality education with material that is informative, and includes content and language that is accessible, suitable and specific to their needs (National Department of Social Development, South Africa, 2015). If adopted, the comprehensive approach to sexuality education will partly address the reproductive violence and injustice, particularly the high risk of death, that young women suffer in the context where they lack access to information.

Last, but not least, empirical findings presented in this chapter have revealed that many countries in southern Africa criminalise termination of pregnancy. This happens in a context where society shuns pregnancy out of wedlock and most governments do not have a child support grant system. The body emerges in this space as a site of struggle for women (young or 'old') who get pregnant out of wedlock, for they are expected to be able to deal with the emotional and financial obligations that come with what the family and society deem to be 'unsupportable immoral pregnancy'. To this day, getting pregnant under these prohibitive circumstances means dealing with the emotional strain and rejection from family and society at large because of the shame the pregnancy attracts; over and above not having the liberty to (legally) terminate the pregnancy, and the subsequent lack of financial support from government. As a result, women either resort to backyard services or risk the effects of the criminal tag attached to termination of pregnancy in Zimbabwe, Botswana and Namibia (Batisai, 2015a; Harries, 2015; Raphuti, 2014; Seleke, 2014) and those who carry the pregnancy to full term unsettle the social norms. Hence the need to further confront cultural and religious factors that govern reproductive health issues often leading: to conscientious objection; lack of support; (intergenerational) stigmatisation; and lack of access to contraception and termination of pregnancy services in southern African. The chapter concludes that an engagement with the moral and legal boundaries that emerge as the state patrols the body has deepened our insight into the meaning and scope of reproductive violence and injustice that women in southern African countries often negotiate through their gendered bodies.

Notes

1 Due to commonality in the participants' lived experiences, the chapter works with the narratives of only six young women whose stories speak to all the thematic discussions.
2 Except for Welma Mukuba whose narrative is drawn from an existing source, already in the public domain.

References

Amnesty International (2017). *Briefing: Barriers to Safe and Legal Abortion in South Africa*. www.amnesty.org/en/documents/afr53/5423/2017/en/ Accessed 9 September 2020.
Appasamy, Y. (2016). Teenage moms shamed by healthworkers and teachers. *Sowetan Live*, 11 March 2016. www.sowetanlive.co.za/news/2016-03-11-teenage-moms-shamed-by-healthworkers-and-teachers/. Accessed 16 November 2021.

Batisai, K. (2013). *Body politics: an illumination of the landscape of sexuality and nationhood? Re-seeing Zimbabwe through elderly women's representations of their sexual and gendered lives.* Doctoral Thesis. University of Cape Town.

Batisai, K. (2014). Policies on abortion: women's experiences of living through a gendered body in Zimbabwe. *AboutGender, International Journal of Gender Studies* 3:5, 174–92.

Batisai, K. (2015a). The politics of control and ownership over women's bodies: discourses that shape reproductive and sexual rights in Zimbabwe. *Perspectives: Bodies, Morals and Politics. Reflections on Sexual and Reproductive Rights in Africa* 2, 6–11.

Batisai, K. (2015b). Being gendered in Africa's flag democracies: narratives of sexual minorities living in the diaspora, *Gender Questions* 3:1, 25–44.

Batisai, K. (2016a). Towards an integrated approach to health and medicine in Africa, *SAHARA-J: Journal of Social Aspects of HIV/AIDS* 13:1, 113–22.

Batisai, K. (2016b). 'Transnational labour migration, intimacy and relationships: how Zimbabwean women navigate the diaspora', *Diaspora Studies* 9:2, 165–78.

Batisai, K. (2020). Understanding health and health systems in southern Africa, in J. Fritz and T. Uys (eds), *Clinical Sociology for Southern Africa*, 245–69. Cape Town: Juta Press.

Batisai, K., Tansey, E. and Muteerwa, T. R. (2010). *Country assessment on HIV-prevention needs of migrants and mobile populations: Lesotho.* Pretoria, International Organization for Migration.

Bene, M. and Darkoh, M. B. K. (2014). The constraints of antiretroviral uptake in rural areas: the case of Thamaga and surrounding villages, Botswana. *SAHARA-J: Journal of Social Aspects of HIV/AIDS*, 11(1), 167–77.

Bennett, J. (2011). 'Subversion and resistance: activist initiatives', in S. Tamale (ed.), *African sexualities: A reader*, 77–100. Cape Town: Pambazuka Press.

CEDAW/Zimbabwe. (1998). *Concluding Observations of the Committee on the Elimination of Discrimination against Women.* Geneva: Office of the United Nations High Commissioner for Human Rights.

Chareka, S., Crankshaw, T. L. and Zambezi, P. (2021). Economic and social dimensions influencing safety of induced abortions amongst young women who sell sex in Zimbabwe. *Sexual and Reproductive Health Matters* 29:1, 1881209.

Chiweshe, M., Mavuso, J. and Macleod, C. (2017). Reproductive justice in context: South African and Zimbabwean women's narratives of their abortion decision. *Feminism and Psychology* 27:2, 203–24.

Chiwire, P. (2016). Factors influencing access to health care in South Africa – PEAH – Policies for Equitable Access to Health. A Project by Daniele

Dionisio. www.peah.it/2016/10/factors-influencing-access-to-health-care-in-south-africa/. Accessed 21 May 2018.

Coovadia, H., Jewkes, R., Barron, P., Sanders, D. and McIntyre, D. (2009). The health and health system of South Africa: historical roots of current public health challenges. *The Lancet* 374: 9692, 817–34.

Courtenay, W. H. (2000). Constructions of masculinity and their influence on men's well-being: a theory of gender and health. *Social Science and Medicine* 50, 1385–401.

Das, M., Angeli, F., Krumeich, A. J. S. M. and van Schayck, O. C. P. (2018). The gendered experience with respect to health-seeking behaviour in an urban slum of Kolkata, India. *International Journal for Equity in Health*, 17:1, 1–14.

Dean, T. (2016). No queues, no fuss, bringing healthcare to your door. www.health24.com/News/Public-Health/no-queues-no-fuss-bringing-healthcare-to-your-door-20161024. Accessed 13 May 2017.

Gerdts, C., DePiñeres, T., Hajri, S., Harries, J., Hossain, A., Puri, M., Vohra, D. and Foster, D. G. (2015). Denial of abortion in legal settings. *Journal of Family Planning and Reproductive Health Care* 41:3, 161–3.

Good, C. M., Hunter, J. M., Katz, S. H. and Katz, S. S. (1979). The interface of dual systems of health care in the developing world: toward health policy initiatives in Africa. *Social Science and Medicine. Part D: Medical Geography* 13:3, 141–54.

Gruskin, S. (2000). The conceptual and practical implications of reproductive and sexual rights: how far have we come? *Health and Human Rights* 4:2, 1–6.

Gudhlanga, E. S. and Makaudze, G. (2012). Indigenous knowledge systems: confirming a legacy of civilisation and culture on the African continent. *Prime Journal of Social Science* 1:4, 72–7.

Guttmacher, S., Kapadia, F., Naude J. T. W. and de Pinho, H. (1998). 'Abortion reform in South Africa: a case study of the 1996 Choice on Termination of Pregnancy Act', *International Family Planning Perspectives* 24:4, 191–4.

Gyasi, R. M., Asante, F., Yeboah, J. Y., Abass, K., Mensah, C. M. and Siaw, L. P. (2016). Pulled in or pushed out? Understanding the complexities of motivation for alternative therapies use in Ghana. *International Journal of Qualitative Studies on Health Well-Being* 11:1, p. 29667.

Harries, J., Gerdts, C., Momberg, M. and Foster, D. G. (2015). An exploratory study of what happens to women who are denied abortions in Cape Town, South Africa. *Reproductive Health* 12:1, 1–6.

Human Rights Watch (2010). Illusions of care. Lack of accountability for reproductive rights in Argentina. www.hrw.org/report/2010/08/10/

illusions-care/lack-accountability-reproductive-rights-argentina. Accessed 6 June 2018.

Jackson, H. (2002). *AIDS Africa: Continent in Crisis.* Harare: SAfAIDS.

Jaiantilal, P., Gutin, S. A., Cummings, B., Mbofana, F. and Rose, C. D. (2015). Acceptability, feasibility and challenges of implementing an HIV prevention intervention for people living with HIV/AIDS among healthcare providers in Mozambique: results of a qualitative study. *SAHARA-J: Journal of Social Aspects of HIV/AIDS* 12:1, 2–9.

Johnson, B. R., Ndhlovu, S., Farr, S. L. and Chipato, T. (2002). Reducing unplanned pregnancy and abortion in Zimbabwe through postabortion contraception. *Studies in Family Planning* 33:2, 195–202.

Kautzky, K. and Tollman, S. M. (2008). A perspective on primary health care in South Africa. In P. Barron and J. Roma-Reardon (eds), *South African Health Review*, 17–30. Durban: Health Systems Trust.

Loi, U. R., Gemzell-Danielsson, K., Faxelid, E. and Klingberg-Allvin, M. (2015). Health care providers' perceptions of and attitudes towards induced abortions in sub-Saharan Africa and Southeast Asia: a systematic literature review of qualitative and quantitative data. *BMC Public Health* 15:139.

Maternowska, M. C., Mashu, A., Moyo, P., Withers, M. and Chipato, T. (2014). Perceptions of Misoprostol among providers and women seeking post-abortion care in Zimbabwe. *Reproductive Health Matters* 44, 16–25.

Macleod, C., Seutlwadi, L. and Steel, G. (2014). Cracks in reproductive health rights: Buffalo City learners' knowledge of abortion legislation. *Health SA Gesondheid* 19:1. DOI:10.4102/hsag.v19i1.743.

Macleod, C., Sigcau, N. and Luwana, P. (2011). Culture as a discursive resource opposing legal abortion. *Critical Public Health* 21:2, 237–45.

Mahomoodally, M. F. (2013). Traditional medicines in Africa: an appraisal of ten potent African medicinal plants, *Evidence-Based Complementary and Alternative Medicine* 1–14.

Mashamba, A. and Robson, E. (2002). Youth reproductive health services in Bulawayo, Zimbabwe. *Health & Place* 8, 273–83.

Moyo, S. Z. (2021). Health provision in Tshitshi, Zimbabwe: A focus on sexual and reproductive health. MA Dissertation. University of Cape Town.

Mutua, M. (2011). Sexual orientation and human rights: Putting homophobia on trial. In S. Tamale (ed.), *African Sexualities: A Reader*, 452–62. Cape Town: Pambazuka Press.

Nair, S., Kirbat, P. and Sarah, S. (2004). A decade after Cairo, women's health in a free market economy. *Women's Global Network for Reproductive Rights and The Corner House, Briefing 31*, Lancashire, RAP Spiderweb.

National Department of Health (2016). *Sexual and Reproductive Health and Rights: Fulfilling our Commitments 2011–2021 and Beyond Final Draft.*

National Department of Social Development, South Africa (2015). *National Adolescent Sexual and Reproductive Health and Rights Framework Strategy*. www.dsd.gov.za/index2.php?option=com_docman&task=doc_view&gid=578&Itemid=3. Accessed 21 June 2018.

National Health Care Facilities Baseline Audit National Summary Report (2013). Health Systems Trust. www.hst.org.za/sites/default/files/NHFA_webready_0.pdf. Accessed 28 November 2016.

O'Brien, S. and Broom, A. (2014). HIV in (and out of) the clinic: biomedicine, traditional medicine and spiritual healing in Harare. *SAHARA-J: Journal of Social Aspects of HIV/AIDS* 11:1, 94–104.

Parker, R. (2010). Reinventing sexual scripts: sexuality and social change in the twenty-first century. (The 2008 John H. Gagnon Distinguished Lecture on Sexuality, Modernity and Change). *Sexuality Research and Social Policy* 7:1, 58–66.

Petchesky, R. P. (2003). *Global Prescriptions: Gendering Health and Human Rights*. London: Zed Books.

Pollock, G., Newbold, K. B., Lafrenière, G. and Edge, S. (2012). Discrimination in the doctor's office: immigrants and refugee experiences. *Critical Social Work* 13:2, 60–79.

Pretorius, E. (1991). 'Traditional and modern medicine working in tandem', *Curationis* 14:4, 10–13.

Ramiyad, D. and Patel, C. J. (2016). Exploring South African adolescents' knowledge of abortion legislation and attitudes to abortion: sexual status and gender differences. *South African Journal of Child Health* 10:2, 105–6.

Raphuti, E. (2014). Should Botswana legalise abortion. *Daily News*. www.dailynews.gov.bw/news-details.php?nid=8049. Accessed 15 May 2018.

Rispel, L. (2016). Analysing the progress and fault lines of health care sector reform in South Africa. In A. Padarath, J. King, E. Mackie and J. Casciola (eds), *South African Health Review*, 83–93. Durban: Health Systems Trust.

Rucell, J. (2017). *Obstetric violence and colonial conditioning in South Africa's reproductive health system*. Doctoral Thesis. University of Leeds.

Saving Mothers (2011–2013). Sixth Report on Confidential Enquiries into Maternal Deaths in South Africa.

Sawyer, S. M., Afifi, R. A., Bearinger, L. H., Blakemore, S. J., Dick, B., Ezeh, A. C. and Patton G. C. (2012). 'Adolescence: a foundation for future health', *Lancet* 37:9826, 1630–40.

Seidman, G. W. (1984). Women in Zimbabwe: post-independence struggles, *Feminist Studies* 10:3, 419–40.

Seleke, T. (2014). Abortion debate in Botswana: the flip side. www.sundaystandard.info/abortion-debate-botswana-flip-side. Accessed 15 June 2017.

Shewamene, Z., Dune, T. and Smith, C. A. (2017). The use of traditional medicine in maternity care among African women in Africa and the diaspora: a systematic review. *BMC Complementary and Alternative Medicine*, 17, pp. 382.

Shisana, O., Rehle, T. M., Simbayi, L. C., Zuma, K., Jooste, S., Zungu, N., Labadarios, N. and Onoya, D. (2012). The national HIV prevalence, incidence and behaviour survey.

Siliwa, L. (2007). Care-giving in times of HIV and AIDS. When hospitality is a threat to African women's lives: a gendered theological examination of the theology of hospitality. *Journal of Constructive Theology* 13:1, 69–82.

Smith, S. (2012). *Perceptions of abortion in contemporary urban Botswana*. Masters Thesis. Centre for Women's Studies, University of York.

Smith, S. S. (2013). The challenges of procuring safe abortion care in Botswana. *African Journal of Reproductive Health* 18:1, 165–7.

Statistics South Africa (2016). Mid-year population estimates – 2016: statistical release, P0302. www.statssa.gov.za/publications/P0302/P03022016.pdf

Steele, L., Iribarne, M. and Carr, R. (2016). Introduction. Medical bodies: gender, justice and medicine. *Australian Feminist Studies* 31:8, 117–24.

Stevens, M. (n.d.). Abortion, girls, young women and gender queer people. Accessed 26 April 2017. www.cal.org.za/wp-content/uploads/2016/10/Intersections-and-continuums-in-reproductive-justice-%E2%80%93-abortion-girls-and-young-women-and-gender-queer-folks-.pdf.

Tamale, S. (2008). The right to culture and the culture of rights: a critical perspective on women's sexual rights in Africa. *Feminist Legal Studies* 16, 47–69.

Tamale, S. (2011). *African Sexualities: A Reader*. Cape Town: Pambazuka Press.

Trueman, K. A. and Magwentshu, M. (2013). Abortion in a progressive legal environment: the need for vigilance in protecting and promoting access to safe abortion services in South Africa. *American Journal of Public Health* 103:3, 397–99.

Umar, K. J., Rabah, A. B., Na'ala, M., Bello, M., Ibrahim, M. L. and Garba, M. (2011). Antibacterial and phytochemical screening of Methanolic extract of Celosia Leptostachya Benth leaves on some selected clinical isolates, *Journal of Medicinal Plants Research* 5:28, 6473–6.

United Nations General Assembly (2001). Implementation of the World Programme of Action for Youth to Year 2000 and Beyond: report of the Secretary-General. Lisbon: United Nations.

Waldman, L. and Stevens, M. (2015). Sexual and reproductive health and rights and health in policy and practice in South Africa. *Reproductive Health Matters* 23, 45–93.

World Bank (2000). *World Bank Development Report 1999/2000*. New York: Oxford University Press.

World Health Organization (2012). *Safe abortion: technical and policy guidance for health systems*. Geneva: WHO.

World Health Organization (2013). *WHO traditional medicine strategy 2014–2023*. Geneva: WHO. www.who.int/medicines/publications/traditional/trm_strategy14_23/en/.

Yeld, J. (2013). Traditional medicine worth billions. *News*, 29 January. www.iol.co.za/news/traditional-medicine-worth-billions-1460531. Accessed 16 May 2018.

Zihindula, G., Meyer-Weitz, A. and Akintola, O. (2015). Lived experiences of Democratic Republic of Congo refugees facing medical xenophobia in Durban, South Africa. *Journal of Asian and African Studies* 52:4, 458–70.

8

The politics of naming: contested vocabularies of birth violence

Rachelle Chadwick

This chapter focuses on the contested vocabularies used to name and conceptualise birth violence across a range of geopolitical contexts. Over the last few decades, several terms have been used to refer to the violations birthers experience during childbirth in healthcare facilities, including: childbirth abuse, mistreatment, disrespectful care, and birth rape. More recently, 'obstetric violence' has emerged as a term used in current debates and activist struggles. The chapter traces the contextual politics of vocabularies about birth violence and the emergence of the notion of 'obstetric violence'. Using a transnational feminist approach, I argue that a tendency towards geopolitical bifurcation (rooted in racist and colonial historical legacies) frames the ways in which birth violence has been approached and conceptualised in different settings. As a result of this bifurcation, separate literatures and vocabularies have developed, which frame the issue of birth violence in distinctive ways depending on geopolitical zones. The conceptual usefulness of the term 'obstetric violence' is thus considered as an alternative, unifying, and transnational vocabulary. However, the limitations of this conceptual lexicon are also discussed, particularly in relation to the ability of the framework to theorise (and address) the multiple modalities of violation that potentially occur during pregnancy, labour, and birth. As such, the question is whether a vocabulary rooted predominantly in a critique of medicalised birth and technology is sufficient to theorise the systemic, normative, and multidimensional violence associated with birthing under global racial capitalism. While the emergence of the critical vocabulary of 'obstetric violence' is an important advance in the feminist theorisation of and struggle against birth violence, I conclude that we need to develop a more sophisticated and explicitly anti-capitalist analysis that recognises the roots of reproductive violence in global capitalocentric (and racist) formations.

Histories of birth violence

Birth violence is not a new phenomenon. However, efforts to explicitly name coercion, mistreatment, and abuse during childbirth as forms of violence are relatively recent. While birth activist Sheila Kitzinger (1992) was ahead of her time, writing about birth violations as a form of violence against women nearly three decades ago, it is only over the last two decades or so that feminist scholars have made more explicit efforts to define, conceptualise, and theorise birth violence (Chadwick, 2017, 2018; Pickles, 2015; Pickles and Herring, 2019; Shabot, 2016, 2018; Wolf, 2013). Abusive practices during birth were reported in American obstetrics from the late 1950s (Goer, 2010). In 1958, an article titled 'Cruelty in the maternity wards' was published in the *Ladies Home Journal*, in which Gladys Denny Schultz (a nurse) exposed the inhumane treatment and 'torture' of women while they laboured under the influence of scopolamine combined with morphine (commonly known as 'Twilight sleep'). This article unleashed a flood of letters from readers describing their experiences of abuse during birth. American women wrote of being strapped down, being left alone for hours, struck and threatened, having episiotomies cut and stitched without anaesthetic, and having their legs held together. This exposé of violation and abuse during birth in the popular American women's magazine was a key moment in the development of what has been termed 'second wave' birth activism (Beckett, 2005), and the Birth Rights movement. In their arguments against the medicalisation of birth in the 1960s and 1970s, Euro-American birth activists, midwives, and feminists used the idea of 'natural childbirth' (developed by British obstetrician Grantly Dick-Read in the 1930s) to advocate for a return to a more 'natural', woman-centred, and drug-free experience of birth. The medicalisation of childbirth had reached a high-point in America during the first three decades of the twentieth century, when new methods of pain relief (i.e. scopolamine, drug cocktails of morphine/

heroin and barbiturates, and full anesthesia) and an interventionist approach to obstetrics combined to produce what has been described as 'an orgy of interference' (Loudon, 1992: 358).

By now well-known, this particular history of medicalisation and birth activism is predominantly a middle-class, whitecentric narrative written from the privileged position of the global north. The so-called 'medicalisation' of birth has been, from its inception, a class- and race-based project and has never applied equally to all women (Oparah and Bonaparte, 2015). For example, the preference for male birth attendants first began to surface among middle- and upper-class women in Europe during the 1750s (Shorter, 1982). The ability to procure a male midwife was regarded as a 'fashion state- ment' (Hanson, 2004) and a sign of high status (Shorter, 1982), likely because they charged higher fees than female midwives (Rothman, 1982). Privileged Euro-American women have thus in many senses been co-constructors of medicalised birth (Arney, 1982; Leavitt, 1986) and were at the forefront of both early twentieth- century campaigns for women's rights to drugs and pain relief during birth and the second-wave of birth activism for less drugs and medical intervention in the 1960s/1970s (Beckett, 2005). Birth activism, until recently, has largely been written from the vantage points and perspectives of middle-class, privileged women. As a result, constructs such as 'control', 'agency', and 'choice' – prominent themes in the broader feminist politics of childbirth (Beckett, 2005) – are arguably premised on privileged positionalities.

The colonial and racist roots and historical legacies of ideas about 'medicalisation' and 'natural birth' remain under-acknowledged in birth scholarship and activisms. Racist colonial mythologies about indigenous women as 'savages' or 'animals', who were 'closer to nature' and experienced childbearing with ease, were rooted in ideologies of racial difference and Social Darwinism (Schiebinger, 2013). These ideas have had destructive material effects and have been used to justify the poor quality of maternal health services for indigenous women in colonial contexts (Jasen, 1997; Searle, 1965). The colonial legacies of these inequalities are often still felt in contemporary (lack of) access to maternal healthcare for many indigenous women (Moffit, 2004; see also chapter 9 below). Myths about easy and painless childbirth for so-called 'primitive' women were also used to frame and legitimise the movement for 'natural childbirth' beginning in the 1930s and 1940s with the publication of obstetrician Grantly Dick-Read's works (1933, 1942). In Dick-Read's philosophy of birth, in which he drew on racist distinctions between 'primitive' and 'civilised' women, pain was regarded as not 'natural' or an essential feature of physiological birth. Low-income women and Black women were construed as 'obstetrically hardy' (Hoberman, 2012) and thus as giving birth effortlessly and without pain (see Dick-Read, 1942). Difficulties and pain during childbirth were seen to be an affliction of middle-class and white women, and regarded as a consequence of civilisation and cultural 'advancement'. Even in contemporary discourse about home birth and unassisted birth, the myth of the 'third-world' woman who births with ease, continues to be used as evidence for women's inherent capacity to birth without medical intervention. According to Cosslett (1994: 9), the 'primitive woman' 'haunts western women's birth stories' as a romanticised ideal and emblem of the power of instinct and the female body. While indigenous women have been seen as hardier, 'savage', closer to nature and able to give birth effortlessly, white and privileged women of the middle classes have been constructed as needing medical intervention and help (even to have a 'natural' birth following Dick-Read and Lamaze) given that so-called European civilisation has made them 'delicate', weak, prone to tension, and sensitive to pain and anxieties (Schiebinger, 2013). The twin process of naturalising and 'ungendering' African and indigenous women (see Chadwick, forthcoming) and 'civilising' white women was a core feature of European modes of gendered coloniality, in which indigenous women became 'savages' and white women became respectable 'ladies' (Lugones, 2007; Mies, 2014).

Attitudes and assumptions about the necessity of medicalisation and pain-relief during birth have thus been framed by racialised and colonial assumptions about how women of different races, nationalities, and class positions give birth. These racist assumptions continue to shape the ways in which women's paining labouring and birthing bodies are treated in healthcare facilities across different settings (Bridges, 2011; Chadwick, 2018; Davis, 2019; Oparah and Bonaparte, 2015). The longstanding racist and imperialist assumption that women in Africa and other areas of the global south give birth easily and without any need of pain relief or medical intervention dates back to traveller's tales of the seventeenth and eighteenth century (Cosslett, 1994; Jasen, 1997). Similar beliefs have also been held about low-income, rural women in wider Europe (Jasen, 1997). While rooted in racist colonial and imperial imaginings, there is evidence of the continued and pervasive legacy of such story lines in birth activist texts (Arms, 1977) and as prominent 'controlling images' (Collins, 1990) that continue to pervade and shape the treatment of Black women in medical/obstetric practice (Bridges, 2011; Davis, 2019). As such, racist conceptions of the reproductive and birthing capacities of Black women (rooted in colonial relations) continue to enable and justify forms of violence and 'obstetric racism' (Davis, 2019) perpetrated against Black birthers (Bridges, 2011; Oparah and Bonaparte, 2015; Owens, 2017). Being cast as more 'animal-like' and as 'breeders', rather than maternal subjects with mother rights, enabled the justification of the commodification of Black reproductive labour under slavery and the use of Black women's bodies as sites of medical and gynaecological experimentation (Barbagallo, 2019; Owens, 2017). Broader forms of reproductive violence (i.e. directed at all aspects of reproduction, including the criminalisation and pathologisation of abortion, forced pregnancy, forced surrogacy, gynaecological violence, birth violence, and the degradation of procreative and maternal labours) has thus been endemic to racial capitalism for hundreds of years (Federici, 2004). These colonial and racist inheritances have historically not been well-recognised within the Birth Rights or 'humanising birth' movements (Chadwick, 2018). However, there are encouraging signs that this is changing. Powerful writing on birth, birth justice, and obstetric racism by Black feminist scholars has radically changed the terms of our conversation/s on these issues (Bridges, 2011; Davis, 2019; Oparah and Bonaparte, 2015). Moreover, the critical lexicon of 'obstetric violence' has also had much to do with critical reappraisals of the racialised politics of birth and the intersectional apects of birth violence (Chadwick, 2018; Dixon, 2015; Smith-Oka, 2015).

Bifurcated vocabularies

Racist mythologies and sociomaterial stratifications continue to shape birthing in the contemporary world, and geopolitical bifurcations continue to persist. For example, a problematic bifurcation is evident in the global rhetoric and politics surrounding birth. While privileged women often push back against high degrees of medicalisation during birth, and some long to return to 'natural' ways of birthing, a lack of basic and adequate medical care in other settings is implicated in unacceptably high rates of maternal and infant death and avoidable complications. There are longstanding historical roots to this bifurcated politics, which are inextricable from colonial exploitation and racism. Dominant narratives of birth (i.e. medical versus natural birth) continue to be written from positions of privilege while the lived experiences and perspectives of women from the global south are all too often missing and silenced. As such, continued and unreflexive valorisation of 'natural' modes of birth (or what is also termed 'physiological birth'), are implicated in the continued mystification of the ideological violences that have 'naturalised' (and appropriated) the labours of Black birthers as 'animal acts' while simultaneously pathologising the birthing labours of white and middle-class women. As such, bifurcated vocabularies are part of the violent machinery that stratifies healthcare resources and technologies according to a stratified logics of profit rather than need/request. This section explores the ways geopolitical bifurcation works to disconnect transnational circuits of birth violence, reproducing a world in which the social and medical realities of minority and majority geopolitical zones are reproduced as separate and unconnected entities (even while deeply interpenetrative).

Literature on birth mistreatment and violence in Euro-American contexts has tended to be conceptualised in relation to childbirth 'trauma' or psychological distress (Elmir etal., 2010; Forssén, 2012; Nilsson, 2014; Thomson and Downe, 2008), while the rhetoric of 'trauma' is rarely used to describe women's experiences of poor treatment in the global south. Recently there has been increasing use of the term 'obstetric violence' across transnational contexts. Researchers working in a wide range of locations have thus adopted the term, including in South Africa (Pickles 2015; Chadwick, 2016; 2017; Dutton and Knight, 2020; Lappaman and Swartz, 2019), India (Chattopadhyay, Mishra and Jacob, 2018), Ethiopia (Mihret, 2019), the US (Diaz Tello, 2016; Garcia, 2020), and Italy (Ravaldi et al., 2018). Typically, however, literature using the concepts of birth abuse, violence, and mistreatment has traditionally been centred on women's experiences in the global south. This is illustrated by two (relatively) recently published reviews. For example, in a mixed-methods systematic review looking at the mistreatment of women during birth 'globally', Bohren et al. (2015) include studies pre-dominantly from African contexts and other settings considered part of the global south (e.g. India, Brazil, the Middle-East). Where countries of the global north are included, studies of mistreatment are based solely on the experiences of immigrant women. Only one study was included which drew on the experiences of privileged women in the global north, namely Sweden (Forssén, 2012). This bifurcated approach to the problem of abuse/mistreatment is interest-ing given that studies have reported patterns of mistreatment during birth among privileged women in the global north (Baker, Choi and Henshaw, 2005; Elmir, Schmied, Wilkes and Jackson, 2010; Forssén, 2012; Nilsson, 2014; Thomson and Downe, 2008). In another systematic review on 'disrespectful intrapartum care', Bradley, McCourt, Rayment and Parmar (2016) purposively limit their analysis only to countries of sub-Saharan Africa. While abuse and mistreatment are clearly urgent problems that need to be addressed in the global south, by delimiting analysis only to these settings, there is a danger of 'Othering' the problem. While we need to understand the distinctive challenges and problems facing women in the global south in relation to maternity care, it is also important that we are careful about reproducing problematic binaries and colonising representations (Mohanty, 1988) that assume birth violence to be predominantly a problem of the global south. It is also critical that we cultivate transnational approaches to the problem of birth violence and avoid only exploring the experiences of women in the global south in terms which might contribute to geopolitical 'Othering'. It is also only by exploring transnational positions and material realities that the entanglements between colonial modes of medicalisation and exploitation and geopolitical materialisations of birth violence in different settings can be adequately acknowledged and debated. It remains dangerous to reproduce binaries between 'western' and 'third-world', 'developed' and 'developing' world and the global 'north' and 'south' (Mohanty, 2002) given tendencies to homogenisa-tion and othering. We need to begin to think of ways of conceptualis-ing birth abuse/mistreatment in relation to both local and global material conditions and transnational legacies of medicalisation, colonialism, and neoliberal global capitalism (Herr, 2014). It is important to explore both the similarities and differences between women's experiences of birth abuse in diverse settings and according to race, class and other socio-material positionalities. As I conclude later in the paper, foregrounding the links between transnational (and historical) relations of capitalism and modes of obstetric (and reproductive) violence, is key to efforts to trace these complex and contradictory entanglements.

A variety of terms have been used to describe violence during childbirth, including mistreatment, disrespectful care, childbirth abuse, birth rape, traumatic birth, and obstetric violence. Literature on 'traumatic birth' has tended to explore distressing birth experiences in relation to privileged women in Euro-American settings. The controversial notion of 'birth rape' has been debated on social media sites, predominantly in relation to middle-class American birth experiences. Public health researchers have favoured the terms mistreatment, disrespectful care, and childbirth abuse. The concept of 'obstetric violence' is relatively new and has a distinctive set of contextual roots. In the following sub-sections, I provide a broad outline of these different vocabularies.

Traumatic birth

Literature on 'traumatic birth' has tended to focus on women in contexts of the global north, including the UK, New Zealand, Australia, the US, Denmark, Holland, and Sweden. The majority of studies on traumatic and psychologically distressing birth experiences have been conducted in the UK (Baker et al., 2005; Elmir et al., 2010; Mozingo, 2002; Thomson and Downe, 2008). There is also a distinctive literature on post-traumatic stress disorder (PTSD) in relation to birth that I do not include as part of the work on distressing or traumatic births. PTSD is a very specific type of psychological disorder that has a particular set of diagnostic criteria and is not relevant to the discussion here. In contexts of the global north, more than one third of women report their experiences of birth to have been traumatic (Baker et al., 2005). There have been virtually no investigations of trauma or PTSD in relation to African women's experiences of childbirth. One known exception is the work by Adewuya et al. (2006) that found the prevalence of PTSD after birth in a group of Nigerian women to be 5.9%. This figure is comparable (on the high-end) with rates of prevalence in the global north. As far as I can deduce, there has been little effort to explore the psychosocial and traumatic impacts of distressing birth experiences for women in African contexts or the global south more broadly.

A meta-ethnography of ten qualitative studies exploring traumatic and distressing birth experiences in the global north found that women reported feeling traumatised during birth largely as a result of unsupportive, disrespectful, and dehumanising treatment by doctors, nurses and other healthcare professionals (Elmir et al., 2010). Traumatic experiences of birth have been found to be linked to feeling invisible, neglected, and ignored during labour (Thomson and Downe, 2008) and to inhumane care which leaves women feeling exposed, degraded, and depersonalised (Beck, 2004; Forssén, 2012; Mozingo, 2002). Women in Scandinavian countries have reported feeling 'nullified' by abuse in maternity settings in which they felt powerless, ignored, humiliated, and suffered through rough treatment and a loss of dignity (Nilsson, 2014; Schroll, Kjaergaard amd Mitgaard, 2013; Swahnberg, Thapar-Bjorkert and Bertero, 2007). Some researchers have used the concept of 'dignity violations' drawn from the work of Jacobsen (2009) to describe women's experiences of distressing birth. According to Jacobsen (2009), being treated with dignity has been found to be the second most important aspect of quality of healthcare (after access to services). Dignity violations in healthcare are described as including a range of interpersonal relations, namely: rudeness, indifference, dismissal, objectification, contempt, intrusion, restriction, revulsion, condescension, and assault. Forssén (2012) shows how several of these themes, including condescension and blame, dismissal (of embodied knowledge and pain) and humiliation were apparent in Swedish women's recollections of disempowering birth experiences. The aftermath of traumatic birth has been associated with long-term emotional and psychological health sequelae, disrupted relationships with infants and partners (Baker et al., 2005; Elmir et al., 2010) and persistent feelings of failure, guilt, and shame (Forssén, 2012). A qualitative study of British women who reported a self-defined traumatic birth, found that trauma was not related to mode of birth (i.e. caesarean section or instrumental delivery) but rather 'to fractured inter-personal relationships with care-givers'

(Thomson and Downe, 2008: 268) in which women felt powerless, isolated, and dehumanised.

Similar themes, highlighting negative interactions with caregivers during labour as triggers for traumatic and distressing birth experiences, have been found in several other studies (Baker et al., 2005; Beck, 2009; Esposito, 1999). Women have described distressing and negative interactions with caregivers during birth as violent and brutal, abusive and like being 'assaulted' or 'tortured' (Thomson and Downe, 2008). Women in other studies have reported that they 'felt raped' and subjected to exposure, violation and invasion (Mozingo, 2002). Further recurrent themes in studies of traumatic birth have included a reported lack of emotional safety during birth (Baker et al., 2005; Nilsson, 2014), loss of control via lack of information (Baker et al., 2005; Thomson and Downe, 2008) and unhappiness with the objectification and depersonalisation that often accompanied technocratic and medicalised modes of birth (Mozingo, 2002; Thomson and Downe, 2008).While the literature on traumatic birth experiences in contexts of the global north contain many similar themes (as will be seen in the following section) to descriptions of birth violence and mistreatment in the global south, there have been limited efforts to explore the interconnected meanings of these continuities (and discontinuities) or to name traumatic births as products of birth violence.

Mistreatment, abuse, and disrespectful care

There is a substantial literature on poor quality of care and abuse during birth in Southern contexts, including Ghana, Egypt, Tanzania, Palestine, Zambia, Turkey, Benin, Nigeria, India, Mexico, Cambodia and South Africa. There are also studies looking on the birth experiences of marginalised, immigrant women in northern settings (Bowes and Domokos, 1996; Varcoe, Brown, Calam, Harvey and Tallio, 2013). Unlike the literature on 'traumatic birth' outlined above, the literature/s on Southern and immigrant experiences of birth abuse do not often refer to the concept of trauma or to the psychological effects of negative birth experiences. Written largely by public health researchers and medical professionals (but with a growing number of anthropological studies), this research is often biomedically framed in relation to 'evidence-based practices', utilisation of maternal health services, and indicators of maternal health. Poor maternal mortality and morbidity rates often frame discussions of abuse and poor quality of care, with mistreatment seen as a barrier to women accessing health services and facilities during birth and thus impacting on poor health outcomes and mortality rates (Mathai, 2011; Van den Brock and Graham, 2009). There is also a growing and discernible trend for studies on birth mistreatment to use a human rights framework and to position such modes of abuse as human rights violations (Bohren et al., 2016).

The substantial body of studies exploring mistreatment and abuse in contexts of the global south collectively point to problems of neglect, lack of support, and poor communication from caregivers, inhumane treatment, non-evidence based practices (routine enemas, lithotomy positions, refusal to allow birth companions, not allowing women to consume food or drink) brutal, aggressive treatment (coercion, physical force and shouting), objectification, and lack of informed consent for procedures, treatments or interventions. Women in the global south have reported wanting friendly, caring staff, humane and professional care, to feel both physically and emotionally safe during labour/birth, have access to medical information and be assured of privacy, dignity and respect (D'Ambruoso, Abbey and Hussein, 2005; El Nemer, Downe and Small, 2006). In women's accounts of mistreatment in Southern settings, negative interpersonal relations with caregivers collectively feature as a prominent concern and problem. Similar to women in northern contexts (see above), women reported being upset by negative attitudes (i.e. impatience, hostility, condescension) from healthcare workers (Cindoglu and Sayan-Cengiz, 2010; D'Ambruoso et al., 2005), being neglected and ignored (Castro and Erviti, 2003; El Nemer et al., 2006), and being inhumanely treated. Inhumane treatment included, for example, having pain denied, being threatened, bullied and coerced into accepting birth control devices, being treated rudely and physically abused (Castro and Erviti, 2003; Cindoglu and Sayan-Cengiz, 2010; El-Nemer et al., 2006).

While it has been argued that 'medicalisation' is only a problem for privileged women (Johnson, 2016), findings from studies conducted with women in the global south hint at a more complex relationship between marginalisation, poverty, and medicalised modes of birth

(Chadwick, 2018). While physical safety was a more prominent concern for Southern women (D'Ambruoso et al., 2005; El Nemer et al., 2006; Spangler, 2011; Varcoe, Brown, Calam, Harvey and Tallio, 2013) than those in contexts of the global north, women were united in desiring a greater sense of emotional safety during birth (El Nemer, et al., 2006; Baker et al., 2005). While hospital or facility-based birth was often regarded as an inevitable necessity for women (Cindoglu and Sayan-Cengiz, 2010), persistent themes of dissatisfaction with elements of medicalised birth (i.e. objectification, cold clinical treatment) are readily apparent from the literature on birth mistreatment in Southern settings (Cindoglu and Sayan-Cengiz, 2010; El Nemer et al., 2006). For example, in El Nemer et al. (2006) an ethnography of birth in an Egyptian hospital, women spoke about their dissatisfaction with what they referred to as 'technical touch', which engendered feelings of depersonalisation and objectification. As one of the Turkish women explained in the study by Cindoglu and Sayan-Cengiz (2010: 231): 'Everyone in hospital is a stranger. We fear doctors and nurses. When you scream they scold you: "Why are you screaming?" … I'm not comfortable in hospitals. They don't value you at all as a human being. It's not as it seems from the outside.'

While women in Southern settings want prompt access to medical technologies when needed and thus do not reject medical modes of birth, they are often dissatisfied with the affective, emotional, and relational dynamics accompanying medicalisation. Not surprisingly, women want to be treated, valued and respected like human beings with feelings and concerns, they want to 'bring back the celebration of life' (Varcoe et al., 2013) and do not want to be objectified, mistreated, or be subject to only cold, impersonal treatment. El Nemer et al. (2006) thus found that Egyptian women were dissatisfied with care that emphasised technology, machines and 'technical touch' (interventions and examinations) at the expense of emotionally supportive 'helping from the heart'. Some women in this study reported that they did not need technology as much as someone that cared for them during labour/birth.

There are thus important and thought-provoking continuities between the negative and distressing birth experiences reported by privileged northern women and women from the global south that hint at similarities in what makes birthing 'good' or distressing across different contexts (see Chadwick, 2019). However, there are also important discontinuities that must be recognised. In Southern settings, women are sometimes subject to harsher forms of physical violence (Bohren et al., 2016; Castro and Erviti, 2003; Cindoglu and Sayan-Cengiz, 2010). Furthermore, related directly to the inequalities inherent in global racial capitalism, medical care in facility-based maternity services are often inadequate and sometimes there is a severe lack of medical treatment so that some women basically give birth unattended and without the expertise of a birth attendant (Chadwick, 2018; 2019; Chadwick, Cooper and Harries, 2014; Moyer et al., 2014). Historically embedded institutional, structural, and systemic inadequacies mean that women giving birth in healthcare facilities in the global south are not always guaranteed proper medical attention and are thus literally at greater physical risk of complications and/or death. While privileged birthers in Euro-American settings might at times feel like they are physically unsafe during labour/ birth (Mozingo, 2002), they generally (however this is also racialised in some settings) receive prompt medical interventions/treatment if needed (hence the dramatically lower rates of maternal mortality and morbidity). Women in Southern contexts, as well as immigrant women in northern settings, also have to deal with legacies of colonisation and inequality, including the fact that a medicalised philosophy of birth is a product of coloniality often imposed on colonised people and which, in some cases, has destroyed traditional birth cultures and local traditions of midwifery. Furthermore, a medicalised approach to birth also at times carries compounding traces of Euro-American patriarchy, racism, Euro-centrism, and class prejudices (Chadwick, 2018). As a result, Southern and immigrant women sometimes complain that traditional practices are dismissed or trivialised by healthcare workers (Varcoe et al., 2013).

As such, there are both discontinuities and continuities in birth violence across transnational settings. Birthers' across a range of contexts report dissatisfaction based on similar themes of feeling disconnected and relationally alienated from healthcare providers. The literatures on traumatic birth and mistreatment, abuse, and disrespectful care point importantly to the key characteristics of distressing birth experiences. However, what is typically missing from these accounts, studies, and reports is an explicit articulation of mistreatment or trauma as rooted in gender/racialised violence and any critical understanding of the global systems of interlocking and historical power relations that produce the conditions for these forms of violence.

Obstetric violence: an alternative critical vocabulary

The concept of obstetric violence emerged in the 2000s in Latin and Central America. Importantly, unlike terms such as mistreatment, abuse, and disrespectful care, the concept of obstetric violence is rooted in birth activist movements to humanise childbirth in the global south (specifically Latin America). As a result, the term obstetric violence is overtly political and provocative and linked to efforts to critique social relations of marginalisation embedded in gender, class and race socio-materialities. According to Dixon (2015: 450), references to obstetric violence are 'unexpected, jarring and provocative' and deliberately used by activists to challenge abusive practices which have often been hidden or normalised during birth. Importantly, the concept of obstetric violence is embedded in legal vocabularies which explicitly name it as a form of gender violence or violence against women. Adopted as a legal term in Venezuela in 2007, followed by Argentina in 2009, and Mexico in 2014, perpetrators of obstetric violence are regarded as guilty of criminal acts and subject to criminal liability (which usually amounts to a fine and a written acknowledgment of wrongdoing on the part of the practitioner and/or institution). In Venezuelan law, published in Article 15 of the Organic Law on the Right of Women to a Life Free of Violence, obstetric violence is identified as one of nineteen different forms of punishable violence against women and is defined as follows:

> The appropriation of the body and reproductive processes of women by health personnel, which is expressed as dehumanized treatment, an abuse of medication, and to convert the natural processes into pathological ones, bringing with it a loss of autonomy and the ability to decide freely about their bodies and sexuality, negatively impacting the quality of life of women. (cited in Perez D'Gregorio, 2010: 201)

Article 51 of the law goes on to outline the following practices as forms of obstetric violence, namely: (a) untimely and insufficient attention to obstetric emergencies (b) forcing women to give birth in a supine position (c) interfering with or blocking the early attachment of mother and baby (d) altering the physiological process of a low-risk delivery via medical interventions (i.e. acceleration techniques) without informed consent and (e) performing unnecessary caesarean sections. Importantly, this definition names abuse during childbirth as a form of gendered violence, including dehumanised treatment, appropriation of women's bodies, unnecessary medicalisation, pathologisation, and loss of autonomy.

When discussing the term obstetric violence, it is important that its roots in the Latin and Central American context are understood. Several countries in Central and Latin America have extremely technocratic, medicalised, and bifurcated obstetric systems (similar to South Africa), with medical interventions and caesarean section rates among the highest in the world. For example, Diniz and Chacham (2004) estimate that in the Brazilian private sector, caesarean section rates are as high as 80–90% of births. In the public sector, caesarean sections are estimated to occur in approximately 30% of births. In Venezuela, the first country to adopt obstetric violence as a legal term, medical practitioners attend all hospital deliveries and midwifery does not exist in obstetric practice (Perez D' Gregorio, 2010). In a cross-national comparison of global caesarean section rates provided by the World Health Organization (WHO) in 2010, Brazil is ranked as the country with the highest caesarean section rate in the world, which is reported as 46%. More recently, the national rate of caesarean section in Brazil has reportedly increased to a figure of 56% (Rudey, Leal and Rego, 2020). Other countries in Central and Latin America also have extremely high caesarean section rates, with Argentina estimated as 35%, Venezuela 25%, Paraguay at 32%, Uruguay as 32%, Mexico 38% and the Dominican Republic as 42% (WHO, 2010). According to the WHO, caesarean section rates above 15% are regarded as potential evidence of unnecessary use of the procedure while rates less than 10% are seen as low and regarded as possible under-utilisation of this potentially life-saving intervention. While the WHO has tempered its statement made in 1985 that 15% was the absolute upper-limit for an acceptable caesarean section rate, they still note that there is no evidence for health benefits to mother or infant in populations with a caesarean section rate of more than 15% (WHO, 2010). In many settings in Latin and Central America, birth is thus highly medicalised and bifurcated along class and status lines (Dixon, 2015; Smith-Oka, 2013; Smith-Oka, 2015). The bodily integrity of both rich and poor women are compromised in different ways in contexts such as Brazil, where middle-class women are subject to astronomical rates of caesarean section (80–90%) and more than 90% of poor women are 'cut below' via episiotomies during childbirth (Diniz and Chacham, 2004). It is thus in contexts of rampant medicalisation, technocratic intervention, and institutional violence directed towards birthers' bodies, that the concept of obstetric violence has emerged. Given the contextual roots of the term, it is thus not surprising that the intersections between abuse, violence, and obstetrics are foregrounded in the articulation of birth violence as specifically embedded in medicalised approaches to birth.

From its roots in Latin and Central America, the concept of obstetric violence has become a travelling concept and is increasingly being debated and taken-up in a range of different contexts, including South Africa (Chadwick, 2016; 2017; 2018; Dutton and Knight, 2020; Lappaman and Swartz, 2019; Pickles, 2015), the US (Diaz-Tello, 2016; Garcia, 2020), India (Chattopadhyay etal., 2018), Ethiopia (Mihret, 2019), and Italy (Ravaldi et al., 2018). Furthermore, since 2014, five obstetric violence observatories (civil rights groups) have been founded in Chile, France, Argentina, Columbia, and Spain (Sadler et al., 2016). Significantly, the concept of obstetric violence originates from birth activist struggles in the global south and contrasts sharply with depoliticising tendencies prevalent in many white and northern-centred debates about the feminist politics of birth (Chadwick, 2018). As noted by Beckett (2005), the Euro-American feminist politics of birth has arguably become stymied by an increasing valorisation of a neoliberal rhetoric of individual 'choice' in relation to birth, which often obfuscates power relations. This is also reflected in the tendency (outlined earlier) for birth violence in Euro-American settings to be framed predominantly in relation to individualist notions of psychological distress and trauma. As a result of this framing, the structural and sociomaterial aspects of birth trauma are sometimes hidden and silenced.

In contrast, activist struggles invoking the term 'obstetric violence' explicitly challenge abuses of medical authority and structural relations of power. Obstetric violence has been theorised as a form of structural or symbolic violence (Sadler et al., 2016). The critique of 'medicalisation' is also prominent in the framing of birth violence as 'obstetric violence'. This runs counter to recent claims that 'medicalisation' is only a problem for privileged women in Euro-American settings (Johnson, 2016). As a result of the contextual roots of the concept of 'obstetric violence' in Latin American settings – often marked by bifurcated maternity systems in which marginalised, low-income women, and privileged women are subject to different forms of medical mistreatment or violence – understandings of 'medicalisation' in relation to 'obstetric violence' are often inherently intersectional. 'Medicalisation' is thus not a singular system that operates on all women's bodies in the same way; instead it intersects with other modalities of socio-material power relations (Chadwick, 2018). As a result, scholars utilising the concept of obstetric violence have often provided rich intersectional analyses that demonstrate the multiple ways in which birth violence and medicalisation materialise in relation to structural inequalities of race, ethnicity, class, and other axes of marginalisation (Chadwick, 2017, 2018; Dixon, 2015; Smith-Oka, 2015).

Obstetric violence in the South African context

As a travelling concept, how well does 'obstetric violence' translate in/to the South African context and potentially to other southern settings such as India (see Chapter 9, this volume). In terms of contextual politics, there are continuities between Latin America and South Africa. For example, rampant social inequality and bifurcated obstetric systems in which rich women and poor women give birth very differently are core features of many Latin American countries (e.g. Brazil and Argentina) and South Africa. South Africa, however, is marked by a very different colonial history and a particular historical legacy of racialised oppression and apartheid, which continues to mark healthcare systems. While medicalisation works differently on the bodies of rich and poor women in Latin American countries (Diniz and Chacham, 2004), interventionist approaches nonetheless seem to dominate obstetric practice in many Latin and Central American settings (Dixon, 2015; Smith-Oka, 2015). Low-income women are thus often subject to unnecessarily high levels of genital cutting via episiotomies, coercive contraceptive and sterilisation practices, and painful and non-evidence based manual revisions of the uterine cavity after birth (Castro and Erviti, 2003; Diniz and Chacham, 2004; Dixon, 2015). Medical practitioners also seem to dominate as birth attendants in Latin American settings (e.g. Venezuela) (Perez D' Gregorio, 2010).

Birth politics are shaped by different dynamics in the South African context. As a result, medicalisation and 'obstetric violence' materialise differently here than in Latin American settings. While the highly resourced private sector in South Africa is highly medicalised, with most women cared for by highly qualified medical specialists (gynecologists or obstetricians) during pregnancy, in the public maternity sector most South African women give birth without a great deal of medical intervention and are usually attended by nurse-midwives. The private and public healthcare sectors are still sharply divided along racial lines, with most white women (and growing numbers of middle-class Black women) giving birth in private, highly medicalised facilities and most Black and impoverished women giving birth in under-resourced public sector settings. Birth is thus riven with racial inequalities in the South African context, with different modes of medicalisation operating according to race/ class dynamics. This is illustrated by deeply unequal maternal mortality rates (MMR): for example, the MMR is estimated to be approximately 40 per 100,000 live births in the private maternity sector (Bateman, 2014). The figure in the public sector is substantially higher, with recent estimates citing an MMR of around 333 deaths per 100,000 live births (Bradshaw, Dorrington and Laubscher, 2012). As a result, low-income and predominantly Black women giving birth in public sector settings are more than seven times as likely to be 'at risk' of death during birth than privileged (white) women in the private sector.

As opposed to many Latin American settings where poor women are subject to high degrees of medical intervention, Kruger and Schoombie (2010) write about the lack of medical surveillance (i.e. absence of the medical gaze) during labour/birth in South African public maternity settings. Instead of receiving high rates of medical intervention, women/girls labouring in public sector maternal obstetric units in South Africa have been found to be left alone, largely unattended, and ignored during labour and (in some cases) even during delivery (Chadwick, 2018; Kruger and Schoombie, 2010). As I have demonstrated elsewhere (Chadwick, 2018), pain relief is not routinely offered in the public sector and Black women are expected to manage pain by themselves and to labour largely without medical intervention or supportive care. Furthermore, sometimes healthcare workers frame the pain and suffering experienced by women and birthers during labour as deserving punishment for being sexually active and pregnant (see Chadwick, 2017). Labouring persons are also at times subject to direct physical violence and emotional abuse in public sector settings (Chadwick et al., 2014). As such, 'medicalisation' plays out differently in the South African context in the sense that modalities of violence in the public healthcare sector are often entangled with a lack of technocratic surveillance and medico-pharmacological interventions. While still broadly rooted in a medical approach, Black birth givers are subject to a different materialisation and optics of power in which invisibility and the lack of technology and monitoring become conduits of violent and distressing relations (Chadwick, 2018). Particular kinds of racist, colonial, and capitalist histories of power interact with medicalisation to produce different modes of birth violence.

More conceptual work thus needs to be done to consider whether the positioning of birth violence as specifically rooted in obstetric medicalisation (even if intersectionally stratified) is the best approach in theorising such forms of violence. What is potentially lost or absent from this overwhelming focus on obstetric institutions, practitioners, and practices? Are efforts to highlight the 'obstetric' nature of birth violence in danger of vilifying technology and framing medical interventions as inherently oppressive? As mentioned, the vocabulary of 'obstetric violence' emerged in obstetric contexts that are highly interventionist. While the definition provided by Perez D' Gregorio (2010) does acknowledge both the use of unnecessary technologies and their absence (when medically needed) as violations, implicit in the conceptualisation is the assumption that 'natural' is best and that efforts to intervene or tranform these 'natural processes' are problematic. As such, implicit in the framework is the idea that non-interventionist modes of birth are ideal and that medical technology should only be applied in situation of 'need'. Entangled in the conceptual lexicon of obstetric violence is a tendency towards technophobia, which potentially marginalises those birthers who choose to opt out of 'natural birth' and find empowerment in medical technologies (Chadwick, 2018). It also fails to recognise the potential violence of the natural (see Emre, 2018) and the ways in which forcing birthers to labour without the free availability of pain-relief, medical intervention, and caesarean section, also amounts to birth violence. As such, more theoretical work needs to be done to explore the complex entanglements between technology, birth violence, biocapitalist medicalisation, and choice. Theorisations of obstetric violence rooted in different transnational and southern contexts (such as South Africa and India) will have different angles, vantage points, perspectives, and insights. These need to be regarded as generative resources as we work towards further developing obstetric violence frameworks. We also need to work towards the articulation of a feminist politics of birth and a critique of birth violence that rejects gynocentrism, the valorisation of 'the natural', uncritical technophobia, *and* that is able to critique and push back against exploitative uses of medical technologies and interventions.

Conclusion

While 'obstetric violence' has been increasingly recognised as a problem in healthcare facilities across geopolitical contexts, there is continued social resistance to thinking of pregnancy, birth, and mothering as sites of (state, medical, socio-economic, gendered, racialised, relational) violence. Many medical professionals and professional associations remain hostile to the rhetoric of 'obstetric violence', and while laws against such violence exist in several Latin American countries, in practice these laws have not been very effective (Kohut, 2020). Feminist scholars have argued that 'obstetric violence' is a form of gender violence against women, which is rooted predominantly in patriarchal social and biomedical relations (Shabot, 2016; Wolf, 2013). Others have emphasised the intersectional dimensions of this violence and the ways it is neces-sarily entangled with racism, ableism, and other forms of structural inequality (Chadwick, 2018; Dixon, 2015). This concluding section argues that obstetric violence is all of these things but is also rooted in (historical, ideological, and transnational) capitalocentric formations. As such, obstetric violence needs to be theorised from an anti-capitalist feminist perspective. Until we recognise the roots (and routes) of such violence in the historical, structural, and affective formations of (patriarchal and racial) capitalism, we will not be able to grasp the logic and complexities of obstetric violence. We will not improve, successfully 'humanise', or radicalise birthing and reproduction more broadly until these labours are fully recognised and respected as life-making work, which is integral and foundational to human societies. Trying to fix obstetric violence and toxic maternal healthcare by targeting individual healthcare providers as problematic and/or punishing individual perpetrators, is not sufficient (see Chapter 9, this volume). Instead, gestation and birthing work needs to be fundamentally recognised and respected as life-making labour. It also needs to be radically reorganised against capitalist profit motives and the individualising, naturalising, stratifying, and desocialising tendencies of capitalocentric medical machineries (Chadwick, forthcoming).

As Marxist feminists have argued (Federici, 2004; Lewis, 2019; Mies, 2014), the degradation of reproductive labour (although always in a stratified sense), is foundational to capitalist social relations; reproductive violence is thus endemic to (racial and patriarchal) capitalism. Silvia Federici (2004) has shown that the rise of capitalism was commensurate with the intensification of efforts to police and regulate reproduction, and to criminalise abortion and contraception use among women in Europe/England. Epistemic authority and control over reproductive processes (as far as possible) were historically and traditionally the realm of women caregivers and healers, birth workers (e.g. midwives), and herbalists, both in Europe, and in the indigineous communities of the Americas, Africa, Asia, and Australasia. This epistemic authority was systematically (and violently) destroyed over hundreds of years by a combination of forces, including: patriarchal and racial capitalism, colonialism, and medicalisation. While feminist scholars such as Federici (2004) have shown that working-class, marginalised, and low-income women in England/Europe were subject to violence (e.g. criminalisation, witch-hunts, and hanging) for social transgressions and/or enacting forms of sexual and reproductive autonomy (i.e. using contraceptives, abortifacients, or practicing gestational healing and birth work), the reproductive labours of enslaved women and colonial subjects in the

'New World' were commodified, exploited, coerced, and violently appropriated (Hartman, 2016; Sharpe, 2014; Weinbaum, 2019). A systemic attack on reproductive labour, particularly on visceral acts/ refusals of procreativity and procreative autonomy (i.e. pregnancy, birthing, abortion, contraception), and a struggle for epistemic control over reproduction and gestationality, was apparent across a range of transnational contexts, and involved the entangled (and at times contradictory) forces of medical science, racism, coloniality, and patriarchy, and capitalocentric forms of social and economic relations. In our efforts to theorise obstetric violence, we need to pay more attention to these entangled socio-economic, historical, and ideological relations.

While the patriarchal, racialised, colonial, and misogynist over-tones of the historical remaking of birthing and birth work into medical affairs must not be minimised or lost, it is also crucial that we recognise the ways in which birth has been territorialised and redefined by the logics of profit (see also Chapter 9, this volume). The commodification of birth work (i.e. midwifery and obstetrics) has always been a central aspect of capitalist medicalisation. The history of obstetrics and gynaecology is deeply entangled with racial capitalism and coloniality (Bridges, 2011; Hoberman, 2012; Owens, 2017). We know that the historical origins of gynaecology, for example, are rooted in violence against Black women (Owens, 2017). Reproductive medicine (i.e. obstetrics and gynaecology) are thus in many senses founded upon and rooted in violence. This requires acknowledgement. Rather than aberrational acts, violence is foundational to the organisation of birth (and gestation) under capitalism. Capitalist and stratified modes of medicalisation are also deeply entangled with profit-motives. While individual medical practitioners practice with different motives and values (and many are caring and supportive), the capitalist-medical machinery is (as larger epistemic and sociomaterial ensemble) founded upon the degradation of life-making and actively enables and reproduces reproductive and birth violence. While the vocabulary of 'obstetric violence' has been critical to the recognition and articulation of multiple modalities of birth violence and their roots in systems of power, future efforts to conceptualise and develop the theoretical lexicon must direct more attention to a critique of transnational capitalism and recognise that violent relations towards acts/refusals of procreative life-making are intrinsic to the reproduction of transnational racial (and patriarchal) capitalisms.

References

Adewuya, A., Ologun, Y., and Ibigbami, O. (2006). Post-traumatic stress disorder after childbirth in Nigerian women: prevalence and risk factors, *BJOG: An International Journal of Obstetrics and Gynecology*, 113, 284–8.

Arney, W. (1982). *Power and the Profession of Obstetrics*. Chicago: Chicago University Press.

Arms, S. (1977). *Immaculate Deception: A New Look at Women and Childbirth in America*. New York: Bantam Books.

Baker, S., Choi, P., Henshaw, C., and Tree, J. (2005). 'I felt as though I'd been in jail': experiences of maternity care during labour, delivery, and the immediate postpartum, *Feminism and Psychology*, 15:3, 315–42.

Barbagallo, C. (2019). Another way home: slavery, motherhood and resistance. In C. Barbagallo, N. Beurat, and D. Harvie (eds), *Commoning with George Caffentzis and Silvia Federici*, 176–91. London: Pluto Press.

Bateman, C. (2014). Dismal obs/gynae training contributing to maternal deaths – Motsoaledi, *South African Medical Journal* 104:10, 656–7.

Beckett, K. (2005). Choosing cesarean: feminism and the politics of childbirth in the United States', *Feminist Theory* 6:3, 251–75.

Bohren, M. A., Vogel, J. P., Hunter, E. C., Lutsiv, O., Makh, S. K., Souza, J. P., Aguiar, C., Coneglian, F. S., Diniz, A. L. A., Tuncalp, O., and Javadi, D. (2015). The mistreatment of women during childbirth in health facilities globally: a mixed-methods systematic review, *PLoS Medicine* 12:6, e1001847.

Bohren, M. A., Vogel, J. P., Tuncalp, O., Fawole, B., Titloye, M. A., Olutayo, A. O., Oyeniran, A. A., Ogunlade, M., Metiboba, L., Osunsan, O. R., and Idris, H. A. (2016). By slapping their laps, the patient will know that you truly care for her: a qualitative study on social norms and acceptability of the mistreatment of women during childbirth in Abuja, Nigeria, *SSM Population Health* 2, 640–55.

Bradley, S., McCourt, C., Rayment, J., and Parmar, D. (2016). Disrespectful intrapartum care during facility-based delivery in sub-Saharan Africa: a qualitative systematic review and thematic synthesis of women's perceptions and experiences, *Social Science and Medicine* 169, 157–70.

Bradshaw, D., Dorrington, R., and Laubscher, R. (2012). Rapid Mortality Surveillance Report 2011. South African Medical Research Council, Cape Town.

Bridges, K. (2011). *Reproducing Race: An Ethnography of Pregnancy as a Site of Racialization*. Berkeley, CA: University of California Press.
Castro, R. and Erviti, J. (2003). Violations of reproductive rights during hospital births in Mexico. *Health and Human Rights* 7:1, 90–110.
Chadwick, R. (2016). Obstetric violence in South Africa, *South African Medical Journal*, 106:5, 423–4.
Chadwick, R. (2017). Ambiguous subjects: obstetric violence, assemblage and South African birth narratives, *Feminism and Psychology* 27:4, 489–509.
Chadwick, R. (2018). *Bodies that Birth: Vitalizing Birth Politics*. London: Routledge.
Chadwick, R. (2019). Good birth narratives: diverse South African women's perspectives, *Midwifery* 77, 1–8.
Chadwick, R. (forthcoming). Visceral acts: gestationality as feminist figuration. *Signs*.
Chadwick, R., Cooper, D., and Harries, J. (2014). Narratives of distress about birth in South African public sector maternity settings: a qualitative study, *Midwifery* 30:7, 862–8.
Chattopadhyay, S., Mishra, A., and Jacob, S. (2018). Safe, yet violent? Women's experiences with obstetric violence during hospital births in Northeast India, *Culture, Health and Sexuality* 20:7, 815–29.
Cindoglu, D. and Sayan-Cengiz, F. (2010). Medicalization discourse and modernity: contested meanings over childbirth in contemporary Turkey, *Health Care for Women International* 31:3, 221–43.
Collins, P. H. (1990). *Black Feminist Thought: Knowledge, Consciousness, and the Politics of Empowerment*. New York: Routledge.
Cosslett, T. (1994). *Women Writing Childbirth: Modern Discourses of Motherhood*. Manchester: Manchester University Press.
D'Ambruoso, L., Abbey, M., and Hussein, J. (2005). Please understand when I cry out in pain: women's accounts of maternity services during labour and delivery in Ghana, *BMC Public Health* 5, 140.
Davis, D. (2019). Obstetric racism: the racial politics of pregnancy, labor, and birthing, *Medical Anthropology* 38:7, 560–73.
Diaz-Tello, F. (2016). Invisible wounds: obstetric violence in the United States, *Reproductive Health Matters* 24, 56–64.
Dick-Read. G. (1933). *Natural Childbirth*. London: Heinemann.
Dick-Read, G. (1942). *Childbirth Without Fear: The Principles and Practice of Natural Childbirth*. London: Heinemann.
Diniz, S. and Chacham, A. (2004). 'The cut above' and the 'cut below': the abuse of caesareans and episiotomy in Sao Paulo, Brazil *Reproductive Health Matters* 12:23, 100–10.
Dixon, L. (2015). Obstetrics in a time of violence: Mexican midwives critique routine hospital practices, *Medical Anthropology Quarterly* 29:4, 437–54.

Dutton, J. and Knight, L. (2020). Reproducing neglect in the place of care: normalised violence within South African midwifery obstetric units, *Agenda* 34:1, 14–22.

Elmir, R., Schmied, V., Wilkes, L., and Jackson, D. (2010). Women's perceptions and experiences of a traumatic birth: a meta-ethnography, *Journal of Advanced Nursing*, 2142–53.

El-Nemer, A., Downe, S., and Small, N. (2006). 'She would help me from the heart': an ethnography of Egyptian women in labour, *Social Science and Medicine* 62, 81–92.

Emre, M. (2018). All reproduction is assisted. *Boston Review*, Forum VII https://bostonreview.net/forum/merve-emre-all-reproduction-assisted. Accessed 1 December 2021.

Esposito, N. (1999). Marginalized women's comparisons of their hospital and free-birth center experiences: a contrast of inner-city birthing systems, *Health Care for Women International*, 20:2, 111–26.

Federici, S. (2004). *Caliban and the Witch: Women, the Body and Primitive Accumulation.* New York: Automedia.

Forssén, A. (2012). Lifelong significance of disempowering experiences in prenatal maternity care: interviews with elderly Swedish women, *Qualitative Health Research* 22:11, 1535–46.

Garcia, L. (2020). A concept analysis of obstetric violence in the United States of America, *Nursing Forum* 53, 634–63.

Goer, H. (2010). Cruelty in maternity wards: fifty years later, *The Journal of Perinatal Education* 19:3, 33–42.

Hanson, C. (2004). *A Cultural History of Pregnancy: Pregnancy, Medicine and Culture, 1750–2000.* Basingstoke: Palgrave Macmillan.

Hartman, S. (2016). The belly of the world: a note on Black women's labours, *Souls* 18:1, 166–73.

Herr, R. (2014). Reclaiming third world feminism: or why transnational feminism needs third world feminism, *Meridians* 12:1, 1–30.

Hoberman, J. (2012). *Black and Blue: The Origins and Consequences of Medical Racism.* Berkeley, CA: University of California Press.

Jacobson, N. (2009). Dignity violation in health care, *Qualitative Health Research* 19:11, 1536–47.

Jasen, P. (1997). Race, culture, and the colonization of childbirth in Northern Canada, *Social History of Medicine* 10:3, 383–400.

Johnson, C. (2016). *Maternal Transition: A North-South Politics of Pregnancy and Childbirth.* New York: Routledge.

Kitzinger, S. (1992). Birth and violence against women: generating hypotheses from women's accounts of unhappiness after childbirth. In H. Roberts (ed.), *Women's Health Matters*, 63–80. London: Routledge.

Kohut, M. (2020). Latin America ponders how to fight 'obstetric violence'. *The Economist.* www.economist.com/the-americas/2020/05/21/

latin-america-ponders-how-to-fight-obstetric-violence. Accessed 9 September 2020.

Kruger, L. M. and Schoombie, C. (2010). The other side of caring: abuse in a South African maternity ward, *Journal of Reproductive and Infant Psychology* 281, 84–101.

Lappaman, M. and Swartz, L. (2019). Rethinking obstetric violence and the 'neglect of neglect': the silence of a labour ward milieu in a South African district hospital, *BMC International Health and Human Rights* 19:30, 1–11.

Leavitt, J. (1986). *Brought to Bed: Childbearing in America, 1750–1950*. New York: Oxford University Press.

Lewis, S. (2019). *Full Surrogacy Now: Feminists against Family*. London: Verso.

Loudon, I. (1992). *Death in Childbirth: An International Study of Maternal Care and Infant Mortality, 1800–1950*. Oxford: Clarendon Press.

Lugones, M. (2007). Heterosexualism and the colonial/modern gender system, *Hypatia* 221, 186–209.

Mathai, M. (2011). To ensure maternal mortality is reduced, quality of care needs to be monitored and improved alongside increasing skilled delivery coverage rates, *BJOG: An International Journal of Obstetrics and Gynaecology* 118:s2, 12–14.

Mies, M. (2014). *Patriarchy and Accumulation on a World Scale: Women in the International Division of Labour*. London: Zed Books.

Mihret, M. (2019). Obstetric violence and its associated factors among postnatal women in a specialized comprehensive hospital, Amhara region, Northwest Ethiopia, *BMC Research Notes* 12, 600.

Mohanty, C. (1988). Under western eyes: feminist scholarship and colonial discourse, *Feminist Review* 30, 61–88.

Mohanty, C. (2002). 'Under western eyes' revisited: feminist solidarity through anticapitalist struggles, *Signs* 28:2, 499–535.

Moffit, P. (2004). Colonization: a health determinant for pregnant Dogrib women, *Journal of Transcultural Nursing* 15:4, 323–30.

Nilsson, C. (2014). The delivery room: is it a safe place? A hermeneutic analysis of women's negative birth experiences, *Sexual & Reproductive Healthcare* 5:4, 199–204.

Oparah, J. and Bonaparte, A. (eds) (2015). *Birthing Justice: Black Women, Pregnancy and Childbirth*. New York: Routledge.

Owens, D. (2017). *Medical Bondage: Race, Gender, and the Origins of American Gynecology*. Athens, GA: University of Georgia Press.

Perez D'Gregorio, R. (2010). Obstetric violence: a new legal term introduced in Venezuala, *International Journal of Gynecology and Obstetrics* 111, 201–2.

Pickles, C. (2015). Eliminating abusive 'care': a criminal law response to obstetric violence in South Africa, *SA Crime Quarterly* 54, 5–15.

Pickles, C. and Herring, J. (eds) (2019). *Childbirth, Vulnerability and Law: Exploring Issues of Violence and Control.* London: Routledge.

Ravaldi, C., Skoko, E., Battisti, A., Cericco, M., and Vannacci, A. (2018). Sociodemographic characteristics of women participating to the LOVE-THEM (Listening to Obstetric Violence Experiences through Enunciations and Measurements) investigation in Italy, *Data in Brief* 19, 226–9.

Rothman, B. (1982). *In Labor: Women and Power in the Birth Place.* New York: W.W. Norton & Company.

Rudey, E., Leal, M., and Rego, G. (2020). Caesarean section rates in Brazil: trend analysis using the Robson classification system, *Medicine (Baltimore)*, 99:17, 1–7.

Sadler, M., Santos, M. J., Ruiz-Berdun, D., Rojas, G. L., Skoko, E., Gillen, P., and Clausen, J. A. (2016). Moving beyond disrespect and abuse: addressing the structural dimensions of obstetric violence, *Reproductive Health Matters* 24, 47–55.

Schiebinger, L. (2013). *Nature's Body: Gender in the Making of Modern Science.* New Brunswick, NJ: Rutgers University Press.

Searle, C. (1965). *The History of the Development of Nursing in South Africa 1652–1960: A Socio-historical Survey.* Pretoria: The South African Nursing Association.

Shabot, S. (2016). Making loud bodies 'feminine': a feminist-phenomenological analysis of obstetric violence, *Human Studies* 39:2, 231–47.

Shabot, S. (2018). Domesticating bodies: the role of shame in obstetric violence, *Hypatia* 33:3, 384–401.

Sharpe, C. (2014). In the wake, *The Black Scholar* 44:2, 59–69.

Shorter, E. (1982). *A History of Women's Bodies.* New York: Basic Books.

Smith-Oka, V. (2013). Managing labor and delivery among impoverished populations in Mexico: cervical examinations as bureaucratic practice, *American Anthropologist* 115:4, 595–607.

Smith-Oka, V. (2015). Microaggressions and the reproduction of social inequalities in medical encounters in Mexico, *Social Science and Medicine* 143, 9–16.

Spangler, S. (2011). 'To open oneself is a poor woman's trouble': embodied inequality and childbirth in south-central Tanzania, *Medical Anthropology Quarterly* 25:4, 479–98.

Swahnberg, K., Thapar-Björkert, B., and Berterö, C. (2007). Nullified: women's perceptions of being abused in health care, *Journal of Psychosomatic Obstetrics and Gynecology* 28:3, 161–7.

Thomson, G. and Downe, S. (2008). Widening the trauma discourse: the link between childbirth and experiences of abuse, *Journal of Psychosomatic Obstetrics and Gynecology* 29:4, 268–73.

Varcoe, C., Brown, H., Calam, B., Harvey, T., and Tallio, M. (2013). Help bring back the celebration of life: a community-based participatory study of rural Aboriginal women's maternity experiences and outcomes, *BMC Pregnancy and Childbirth* 13:1, 1–10.

Weinbaum, A. (2019). *The Afterlife of Reproductive Slavery: Biocapitalism and Black Feminism's Philosophy of History*. Durham, NC: Duke University Press.

Wolf, A. (2013). Metaphysical violence and medicalized childbirth, *International Journal of Applied Philosophy* 27:1, 101–11.

World Health Organization (2010). The global numbers and costs of additionally needed and unnecessary caesarean sections performed per year: overuse as a barrier to universal coverage. Background paper, 30, 1–31.

9

Individuals, institutions, and the global political economy: unpacking intentionality in obstetric violence

Sreeparna Chattopadhyay

Just another day in a labour ward in rural India

On a pleasant December morning a few years ago, my colleague, an obstetrician, and I, an anthropologist, visited a busy teaching hospital in a disadvantaged district in south India.[1] The hospital is located more than 200 kilometres away from the nearest metropolitan city. It is a 750-bed tertiary facility with 10 beds allocated to obstetrics and gynaecology, which also handles complicated referrals. Our plan was to interview physicians, nurses, and interns involved with deliveries to understand the drivers of disrespectful and abusive behaviour that pregnant women routinely encounter in public facilities in India.[2] This public facility was newly (and hurriedly) constructed to coincide with the state elections, as proof of the ruling party's prioritisation of health. It was a large eight-storeyed building, where several empty rooms, peeling plasters, and already damp walls were telling us a story that did not spell unqualified success. Of the two sets of elevators, one was out of order and the other was so busy that we found it easier to climb the stairs to the fourth floor where the labour room was located. We noticed walls stained with *pan* (betel-leaves eaten with areca nut in some parts of India) along the staircase and commented on how quickly public infrastructure becomes decrepit in India from a lack of regular cleaning and intractable behaviours like public spitting.

My colleague headed to the pre-eclampsia ward to speak to doctors while I walked into a large room with eight beds which functioned as the labour and recovery ward for women who had uncomplicated, normal births. I had been examining obstetric violence for over four years and this was my second stint at fieldwork. I was accustomed to the smells, sights, and sounds in the labour ward – the pungent aroma that is often a cocktail of blood, fluids, and antiseptic, the sight of labouring women in a state of undress with seldom a curtain to guard their privacy, and their whimpers of pain. Plastic buckets filled with body fluids stood guard, next to thin metal beds with skinny mattresses. Bloodied and tired surgical instruments lay on trays on side tables, having ushered new lives into this world. Doctors and nurses often moved at break-neck speeds, rarely pausing to catch breath, especially if women in active stages of labour occupied all available beds, while irritably trying (and often failing), to mollify anxious relatives awaiting their turn for an update outside the room.

I pulled up a chair at the far end of the well-lit room and said a quiet prayer of gratitude that there were only three women in the room that morning. The hospital allowed pregnant women inside the labour ward only after they were nearly fully dilated because of space constraints. Until then they laboured in the neighbouring room, which had beds more closely spaced together and allowed relatives to attend, unlike the labour ward, which as the attending obstetrician Dr Vikas[3] remarked, was a 'relative-free' zone. Typically four to five relatives or 'attendants' in local terms accompanied pregnant relatives and insisted on staying in the room. But this was a constant source of irritation for healthcare providers who believed that relatives needed to be kept at bay, otherwise they interfered with medical decision making. But relatives were needed for various tasks – to procure prescribed medications from private sources when government pharmacies didn't have them, which happened often enough; to arrange for blood when the blood bank did not have their type, and also to donate their own blood to substitute one unit that they took, which was the informal requirement in most institutions; and to care post-delivery. I observed that relatives, though well-meaning, often tested providers' patience, stretching already exhausted personnel by repeated questions since they had limited understanding of western biomedical practices.

Doctors needed relatives to 'counsel' women into medical compliance. Sometimes providers invited female relatives into the labour room to encourage a woman to push, if she was exhausted, or to apply fundal pressure (pressure on the abdomen) to speed up the birth. The latter is an iatrogenic practice, but is still widely used in many Indian facilities (Sharma, et al., 2019). However, most providers, except for staff nurses, typically do not admit to using fundal pressure. Pregnant women had little autonomy, and providers typically consulted husbands or, in their absence, fathers, and obtained consent from them for procedures. From my decade-long experience conducting observations in Indian hospitals, I knew this wasn't particular to pregnant women but rather individuals inhabiting the sick role.

Dr Vikas was from a nearby town and had finished his first medical degree at a medical college in north-east India. Since we had common ground because of my familiarity with north-east India, conversation flowed freely. Dr Vikas often commented about under-development in north-east India compared to south India, which he thought was responsible for poor outcomes in the former. Recounting his experience of his first maternal death he said 'We could do nothing to save her. I felt so bad. Such a young life, lost because of delay'. The first-time adolescent mother had died from haemorrhage due to obstructed labour.[4]

While Dr Vikas had a thriving private practice, he attended the teaching hospital as a favour to a politically well-connected friend. He complained about the patient load and the absence of good infrastructure in the hospital. From our observations and interviews we knew that the hospital lacked basic facilities like hand soap and disinfectant for cleaning. In the middle of one conversation, I noticed that a heavily pregnant women had walked in, complaining of pain to the nurse. She directed him to Dr Vikas who dismissed her pain and began an internal exam by rudely asking her to take off her *salwar* (loose trousers worn by women in South Asia) and panties, took details of how many past births she had (three), and signalled for the staff nurse to get her ready for the operating theatre and to inform her 'attendants'. While I surmised from the exchange that she would have a c-section, Dr Vikas did not share this information with her; nor was she prepped mentally for the internal exam that he had just finished. Her clothes suggested that she belonged to a religious minority. I did not know why Dr Vikas was disrespectful towards her – whether it was because she had multiple children or belonged to a religious minority or she was poor, or that was his general demeanour with all the users of the facilities, or a combination of these or something else.

Soon after, Dr Vikas grumbled about how many 'poor and illiterate' patients he had to attend to in this facility in contrast to the institution in the more developed Indian state where he completed his postgraduate training. While he marvelled at the public health infrastructure and clinical competency of healthcare personnel in that state, he also complained about patients being too demanding. He reported that they did not tolerate even small slips and were quick to take the offending personnel to task. For example, he conducted a cervical smear on a patient who complained about being in pain first to him. When he wasn't responsive, she formally complained to the Chair of the Department. He said, partly in jest but also seriously, that the training in that facility had prepared him for his patients in private practice who demanded greater accountability from providers.

Doctors in the teaching hospital had a very large patient load because it was the largest tertiary hospital at the border of two states in a poor area that received complicated and emergency referrals. On a different day, we had followed one such patient – Mrs P, barely an adult, and a first-time mother, who had been referred by the attending doctor, a paediatrician from a community health centre (CHC) in a rural area, 40 kilometres from the tertiary facility. We had seen her labouring for several hours in that rural CHC, with a female relative, a staff nurse, and an *ayah* (hospital helper) assisting her. This CHC had one room for births, and another with five beds for post-partum women. Other than deviating from medical protocol where with three centimetres dilation, the staff nurse was asking her to push the baby, we did not observe any instances of abuse or discrimination against Mrs P at the CHC. The CHC did not have an obstetrician on duty on that day because she was able to visit only three times a week since they dumped other 'duties' on her such as sterilisation camps in the district. The paediatrician did not want to risk a complicated birth or a maternal death, a possibility because the CHC did not have a blood bank or facilities for a c-section, both of which he believed Mrs P would need. After a few hours of labouring, an ambulance drove Mrs P to the tertiary facility where we caught up with her. The next day when we visited the hospital, we saw that she had given birth to a healthy baby, vaginally, but did need one unit of blood. The paediatrician was correct in his risk assessment. However, had there been a blood bank at the CHC, which there should according to government mandates for CHC infrastructure, and Mrs P has been allowed to labour normally, she could have given birth closer to her home, instead of being transported to an unfamiliar place far away, birthing alone. While providers at the tertiary facility often complained about CHCs not being 'able to handle even simple cases', the shortage of personnel and infrastructure meant that the outcomes for even so called low-risk patients were unpredictable. Dr Vikas' patient load was especially high because the tertiary facility, being a new medical college, did not (yet) offer postgraduate training programmes in obstetrics to recent medical graduates, such as an MD or a DNB, mandatory qualifications in India for an obstetrician. Had this cadre been present, much of the work of instructing interns, handling patients, and the daily uncomplicated clinical work in the labour ward would have fallen to them and Dr Vikas' expertise and experience would be called on only for complicated cases.

On one occasion, I noticed that Dr Vikas reprimanded a male intern who was part of a group doing a two-week rotation in gynaecology. The intern was conducting a pelvic exam incorrectly and Dr Vikas said, 'don't keep putting one finger, then another. Examine the cervix, write your observations. Just because it is lose enough for one finger, don't put another finger to try to see whether that fits or not'. He also instructed them on how to identify high risk 'patients', so that timely treatment can avoid obstetric emergencies. I noticed that he was more actively engaged in teaching male interns than female interns. Female interns were often left to communicate with the patients, as if being female meant that this had naturally become their role in the busy labour ward.

Providers reported that many women who visited this tertiary care facility were 'unbooked' patients. Unbooked patients are women who arrive at the hospital for the first time during delivery or are referred by other facilities or because it is an emergency. Providers must often make quick and intuitive assessments about whether pregnant women could need blood transfusions based on their clinical judgements (checking the eyes or skin for pallor). Over 50% of Indian women enter pregnancy with anaemia (NFHS-4, 2014–2015). India has the highest global burden of anaemia in terms of absolute numbers of women and children who are anaemic, despite efforts to improve haemoglobin levels (through fortification and supplementation) (Nguyen et al., 2018). Sometimes unbooked women did not know their blood type, which made it difficult to reserve blood, even when blood banks were available at the facilities. Furthermore, unbooked women did not have a prior relationship with the providers, affecting rapport and communication during labour. This facility, as the largest tertiary facility in a poor, rural area, attracted a large number of unbooked women who had multiple intersectional disadvantages – poor, migrant workers, or those from nomadic tribal communities or religious communities. This is common in many Indian public tertiary facilities, where most women who arrive to give birth are vulnerable, unbooked women (Bangera et al., 2020; Madan et al., 2020), and many have poor obstetric outcomes, often due to a lack of antenatal care, high levels of anaemia, postpartum haemorrhage, eclampsia, or other complications (Bulsara et al., 2019). In such cases there isn't enough documentation or time to ensure that tenets of respectful care such as good communication and patient autonomy can be adhered to. Unbooked women were often the most vulnerable of all pregnant women, and these contextual constraints had direct and indirect impacts on the probability of encountering unconsented care and the routinisation of disrespectful behaviour.

Some providers at this facility complained that women's families strategically used government facilities – using private care for antenatal visits but delivering at a state facility because private providers (either correctly or for profiteering) recommended a caesarean birth. This infuriated state providers because they viewed it as an opportunistic use of government entitlement by users – that these users could pay for care but chose not to spend the additional money required for a c-section delivery in a private clinic. While technically not unbooked, providers said that these families were reluctant to share prior medical information because they expected to be reprimanded for gaming the system. Dr Vikas said a c-section in a sub-standard private clinic in the area would cost at least 700 USD, almost equivalent to the annual income of a family in that area. Even with the inevitable out-of-pocket expenses that patients incur for drugs and consumables in public facilities in India, c-section costs are much lower in state hospitals. Childbirth in private facilities is on average nine times more expensive and can lead to catastrophic medical expenses that can impoverish families (Tripathy et al., 2017).

It wasn't apparent to me that state providers were aware of these issues and this influenced their attitudes and behaviours towards some pregnant women.

Individual responsibility, institutional constraints, and systemic problems

This vignette demonstrates that several factors particular to the Indian context, and perhaps other low- and middle-income country (LMIC) contexts drive disrespectful and abusive care. Women in LMICs experience multiple forms of disrespectful and abusive behaviour, including verbal or physical, unconsented care, poor communication, withholding pain relief medications, deviating from established medical protocols, and coercion around contraception immediately after birth. Some of these are rooted in provider bias against a group of users based on their social identities (Perera et al., 2018). Disempowered groups, who are often the users of state facilities, may not recognise certain behaviours as disrespectful and may either normalise them or feel unable to challenge them (Sen et al., 2018). Linguistic and cultural barriers between providers and users can also lead to disrespectful care, particularly in institutions like the one described here, which are multilingual, with users possessing low literacy levels and who potentially misunderstand medical advice, frustrating overworked health providers. Weak accountability systems within these institutions imply that there are few redressal mechanisms for aggrieved groups (Sen et al., 2020).

Another cluster of factors that influence the likelihood of experiencing obstetric violence are linked to institutional cultures and constraints – the ways in which labour rooms are designed and the 'internal logic of the institution', often driven by structural constraints such as a lack of nurses or helpers, create situations where male relatives arranged for consumables, robbing women of privacy in labour wards in urban (state) facilities in India (Madhiwalla et al., 2018). Also, the organisation and practices of western biomedical obstetrics in LMICs like India with a hierarchical and a punitive system imply that there is little mentoring and interprofessional learning, but plenty of blaming and distrust between different cadres of providers. Female staff nurses often informally 'teach' interns in most public facilities, especially in rural India, where they also conduct deliveries alongside interns given the perennial shortage of obstetricians in these areas. Yet they are not acknowledged, and must defer to the authority of physicians because of rigid professional and gender hierarchies within institutions. In many LMICs like India, the social determinants of health are not embedded in the medical education curriculum. Disrespectful practices are reproduced through formal and informal learning channels in top-down institutions where heads of departments hold unquestioned authority, normalise such behaviour which are imbibed by generations of health providers (Sen et al., 2018). While unconsented care, lack of autonomy, organisational hierarchy, and the internal logic of western biomedical practice that are arranged and managed for the convenience of providers and institutions are common experiences for women in both LMICs and high-income countries, the biomedical and non-clinical complexities that providers have to tackle in an LMIC context are vastly different given the large numbers of unbooked women and/ or women who are chronically malnourished with serious anaemia and who are also the group more likely to have poor obstetric outcomes.

Problematising obstetric violence as a conceptual category

Given these important contextual differences, we need to question whether obstetric violence as an overarching conceptual category is helpful for describing all forms of poor care that pregnant women experience in contexts like India. Obstetric violence has animated feminists for more than fifteen years, especially in Latin American countries, where the term first emerged to describe specific forms of abuse, violence, and discrimination that women, especially low-income, indigenous, or Black women experienced in these countries. Sadler et al. (2016), translating from the Spanish, define obstetric violence as:

> The appropriation of women's body and reproductive processes by health personnel, which is expressed by a dehumanising treatment, an abuse of medicalisation and pathologisation of natural processes, resulting in a loss of autonomy and ability to decide freely about their bodies and sexuality, negatively impacting their quality of life.

This definition explicitly makes health personnel responsible for perpetrating obstetric violence. However, as a recent special issue on obstetric violence in the journal *Violence Against Women* indicates, there isn't consensus on this in LMICs like South Africa. Lappeman and Swartz (2021) argue that as a conceptual category obstetric violence or its counterparts (for example the concept of gentle violence in Chadwick, 2018) is unhelpful in changing care provision in South Africa because it overemphasises provider responsibility and intentionality and puts women in a permanent state of disempowerment in relation to providers. In response, many feminists have argued that the 'silence' of women in labour wards or labouring alone must be categorised as a form of obstetric violence (Salter et al., 2021). Swartz and Lappeman (2021: 5) in their rejoinder contended that blaming individual providers is counterproductive and in fact using obstetric violence in this manner is a form of epistemic violence because it is blind to the contextual realities in many non-western settings. Instead they suggest using a feminist ethics of care that is attentive not to 'who is good and who is bad, but how different kinds of relational engagements and interventions may lead to different outcomes in terms of the welfare' of mothers and infants. While scholarship and activism in countries like Venezuela have demanded that obstetric violence be criminalised and recognised as a form of gender-based violence, these (and other) debates suggest that obstetric violence is a highly divisive term, pitting healthcare providers and scholars in the global south against Euro-American feminists.

Why has obstetric violence become so polarising and why the sudden interest in it? Firstly, as Sen et al. (2018) posit, current research and policy interest in examining disrespectful care during childbirth have been partly triggered by a systematic engagement by the World Health Organization (WHO)'s Department of Reproductive Health, especially the 2014 statement that has led to a flurry of empirical work in LMICs. The WHO, however, expects that we should use the term Respectful Maternity Care (RMC), under the ambit of quality of care, while recognising that it is a human rights violation and suggests that 'abuse' should be replaced by 'mistreatment', 'a term that is not only more acceptable and less provocative, but further separates the issues from individual intentionality and links it to the realm of healthcare quality' (Sen et al., 2018: 8). While RMC allows for provider buy-in, it also conceals intentional examples of disrespectful care and masks socio-economic inequalities that create asymmetric relationships between users and providers of maternity services.

Secondly, in many LMICs, particularly in South Asia and sub-Saharan Africa, which have the highest burdens of maternal death, institutional births were massively scaled between 2010 and 2020. This expansion has typically followed a western blueprint where western biomedical interventions, physicians, and nurses have been empowered, but traditional birth attendants and home-based births have been actively discouraged in a bid to promote 'safe births'. It is worth acknowledging that in many LMIC contexts, western biomedicine has a fundamentally colonial origin, which explains some of the distrust and asymmetric power relationships in these systems and, as discussed earlier, western biomedicine has the tendency to embed, routinise, and normalise disrespectful behaviours into the system.

In recent times, labour room violence, disrespectful and abusive care, (lack of) RMC, and poor quality of care have all been used to describe women's negative childbirth experiences. The Sapir-Whorf hypothesis suggests that labels are important – these terms are not interchangeable and each may convey a different reality and influence our perception of that reality (Werner, 1994). Figure 9.1 shows that each term is political and polarising to a different degree. While I do not intend to precisely depict the degree of polarisation or politicisation of each term, and have joined some together for categorisation, the picture clarifies that these debates are not settled and the naming and meanings ascribed to these experiences depend on who's doing the naming, what's the agenda, and for whom is this being done?

Following Swartz and Lappeman (2021), I argue for a feminist ethic of care that can be applied to RMC for LMICs like India where health systems and user characteristics are so vastly different from western countries that they require a different framework. I argue that a feminist ethic of care must do two things: firstly engage with a process of *re-centring*, moving away from the rather instrumental ways in which many stakeholders have approached this issue. Secondly, it needs to be firmly embedded within feminist and decolonial approaches that not only make individual providers or institutions accountable, but uncover historical and transnational

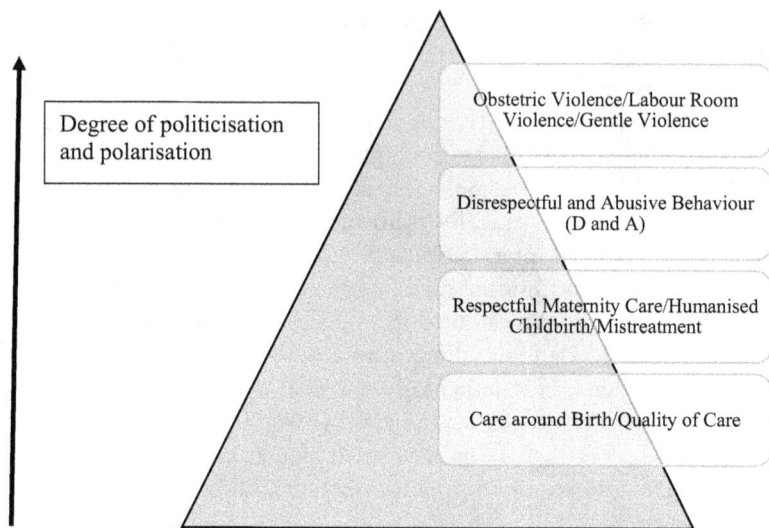

Figure 9.1 The politicisation and polarisation of obstetric violence

forces that have shaped both discursive and material practices around respectful care and maternal health more generally, with spill-over effects on the propensity to encounter obstetric violence. To do this, we need to i) unpack ways by which institutional births became normative; ii) analyse the current practices that engage (or not) with respectful care and identify the reasons; iii) imagine possibilities that do not reproduce the problems of the current systems of care.

Unpacking the trajectory of institutional births in India

Before 2005, less than half of all Indian babies were born in facilities, and the majority of rural Indian women had home births (Joe et al., 2018: 649). The slow move towards institutional deliveries was disconcerting to many, with warnings like, 'it will take until 2025, for half of all rural births to be institutional and mid-century before 75% coverage is reached' (Kesterton et al., 2010: 7). Recent figures prove that these fears were unfounded, with over 75% of all births in most Indian states now occurring in institutions. The Government of India (GoI) launched the National Rural Health Mission (NRHM) in 2005 with the goal of providing safer, good quality maternal and child health services, and also sponsored the Janani Suraksha Yojana, a scheme that financially incentivised deliveries in state institutions through conditional cash transfers to pregnant mothers and healthcare workers (WHO, 2008). The private sector is a small player where deliveries are concerned, especially in rural India, and the majority of low-income Indian women have births in state facilities because private births can be prohibitively expensive. Notwithstanding inter-state, intra-state, inter-district, and intra-district disparities in facility births, currently nearly all pregnant women in south India, and the majority of urban Indian women, deliver in facilities, and the expansion of institutional access has occurred at a stunning rate for rural India (NFHS-5, 2019–2021).

Why did institutional births become such a pressing priority for India? Why weren't other programmes, such as strengthening the midwifery and Traditional Birth Attendant programmes or scaling up the training of Auxiliary Nurse Midwives (ANMs), who were less expensive than nurses and physicians and were already embedded in the system, considered seriously? Why were there no significant efforts to reduce the inequitable risks of maternal deaths by geography, caste, class, and other stratifiers by focusing on improving income and livelihood support, increasing age at marriage for women by expanding educational and work opportunities for them, so that these inequities can be addressed (Qadeer, 2005)? India has one of the highest numbers of underage marriages (UNICEF, 2019) and consequently early childbearing with its subsequent effects on adolescents, one of the lowest (and diminishing) participation of women working in paid employment (World Bank, 2019) and, while levels of acute poverty have diminished, anaemia and malnutrition continue to be persistently high (OPHI, 2020). All of these have biological, medical, psychological, economic, and social impacts for women in the reproductive age group, including their ability to negotiate better care for themselves and the probability of experiencing disrespectful or abusive care.

There was a wealth of evidence around what matters for maternal and child health before the NRHM was established in 2005 and before institutional deliveries achieved scale. Studies had indicated: that low-income or tribal women experienced disrespectful care, which encouraged home births (Soman, 1997); that consistent and good quality ante-natal care encouraged women to have institutional births (Sugathan et al., 2001); and that even in rural and remote areas while 45% needed emergency medical attention, primarily post-partum, which could be delivered at home by trained health workers, 15.3% needed access to emergency institutional obstetric care because of life-threatening complications, consistent with WHO expectations (Bang et al., 2004).

I argue that there are two major reasons why India moved towards institutional deliveries along with other technocratic fixes such as Iron Folic Acid (IFA) supplementation – which have done little to address problems like anaemia over the years, a major cause of poor maternal health outcomes – as the silver bullets to tackle maternal deaths in the country, with clear knock-on effects for obstetric violence and poor quality of care that we see in institutional deliveries today. The first is embedded in the colonial and early postcolonial history of institutional births in India, the development of modern biomedicine that empowered physicians trained in western medicine, rather than traditional midwives (Chattopadhyay and Jacob, 2022). The second is linked to the emphasis placed by transnational Global Health Initiatives (GHIs) on Evidence Based Advocacy, which has narrowed safe motherhood to a limited set of measurable outcomes (Storeng and Béhague, 2014) and naturally deprioritises women's experiences of childbirth since these cannot be easily enumerated, spliced, and analysed into neat charts and figures, notwithstanding valiant attempts to measure quality of care during deliveries in recent years (Brizuela et al., 2019).

In pre-colonial India, childbirths occurred at home facilitated by *dais* (traditional midwives). Modern biomedicine made incursions into India for two reasons: firstly, colonial governments were forced to reckon with tricky inheritance issues that emerged, when a (male) baby, also a potential heir died during childbirth. When the first lying-in hospitals were established through the auspices of the Lady Dufferin Fund in 1885, they were primarily intended for, and used by, women of landed families (Forbes, 2005: 123). Secondly, while European female doctors found employment difficult at home, it was possible to find work in colonies like India where there was a reluctance for women to seek intimate medical care from male doctors (Guha, 1998). Colonial-era interventions did not try to strengthen *dais*, instead viewing them as 'dirty', 'unclean', and 'ignorant', posing risks to mothers and babies, a view that persisted into the postcolonial period (Lang, 2005). British attempts to modernise the Indian system were supported by many Indian reformers as well as upper-class Indians and slowly a dominant discourse privileging western bio-medicine emerged (Guha, 1998).

Yet home birthing continued after Independence, which led to the Bhore committee (an important health committee formed in the 1940s) to recommend that *dais* be integrated into the new modern Indian healthcare system. But this did not find much traction because of the new postcolonial government's anxieties, partly fuelled by western discourses around 'population explosion' in India so that a target-driven family planning programme, inimical to women's reproductive rights, took centre stage instead of human rights oriented reproductive reforms (Qadeer, 1998). The second phase of India's Reproductive and Child Health Programme excluded *dais* and stopped their training (Sharma, et al., 2013), in favour of biomedically trained doctors and nurses through Skilled Birth Attendant training, increasing access to emergency obstetric care to prevent deaths from post-partum haemorrhage, infections, and obstructed labour along with the rapid scaling of institutional access.

One reason for the deterioration of the quality of care in under-resourced state facilities is due to the mismatch between demand for biomedical care and the ability of the system to supply quality services (Chattopadhyay et al., 2018). Except for Kerala and Tamil Nadu in south India, which have better quality primary healthcare and a robust system of accountability (Balabanova et al., 2013; Das Gupta et al., 2020), in most Indian states, there has been a flight towards private healthcare in areas outside of maternal healthcare because of both real and perceived improvements in the quality of care in the sector (Mohanty and Kastor, 2017). It is not as if women do not experience unconsented care or medically unnecessary and costly interventions in private facilities such as c-sections. However, due to the customer orientation of these institutions, and competition from other providers, users are often treated more politely and feel more empowered to demand respectful care (Bruce et al., 2015). These developments suggest that those users who may have had the most social, cultural, and economic capital to demand greater accountability from state institutions have moved to the private sector, weakening these institutions, and allowing them to become less responsive to complaints of poor care (Drèze and Sen, 2013). Nevertheless, there is agreement that the GoI's scaling of institutional births has reduced maternal and neonatal deaths, especially for disadvantaged women who need emergency obstetric care (Altman, et al., 2017).

In recent years, it may seem as if the scope of India's maternal health strategy has widened through its focus on RMNCH+A (Reproductive, Maternal, Neonatal, Child Health and Adolescents), launched in 2013 during the National Summit on Call to Action for Child Survival and Development 'guided by the central tenets of universal care, entitlement and accountability (there has been) ... a renewed emphasis on high-impact health interventions and addressed strengthening of healthcare services especially in the poor-performing geographies of the country' (Taneja et al., 2019: 2). This programme used maternal mortality ratios, safe deliveries (equated to institutional births), infant mortality rates, immunisation rates, fertility rates, and contraceptive prevalence rates to identify 184 high-priority districts. The Ministry of Health and Family Welfare with local and international partners such as the US Agency for International Development (USAID) created a 5 x 5 matrix comprising monitoring indicators for reproductive, maternal, neonatal, child, and adolescent health. However, in this tool just one component was not a technocratic intervention in maternal health, that is, incentivisation of Auxiliary Nurse Midwives for home deliveries. Joint GoI and USAID funded programmes like Vriddhi evaluated the availability of essential medicines and commodities, and practices in the labour room such as recording foetal heart rate, partographs to monitor labour, administering uterotonic after birth, and using magnesium sulfate to manage eclampsia. While all of these contribute to reducing maternal and neonatal mortality, they are biomedically derived clinical indicators, and none concern the behavioural aspects of RMC.

The GoI recognises that poor quality of care is a serious problem, especially since institutional births have been scaled. In December 2017, the GoI launched the ambitious Labour Room Quality Improvement Initiative (LaQshya) programme. LaQshya in many Indian languages means a goal or an objective. The preamble to the 144-page document drafted by the Minister of Health and Family Welfare states:

> Every pregnant woman and her family desires to have a joyful birthing experience with a safe and healthy mother and new-born. The Ministry

of Health and Family Welfare is committed to supporting the public health system in creating such an environment within the health facilities to ensure every mother and her new-born are cared for most appropriately and that such care is respectful of the woman and her family. (GoI, 2017: 5)

While this seems promising, as we go down the chain of command, elements of RMC keep getting diluted in the document. For example, two rungs down, the Additional Secretary and Mission Director says, 'A transformational improvement in the quality of care around child-birth relating to intra-partum and immediate post-partum care can dramatically improve maternal and newborn outcome' with an emphasis on the cognitive development of babies. By the time it reaches the Programme Officer, who is also the Deputy Commissioner of Maternal Health, LaQshya has been reduced to a set of targeted interventions with checklists that medical college hospitals and other facilities should implement and the word 'respect' or 'RMC' is altogether absent. If this emphasis has been lost within the official document, one can only imagine its further dilution during the implementation stage in primary health centres, the smallest institutional unit where rural women have uncomplicated births.

This is not to deny that the scope of LaQshya includes respectful care – LaQshya prohibits certain procedures such as routine shaving of pubic area, enemas, episiotomies, and fundal pressure and encourages providers to allow a birthing companion, privacy, psychosocial support for the mother by providers, and a choice of labour position. However, the scope of LaQshya is so ambitious with 160 items in a checklist for labour rooms and over 100 items for the operating theatre, and an impossible 12-month implementation period, that it is likely that clinical components and infrastructural upgradation will be prioritised over changing attitudes, building provider competencies, or changing medical education around RMC.

Instrumentalising women's health: the role of global health initiatives

Several studies have highlighted the links between disrespectful behaviour and obstetric complications (Bhattacharya and Ravindran, 2018; Raj et al., 2017) and between 10% and 100% prevalence rate of disrespectful and abusive during births in India (Ansari and

Yeravedkar, 2020; Jungari et al., 2019). However, most studies typically do not include qualitative tools and use the term obstetric violence/labour room violence, with the exception of two empirical Indian studies (Chattopadhyay et al., 2018; Goli et al., 2019). It appears that, generally, global health practitioners prefer to use the more depoliticised and therefore more palatable RMC with clear measurable elements, instead of the more political and feminist term obstetric violence as a descriptor for poor birth experiences. The tendency to characterise abuse that women experience during labour as RMC instead of obstetric violence is reminiscent of the ways by which GHIs used Evidence Based Advocacy to narrow safe mother-hood to a set of measurable indicators and technocratic interventions such as a single disease focus, immunisations, IFA supplementation, antibiotics, and hospital-based births (Béhague and Storeng, 2008; Storeng and Béhague, 2014; Storeng, 2014).

Béhague and Storeng's trenchant critique reveals that dominant GHIs, particularly those funded by the Gates Foundation and the USAID, became so powerful that they not only changed the discursive, but also the material practices, including practical interventions for Safe Motherhood Initiatives (SMIs). While GHIs greatly expanded the resource base available to global health practitioners, policies were guided by cost-effectiveness, an audit-based system of govern-ance, and a narrowing of what qualified as evidence, including the use of experimental methods such as randomised controlled trials, which were expected to identify and measure factors to reduce maternal mortality. This approach seems puzzling because there is a mountain of evidence that demonstrates that mothers and infants die during or soon after childbirth, not only due to an absence of technologically driven commodities such as immunisations or antibiot-ics, but also due to inequities emanating from within and outside of health systems. Further, research has shown that the risks of dying during childbirth were not shared equally by all women, even in wealthy countries such as the US.[5]

Béhague and Storeng argue that in its early years, SMIs, drawing from the 1994 Beijing ICPD Conference, embedded feminist advocacy that emphasised poor maternal health as an outcome of gendered, classed, racialised, and other forms of intersectional inequities. But when funders started mandating that SMIs statistically prove the effectiveness of interventions, SMIs were compelled to change strategies, such as including neonatal and child health within the ambit of maternal health, emphasising the negative spill overs of maternal deaths such as macroeconomic losses to the economy and the household, and indirect impacts on children's health when mothers died during childbirth, despite recognising that this strategy narrowed their focus considerably.

Evaluations of programmes like Vriddhi demonstrate that in many Indian states with weak health systems, and a constant shortage of skilled personnel and poor infrastructure, implementing targeted interventions is problematic (Jayakumar et al., 2018). It is noteworthy that obstetric violence does not appear anywhere in Vriddhi's evaluation, and abuse appears only once in the context of RMC, which the authors acknowledge is a 'nascent' concept in India. In fact, Vriddhi's Care around Birth approach seems to be focused on reducing infant and maternal mortality through Technical Intervention Packages aimed at building provider competencies on routine obstetric and newborn interventions. The evaluators' admission that 'There is no evidence to support the inference that improved quality of services will lead to reductions in mortality and morbidity without concomitant efforts to reach the most vulnerable who are furthest from care' (Jayakumar et al., vii), indicate that despite recognising that poor health outcomes are inextricably linked to inequities, organisations like USAID invest most of their resources in uncontroversial, technical measures that can be delivered, measured, and evaluated so they can be fed back into the policy and programme implementation cycle, for this to be repeated again.

Vousden et al. (2020: 1087), in their multicountry intervention to tackle maternal mortality using a randomised controlled trial, precisely the method that GHIs prefer, concluded:

> Our data suggest that the vast majority of deaths occurred in hospital, despite relatively good availability of resources, probably through a combination of women who arrive too unwell to benefit from emergency care, women with complications who could have been treated with timely effective interventions and women who develop serious complications whilst in hospital.

While in recent years GHIs like GAVI (Global Vaccine Alliance) have expanded to strengthen health systems, acknowledging that the successful delivery of commodities is only possible within a well-functioning system, Storeng argues that the interpretation is far removed 'both conceptually and ideologically from earlier, broader reinterpretations of health systems, particularly, the commitment to publicly funded health systems' that were enshrined in the Alma-Ata Declaration of 1978 (2014: 866). Such an instrumentalist approach towards women's health is not new – we see a similar framing of the problem of domestic violence, especially within global health where domestic violence seems intervention worthy only because of its impacts on a range of outcomes, including reproductive health, HIV/AIDS risks, child immunisation and nutrition status, and myriad development outcomes in LMICs (Yount et al., 2011; Mukanangana et al., 2014; Patrikar et al., 2017). It is as if centering *women* in women's health does not qualify as a valuable developmental agenda unless there are negative impacts on their abilities to reproduce healthy offspring, families, communities, and the nation state.

I believe that a similar set of events appear to be unfolding in the contested terrain around the naming of obstetric violence, disrespect, and abuse or mistreatment of women. A dominant section of the global health community, particularly those funded by wealthy international organisations may deploy the rhetoric of gender equity in theory, but in practice follow a depoliticised, number-centric approach. Engaging with issues of violence and discrimination that women encounter during childbirth would require an epistemic overhaul – moving away from solution-centric approaches to foregrounding power asymmetries not only between providers and users of health services, but the organisation of care in its most expansive sense.

The giving and receipt of care is highly gendered and classed, both within households and within health systems. In India, like elsewhere, women are the primary caregivers in their households; yet resources such as food, healthcare, and education, and opportunities are not distributed equally between male and female children. Some of these decisions are made by women not necessarily as victims of patriarchy, but because such decisions can potentially strengthen their positions in a deeply misogynistic system (Kandiyoti, 1988). Within health systems, women tend to have the least paid, and most laborious roles, and rarely occupy leadership positions that permit real decision-making power. However, female health workers' disempowerment does not automatically translate into empathy and sensitivity for female users – several studies show that midwives and nurses are often disrespectful and/or abusive in both LMICs and in high-income countries (Amole et al., 2019; Chattopadhyay et al., 2018; van der Pijl et al., 2020).

A different model

Shaheed Hospital, established in 1983 in the central Indian state of present-day Chhattisgarh, the largest producer of iron ore in India, may offer a different model for respectful care, not limited to maternal health alone. Chhattisgarh state has a long history of tribal dispossession through extractive industries like mining, is highly militarised with poor human development indicators and, since 1967, has been at the centre of anti-state violent struggle by Maoist and/or Naxalite groups. The hospital is located in a town with a large steel plant – the Bhilai Steel Plant, and there are several mines on the outskirts that serve as the primary source of employment.

In the 1970s and 1980s, when work conditions were deplorable, a labour movement began to advocate for contractual workers. Shankar Guha Niyogi, a trade union activist provided inspiring early leadership to the Chattisgarh Mukti Morcha, which fought to improve the working conditions of contractual workers and their healthcare (Video Volunteers, 2017). Though an outsider, he had worked as a miner and was married to a local tribal miner. During that period, a pregnant miner who was also the vice-president of the union died during childbirth because she was refused entry into the Bhilai Steel Plant hospital for being 'a dirty mine worker' (PSBT, 00:14:00–00–15:00). This incident, along with the workers' movement, became the springboard for the establishment of a small clinic, which started with just 2000 Rupees (roughly equivalent to 40,000 Rupees in current value or USD 530) in a disused garage with a few committed doctors and miners trained as voluntary health workers. The clinic subsequently became a 120-bed hospital through financial contributions and the labour of workers, and possessed a single capital asset, a truck that paid for the running expenses of the hospital.

Instead of importing a capital-intensive model, Shaheed Hospital emphasised community health education, training workers to become frontline health workers, and providing generic medicines in a system that was not overly biomedicalised. There were several formal and informal ways in which the ethic of care was deeply embedded in their model, both between patients and between providers and patients – a nurse reported that lactating mothers were urged to nurse infants of malnourished new mothers as an act of generosity, and none had ever refused (PSBT, 0043:00–0045:00). In its formative years, Dr Kundu, the only surgeon reported donating blood for a pregnant woman during an emergency c-section for obstructed labour (PSBT, 0046:00–0048:00). Despite its need, the hospital only accepts individual contributions from workers and donors and refuses funding from any domestic or international organisations, presumably because such aid might come with strings attached.

Khare and Varman (2017) in an analysis argue that Shaheed Hospital succeeded because of systems of leadership and governance, accountability, financing, a social determinants of health framework, and a rights-based ideology of health. Unlike other institutions with huge economic and cultural distance between health providers and users, at Shaheed Hospital, the doctors were moved by left-wing causes and had opted to work in this disadvantaged area. Frontline healthcare workers such as nurses were recruited from the local population. Health promotion messages clarified the links between the larger political economy and poor health, and active worker health committees created robust accountability systems. The hospital had minimal charges for beds and laboratory testing, as well as for normal deliveries and c-sections because it did not follow a profit-oriented model of healthcare. Hospital users were treated with respect and while Shaheed Hospital was not able to completely erase medical hierarchy, it was more flexible than other institutions. Most health workers were paid the same whether they were cleaners or pharmacists and the wage gap between doctors and other workers were minimal (PSBT, 2016). Further, they allowed harmless cultural practices such as consumption of herbal beverages by new mothers, and warm compresses for neonates, while educating against harmful traditional practices such as throwing away colostrum.

But the hospital has begun to decline since the 1990s for several reasons – firstly in 1991, Niyogi was murdered by a local businessman when he began to organise workers outside of mining. Secondly, Dr Jena reported that 'Shaheed Hospital was founded through a social movement rooted in workers' wellbeing and the weakening of the movement means that it has become much harder to get volunteers and health providers who want to live there for more than four to six years' (Video Volunteers, 2017: 7:30–8:00 minutes). Simultaneously during the 1990s–2000s, the GoI introduced mandates related to medical education such as formal nursing degrees for nursing staff, that only qualified obstetricians could conduct c-sections, and others which affected resourcing of health personnel. Formally qualified providers were both prohibitively expensive and scarce for organisations like Shaheed Hospital. A recent video showed over-crowding at the hospital, though the providers still provide respectful and quality care (Video Volunteers, 2017).

The successes and failures of Shaheed Hospital demonstrate the possibilities for a model of healthcare provision that is neither market oriented nor state funded, but an outcome of collectivisation. However, such models are often hard to scale, and with huge changes in the macroeconomy, including standardisation of provider qualifica-tions, the institution may not have the ability to absorb these shocks. However, what it does demonstrate is that low-cost healthcare rooted in social epidemiology is possible when embedded within social movements such as those for workers' rights. It allows us to think of the ways in which advocates for ending obstetric violence can align themselves with other collectives so that the problem of poor treatment during childbirth is viewed as an extension of wider discriminatory practices within and outside of health systems, which are also interwoven with the domestic and the transnational politics of global health. Such solidarities will foreground women in women's health, rather than instrumentalising outcomes for children, families, communities, and countries.[6]

Conclusion

In this chapter, I argue that while it is helpful to conceptualise obstetric violence as a type of gender-based reproductive violence, not all forms of mistreatment, neglect, or poor quality of care that women encounter in Indian health facilities or similar LMIC contexts can be helpfully captured using the term obstetric violence. It is important to develop multiple categories to describe levels of mistreatment that inhere in the care that women receive during childbirth because the genesis of such poor treatment varies significantly. While individual providers must continue to be held responsible if they abuse women during childbirth or discriminate against them, the question remains as to how we apportion blame when the perpetrator(s) are amorphous like transnational GHIs that have done little to address the fundamental causes of poor maternal health such as poverty and poor nutrition and have only recently started engaging with quality of care because of its impacts on infant and maternal mortality. While the term slow violence, drawing from Nixon's work on environmental pollution found resonance for some scholars, or the term structural violence has been used to emphasise elements of the local political economy that disadvantage (some) women in the context of childbirth, they cannot fully capture the complex exchanges between local policies and global and transnational initiatives, which may be well-intentioned but do not tackle the fundamental causes of poor health. Unlike the dumping of environmental toxins, where organisations are cognisant of the consequences of their actions, though they may unfold over a much longer period of time, I am not confident that nebulous entities like transnational GHIs and especially the engagements with local health systems, themselves a product of colonial governance and postcolonial inequities in many LMICs, possess complete knowledge of the consequences of their actions, or in some instances the absence of their interventions in areas which matter for maternal health and the quality of care that pregnant women receive.

The focus on technocratic fixes such as iron folic acid supplementation, even if they are ineffective, is politically expedient, cost-effective, and is influenced by both the logic of the market and a culture of accounting, which privileges a specific form of knowledge categorising it as 'evidence' that can be fed back into the policy cycle. It also limits our imagination, vocabulary, and taxonomy of what is needed and possible for just and equitable health. Tsing, writing about the importance of the different forms of environmental activism in Indonesia makes an important observation 'Difference within common cause: Perhaps this is more important than we ordinarily think' (Tsing, 2004: 246). Pluralising the debate around obstetric violence and disrespectful care will ultimately be productive in identifying the mechanisms by which local, transnational, and global forces create visible and invisible force fields within which concerns over women's health are articulated and concretely addressed or alternatively invisibilised. Rather than restricting ourselves to apportioning blame to institutions, intentions, and providers, it is important to imaginatively build solidarities between advocates and movements for ending disrespectful and/or abusive care and other social movements in LMIC contexts that focus on social justice.

Notes

1 To retain the anonymity of the providers and the institution, I have concealed the name of the state and the district where the fieldwork was undertaken but have provided supplementary information. This district was in a state in the southern part of India, which has better human development indicators than north or north-east India. However, the district had several markers of disadvantage – higher infant deaths, lower immunisation rates, lower female literacy rates, higher levels of landlessness, water shortage and regular droughts, shortage of public infrastructure such as clean drinking water, lack of access to public health infrastructure, and several tribal groups (Scheduled Tribes) living in remote areas of the district. These were some of the reasons that contributed to large disparities in health outcomes within the district.

2 The study was conducted when I was employed by the Public Health Foundation of India and was funded by the Bill and Melinda Gates Foundation to understand the institutional drivers of mistreatment during childbirth using mixed methods. While the overall scope had been decided, I had a significant role to play in selecting districts, constructing research instruments, and fieldwork. I am no longer formally affiliated with the institution, and research and publications continue at the time of writing.

3 Not his real name.

4 Post-partum haemorrhage and factors associated with obstructed labour contribute to more than half of all maternal deaths in India. The risks of death are higher for women if they live in rural areas, belong to a marginalised group, and also are not part of health schemes that provide good prenatal care (Horwood et al., 2020).

5 Owens and Fett (2019) argue that the legacy of slavery and continued systemic and systematic violence, plus racism that Black communities experience in the US have contributed to disproportionately high rates of maternal and infant mortality among Black mothers.

6 I use the word woman to mean females who have been born with the X and the Y chromosomes and are capable of biological reproduction.

While trans women in the distant future may be able to birth children through uterine transplants, such procedures currently remain in the realm of theory (Maron, 2016).

References

Altman, R., Sidney, K., De Costa, A., Vora, K., and Salazar, M. (2017). Is institutional delivery protective against neonatal mortality among poor or tribal women? A cohort study from Gujarat, India, *Maternal and Child Health Journal* 21:5, 1065–72.

Amole, T. G., M. J. Tukur, S. L. Farouk, and A. O. Ashimi (2019). Disrespect and abuse during facility based childbirth: the experience of mothers in Kano, Northern Nigeria, *Tropical Journal of Obstetrics and Gynaecology* 36:1, 21–7.

Ansari, H., and Yeravdekar, R. (2020). Respectful maternity care during childbirth in India: a systematic review and meta-analysis, *Journal of Postgraduate Medicine* 66:3, 133.

Balabanova, D., Mills, A., Conteh, L., Akkazieva, B., Banteyerga, H., Dash, U. Gilson, L., et al. (2013). Good health at low cost 25 years on: lessons for the future of health systems strengthening, *The Lancet* 381:9883, 2118–33.

Bang, R. A., Bang, A. T., Hanimi Reddy, M., Deshmukh, M. D., Baitule, S. B., and Filippi, V. (2004). Maternal morbidity during labour and the puerperium in rural homes and the need for medical attention: a prospective observational study in Gadchiroli, India, *BJOG: An International Journal of Obstetrics & Gynaecology* 111:3, 231–8.

Bangera, T. R., Bhavani, K., Padmavathi, T. Anuradha (2020). Comparative study of outcome of high risk pregnancies in unbooked and booked cases in tertiary care centre, *IAIM* 7:1, 53–60.

Béhague, D. P. and Storeng, K. T. (2008). Collapsing the vertical–horizontal divide: an ethnographic study of evidence-based policymaking in maternal health. *American Journal of Public Health* 98:4, 644–9.

Bhattacharya, S. and Sundari Ravindran, T. K. (2018). Silent voices: institutional disrespect and abuse during delivery among women of Varanasi district, northern India, *BMC Pregnancy and Childbirth* 18:1, 1–8.

Brizuela, V., Leslie, H. H., Sharma, J., Langer, A., and Tunçalp, Ö. (2019). Measuring quality of care for all women and newborns: how do we know if we are doing it right? A review of facility assessment tools, *The Lancet Global Health* 7:5, e624–32.

Bruce, S. G., Blanchard, A. K., Gurav, K., Roy, A., Jayanna, K., Mohan, H.L., Ramesh, B. M., Blanchard, J. F., Moses, S., and Avery, L. (2015).

Preferences for infant delivery site among pregnant women and new mothers in Northern Karnataka, India, *BMC pregnancy and Childbirth* 15:1, 1–10.

Bulsara, N. M. and Bhatia, S. G. (2019). Study of feto-maternal outcome of pregnancy in booked versus unbooked patients, *Indian Journal of Obstetrics and Gynecology* 7:2, 190–5.

Chadwick, R. (2018). *Bodies that Birth: Vitalizing Birth Politics*. London: Routledge.

Chattopadhyay, S., and Jacob, S. (forthcoming). 'Oils, Oxytocin, and Obstetrics: Narratives of Changing Birth Practices in India, *South Asia Research* 42:3.

Chattopadhyay, S., Mishra, A., and Jacob, S. (2018). 'Safe', yet violent? Women's experiences with obstetric violence during hospital births in rural Northeast India, *Culture, Health and Sexuality* 20:7, 815–29.

Das Gupta, M., Dasgupta, R., Kugananthan, P., Rao, V., Somanathan, T.V., and Tewari, K. N. (2020). Flies without borders: lessons from Chennai on improving India's municipal public health services, *The Journal of Development Studies* 56:5, 907–28.

Drèze, J. and Sen, A. (2013). *An uncertain glory: the contradictions of modern India*. London: Allen Lane.

Forbes, G.H., 2005. *Women in Colonial India: Essays on Politics, Medicine, and Historiography*. New Delhi: Orient Blackswan.

GoI (2017). LaQshya Guidelines National Health Systems Resource Centre Technical Support Institute with National Health Mission. http://qi.nhsrcindia.org/cms-detail/laqshya-guidelines/MjI4. Accessed 18 November 2021.

Goli, S., Dibyasree, D., Chakravorty, S., Siddiqui, M. Z., Ram, H., Rammohan, A., and Sheel Acharya, S. (2019). Labour room violence in Uttar Pradesh, India: evidence from longitudinal study of pregnancy and childbirth, *BMJ Open* 9:7, e028688.

Guha, S. (1998). From dais to doctors: the medicalisation of childbirth in colonial India. In *Understanding Women's Health Issues: A Reader*. New Delhi: Kali for Women.

Horwood, G., Opondo, C., Choudhury, S.S., Rani, A., and Nair, M., 2020. Risk factors for maternal mortality among 1.9 million women in nine empowered action group states in India: secondary analysis of Annual Health Survey data, *BMJ Open* 10:8, p.e038910.

Jayakumar, B., Feenstra, M., Ghoston, L., and Raj, F. (2018). Evaluation report USAID/India Vriddhi: Scaling up interventions in RMNSCH+A. Mid-term performance evaluation. Report. USAID. June. https://pdf.usaid.gov/pdf_docs/PA00T556.pdf. Accessed 1 May 2021.

Joe, W., Perkins, J. M., Kumar, S., Rajpal, S., and Subramanian S. V. (2018). Institutional delivery in India, 2004–14: unravelling the equity-enhancing contributions of the public sector, *Health Policy and Planning* 33:5, 645–53.

Jungari, S., Sharma, B., and Wagh, D. (2019). Beyond maternal mortality: a systematic review of evidences on mistreatment and disrespect during childbirth in health facilities in India, *Trauma, Violence, and Abuse*. DOI:1524838019881719.

Kandiyoti, D. (1988). Bargaining with patriarchy, *Gender and Society* 2:3, 274–90.

Kesterton, A. J., Cleland, J., Sloggett, A., and Ronsmans, C. (2010). Institutional delivery in rural India: the relative importance of accessibility and economic status, *BMC Pregnancy and Childbirth* 10:1, 1–9.

Khare, A. and Varman, R. (2017). Subalterns, empowerment and the failed imagination of markets, *Journal of Marketing Management* 33:17–18, 1593–1602.

Lang, S. (2005). Drop the demon dai: maternal mortality and the state in colonial Madras, 1840–1875, *Social History of Medicine* 18, 357–78.

Lappeman, M. and Swartz, L. (2021). How gentle must violence against women be in order to not be violent? Rethinking the word 'violence' in obstetric settings, *Violence Against Women*. DOI:1077801221996444.

Madan, A., Kaur, J., Meena, S., and Puri, A. (2020). Maternal and fetal outcome in multiple pregnancy, *International Journal of Health and Clinical Research* 3:12, 221–6.

Maron, D. F. (2016). How a transgender woman could get pregnant, *Scientific American*, 15 June www.scientificamerican.com/article/how-a-transgender-woman-could-get-pregnant/. Accessed 5 May 2021.

Mohanty, S. K. and Kastor, A. (2017). Out-of-pocket expenditure and catastrophic health spending on maternal care in public and private health centres in India: a comparative study of pre and post national health mission period, *Health Economics Review* 7:1, 1–15.

Mukanangana, F., Moyo, S., Zvoushe, A., and Rusinga, O. (2014). Gender based violence and its effects on women's reproductive health: the case of Hatcliffe, Harare, Zimbabwe, *African Journal of Reproductive Health* 18:1, 110–22.

NFHS-4 (National Family Health Survey, India) (2014–2015). http://rchiips.org/nfhs/nfhs4.shtml. Accessed 18 November 2021.

NFHS-5 (National Family Health Survey, India) (2019–2021). http://rchiips.org/nfhs/factsheet_NFHS-5.shtml. Accessed 18 November 2021.

Nguyen, P. H., Scott, S., Avula, R., Tran, L. M., and Menon, P. (2018). Trends and drivers of change in the prevalence of anaemia among 1 million women and children in India, 2006 to 2016, *BMJ Global Health* 3:5.

OPHI (Oxford Poverty and Human Development Initiative) (2020). https://
ophi.org.uk/global-mpi-report-2020/. Accessed 16 November 2021.

Owens, D. C. and Fett, S. M. (2019). Black maternal and infant health:
historical legacies of slavery, *American Journal of Public Health* 109:10,
1342–5.

Patrikar, S., Basannar, D., Bhatti, V., Chatterjee, K., and Mahen, A. (2017)
Association between intimate partner violence and HIV/AIDS: exploring
the pathways in Indian context, *The Indian Journal of Medical Research*
145:6, 815.

Perera, D., Lund, R., Swahnberg, K., Schei, B., and Infanti, J. J. (2018).
'When helpers hurt': women's and midwives' stories of obstetric violence
in state health institutions, Colombo district, Sri Lanka, *BMC Pregnancy
and Childbirth* 18:1, 1–12.

PSBT (2016). First Cry, Ajay T. G. www.youtube.com/watch?v=I8iI4oQbSXw.
Accessed 16 November 2021.

Qadeer, I. (1998). Reproductive health: a public health perspective, *Economic
& Political Weekly* 2675–84.

Qadeer, I. (2005). Unpacking the myths: inequities and maternal mortality
in South Asia, *Development* 48:4, 120–6.

Raj, A., Dey, A., Boyce, S., Seth, A., Bora, S., Chandurkar, D., Hay K.,
et al. (2017). Associations between mistreatment by a provider during
childbirth and maternal health complications in Uttar Pradesh, India,
Maternal and Child Health Journal 21:9, 1821–33.

Salter, C. L., Abisola Olaniyan, A., Mendez, D. D., and Judy C. Chang,
J. C. (2021). Naming silence and inadequate obstetric care as obstetric
violence is a necessary step for change, *Violence Against Women*. DOI:
1077801221996443.

Sen, G., Iyer, A., Chattopadhyay, S., and Khosla, R. (2020). When accountability meets power: realizing sexual and reproductive health and rights,
International Journal for Equity in Health 19:1, 1–11.

Sen, G., Reddy, B., and Iyer, A. (2018). Beyond measurement: the drivers
of disrespect and abuse in obstetric care, *Reproductive Health Matters*
26:53, 6–18.

Sharma, B., Giri, G., Christensson, K., Ramani KV, and Johansson, A.
(2013). The transition of childbirth practices among tribal women in
Gujarat, India: a grounded theory approach, *BMC International Health
and Human Rights* 13, 41.

Sharma, G., Penn-Kekana, L., Halder, K., and Véronique Filippi, V. (2019).
An investigation into mistreatment of women during labour and childbirth
in maternity care facilities in Uttar Pradesh, India: a mixed methods
study, *Reproductive Health* 16:1, 1–16.

Soman, K. (1997). *Social dynamics of women's health - a study of Bolpur Block in the district of Birbhum.* Unpublished Doctoral Thesis. Jawaharlal University, New Delhi, India.

Storeng, K. T. (2014). The GAVI Alliance and the 'Gates approach'to health system strengthening. *Global Public Health* 9:8, 865–879.

Storeng, K. T. and Béhague, D. P. (2014). 'Playing the numbers game': evidence-based advocacy and the technocratic narrowing of the safe motherhood initiative, *Medical Anthropology Quarterly* 28:2, 260–79.

Sugathan, K. S., Vinod K. Mishra, V. K., Robert D., and Retherford, R. D. (2001). *Promoting Institutional Deliveries in Rural India: The role of Antenatal-Care Services.* Mumbai: International Institute for Population Sciences and Honolulu: East-West Center.

Swartz, L. and Lappeman, M. (2021) Making care better in the context of violence: the limits of blame, *Violence* against women. DOI:1077801221996468.

Taneja, G., Suryanarayana-Rao Sridhar, V., Swarup Mohanty, J., Joshi, A., Bhushan, P., Jain, M., Gupta, S., Khera, A., Kumar, R., and Gera, R. (2019). India's RMNCH+A strategy: approach, learnings and limitations, *BMJ Global Health* 4:3, e001162.

Tripathy, J. P., Shewade, H. D., Mishra, S., Kumar, A. M. V., and Harries, A. D. (2017). Cost of hospitalization for childbirth in India: how equitable it is in the post-NRHM era? *BMC research notes* 10:1, 1–9.

Tsing, A. F. (2004). *An Ethnography of Global Connection.* Princeton, NJ: Princeton University Press.

UNICEF (2019). Ending child marriage: a profile of progress in India. https://data.unicef.org/resources/ending-child-marriage-a-profile-of-progress-in-india/. Accessed 16 November 2021.

van der Pijl, M. SG., Hollander, M. H., van der Linden, T., Verweij, R., Holten, L., Kingma, E., de Jonge, A., and Verhoeven, C. JM. (2020). Left powerless: a qualitative social media content analysis of the Dutch #breakthesilence campaign on negative and traumatic experiences of labour and birth, *PloS one* 15:5, e0233114.

Video Volunteers (2017). Shaheed Hospital: The Story of a Revolution. www.youtube.com/watch?v=2caOJz_lVeU. Accessd 16 November 2021.

Vousden, N., Holmes, E., Seed, P. T., Gidiri, M. F., Goudar, S., Sandall, J., Chinkoyo, S., et al. (2020). Incidence and characteristics of pregnancy-related death across ten low-and middle-income geographical regions: secondary analysis of a cluster randomised controlled trial, *BJOG: An International Journal of Obstetrics and Gynaecology* 127:9, 1082–9.

Werner, O. (1994). Sapir-Whorf Hypothesis, The *Encyclopedia of Language and Linguistics* 7, 3656–62.

World Bank (2019). https://data.worldbank.org/indicator/SL.TLF.TOTL.FE.ZS. Accessed 16 November 2021.

World Health Organization (2008). *Skilled Birth Attendants, Factsheet.* Geneva: World Health Organization.

Yount, K. M., DiGirolamo, A. M., and Ramakrishnan, U. (2011). Impacts of domestic violence on child growth and nutrition: a conceptual review of the pathways of influence, *Social Science and Medicine* 72:9, 1534–54.

Part III

Birth assisted

10

Caste and the stratification of reproductive labour: Dalit feminist voices from the field

Johanna Gondouin, Suruchi Thapar-Björkert, Mohan Rao

Transnational commercial surrogacy and the 'outsourcing' of reproductive labour to women of the global south is arguably the most controversial practice in an expanding market in body parts and reproductive labour. The central role of India in this market represents a particularly challenging example, given the historical symbiosis between reproductive policies and population control in the country. For roughly a decade, India was a hub for commercial surrogacy and 'biocrossings' (Bharadwaj, 2008; Rao and Sexton, 2010), facilitated through the global assemblages of a liberalised capitalist economy. Within this global fertility market, bodies of underprivileged Indian women – formerly seen as 'waste' and their reproduction as something to be 'controlled' (Rao, 2004a; 2010) – were transformed into sites of profit generation within the reproductive industry of the neoliberal Indian state, but still remaining within the frame of 'non-valuable breeders' for the embryos of 'valuable' women (Corea, 1985: 276).

The present bioeconomy operates through gendered bodies, stratified in accordance to hierarchies of class, race, ethnicity and migration status, creating an international division of reproductive labour (Vora, 2008, 2012; Sangari, 2015; Twine, 2015). Indeed, reproduction is in itself stratified, that is, the reproductive choices of privileged women and men are made through the bodies of less privileged women (Gupta, 2006). While previous research on surrogacy has addressed the 'stratified reproduction' (Colen, 1995) of Indian women in terms of class and economic status (Deomampo, 2016; Pande, 2014b; Rudrappa 2015; Vora 2015), the question of caste has received little attention (Madge, 2015). Responding to the lack of research on assisted reproductive technologies (ARTs) and caste, the aim of this chapter is to explore the significance of this intersection with ARTs in general and commercial surrogacy and egg donation in particular. We draw on in-depth interviews with Dalit feminists whose perspectives on ARTs are uncharted. Our analysis explicates the need to connect Dalit women's reproductive lives with broader questions of social inequalities that we theorise through the framework of *reproductive justice*: an understanding which challenges dominant articulations of ARTs centred on *reproductive rights*.

Surrogacy in India: trends and transitions

Surrogacy was legalised in India, a world leading destination for medical tourism (Deomampo, 2016; Pande, 2011; Rudrappa, 2014), in 2002 and benefited from the active promotion by the Indian government (Rudrappa, 2015; Deompampo, 2016). As Amrita Pande (2014a: 13) notes, 'Clinics in India […], not only operate without state interference but often benefit from explicit state support for clinics catering to medical and reproductive travelers'. Low costs, the availability of highly qualified English-speaking medical doctors, women willing to work as surrogates, and the lack of legal regulation surrounding surrogacy arrangements are factors that contributed to India's flourishing fertility industry (Bhatia, 2012; Nayak, 2014).

In 2005, *the National Guidelines for the Accreditation, Supervision and Regulation of ART Clinics in India*, developed by the Indian Council of Medical Research (ICMR) and the Ministry of Health and Family Welfare (MoHFW), were published (ICMR, 2005). However, through cases such as the Baby Manji Yamada case and the Jan Balaz case in 2008 (Saravanan, 2018), insufficient guidelines regarding citizenship of children born through surrogacy or parentage were brought to public attention. Responding to the growing pressure on the Indian government from stakeholders within the ART industry to provide a legal framework, the ICMR and the MoHFW outlined the Draft Assisted Reproductive Technologies (Regulation) Bill and Rules in 2008, which was revised in 2010 and 2013. Both the 2008 and 2010 versions of the draft were criticised for harboring a bias towards the private sector and for promoting the interests of the industry, while failing to address the vulnerability of surrogate mothers (Sama, 2012). The 2013 draft restricted the issuing of surrogacy visas to married couples, thus excluding single and gay parents. The ART (Regulation) Bill 2014, banned foreign nationals from hiring commercial surrogates in India and revoked the provision of a surrogacy visa, progressively clamping down on, and narrowing the scope of, what was legally accepted around ART in India. As a consequence, parts of the business moved to Nepal. However, as Nepal banned its female citizens from being hired as surrogates, but permitted foreign women, Indian and Bangladeshi women were taken to Nepal. A number of highly mediatised cases contributed to the present Indian regulation of surrogacy. One pertains to the 2015 earthquake in Nepal, when the Israeli government arranged a rescue mission to bring back intended parents and their babies from Kathmandu. The complete disregard of the surrogate mothers in the surrounding media coverage is a clear indication of whose bodies matter in this transaction (Kamin, 2015; Shalev et al., 2017).

Almost simultaneously, Thailand, another hub for transnational surrogacy arrangements, banned commercial surrogacy for foreigners in 2015, in the aftermath of the Baby Gammy case and the Mitsutoki Shigeta case in 2014. In 2016, the Indian Surrogacy (Regulation) Bill was approved by the Union Cabinet,[1] which banned all commercial surrogacy, and prohibited foreigners from accessing surrogacy in the country, while permitting altruistic surrogacy for married couples with documented infertility, provided they use a close relative for the procedure (*The Hindu*, 2016). Arguably, the intent of this bill was to prevent the oppression embedded in the idea of 'rent a womb' while simultaneously strengthening cultural nationalism. In the current political landscape, the alliance between neoliberal capitalism and patriarchal Hindutva ideology, represented by the BJP, intertwines 'virulent Islamophobia, caste supremacism and patriarchal values' and 'a commitment to supporting the interests of neoliberal corporate capital through the intensification of gendered processes of exploitation, displacement and dispossession' (Wilson et al., 2018: 2). The implications this has for gendered forms of reproductive labour and structural subordination of women from impoverished and marginalised communities is noteworthy and subject of further investigation.

Reproductive rights vs. reproductive justice

Analysing reproductive work through the lens of reproductive justice means putting the above mentioned structural conditions centre stage. The concept was coined in the 1990s by SisterSong, a US based grassroots collective of women of colour, which situates women's reproductive lives within the broader contexts of social justice and human rights (Ross and Solinger 2017; Ross et al., 2017). As opposed to dominant western discourses on reproductive rights and the associated liberal rhetoric of bodily autonomy and individual choice, the conversation is extended to address how the intersections of race and class have exposed women of colour and their communities to abusive population policies such as forced sterilisation, high-risk contraception, environmental pollution and discriminatory adoption industries and foster care systems (Briggs, 2002; Briggs, 2012). Going beyond the pro-choice/pro-life divide, this perspective highlights how policies on housing, education, living-wages, migration and incarceration shape women's reproductive options. The historical and ongoing violence against Black women's bodies in the US is fundamental for the formation of the reproductive justice movement (Ross and Solinger 2017; Ross et al., 2017). Addressing this legacy, Black legal scholar Dorothy Roberts asks: 'What does it mean that we live in a country in which white women disproportionately use expensive technologies to enable them to bear children, while black women disproportionately undergo surgery that prevents them from being able to bear any?' (Roberts 1996: 944).

Roberts' words illustrate the particular relevance that a reproductive justice approach has to India, where the eugenic and neo-Malthusian notion of 'over-population' has shaped reproductive politics since the early twentieth century. Importantly, neo-Malthusian concerns were transformed into upper-caste anxieties about the lower castes. An upper-caste neo-Malthusian agenda interweaved with the upper-caste agenda of Brahminical Hinduism to reduce women to merely reproductive bodies requiring male control, in a reimbrication of patriarchy (Anandhi, 1998). In the initial debates on birth control, the seamless welding of 'Hindu' with upper castes, and the conflation of upper-caste practices and norms as Hindu was achieved (Rao, 2004b: 3602). Central arguments concerned the reproductive excesses of the lower castes and religious minorities, in particular Muslims.

Thus, in this setting, birth control clearly means 'a selective control by which some births are restricted and others encouraged' (Connelly, 2008: 103). Anandhi points out that several political groups articulated the opposition between 'desexualised' reproductive bodies as the ideal norm of 'respectable' female sexuality and 'sexual bodies' as representing 'immoral' and 'disreputable' sexuality (Anandhi, 1998: 145).

In the cold war period, the international community began to see former colonies, in particular India and communist China, as geopolitical threats. The idea of low-income women's reproduction as wasteful was embraced by both the post-independence Indian state and policy makers in the global north (Rao, 2010; Wilson et al., 2018). Negative eugenics has been aggressively practised in India and targeted towards vulnerable communities. The widespread use and abuse of sterilisation is a case in point, as exemplified by the Chhattisgarh sterilisation scandal in 2014 (Ghose, 2018). With the exception of a short period of forced mass vasectomies between 1975 and 1977, female sterilisation has been the main instrument of India's population policies and has been the most common form of contraception available since the late 1970s (Deomampo 2016: 40). Thus, with the advent of the ART industry, what was formerly considered as waste is now transformed into sites of profit generation.

Framing the conversation: previous research and ARTs

As the emblem of reproductive outsourcing, Indian commercial surrogacy has attracted ample scholarly attention. Feminist ethnographic research has centred on the lived reality of surrogate mothers and highlighted the agency and resistance of women living under constrained and exploitative conditions (Pande, 2014a, 2014b; Rudrappa, 2015; Vora, 2015). This research demonstrates the need to go beyond western moral frameworks of autonomy, choice and coercion for understanding commercial reproductive labour as it is practised in the global south (Bailey, 2011). As an example, Amrita Pande observes that these women explicitly reject the category of choice, speaking instead of *majboori* (a compulsion) and loyalty with their families (Pande, 2014a). Her ethnographic accounts add a complexity which makes it impossible to see surrogacy as either a win-win situation or one that transforms surrogate mothers into passive victims of exploitation.

Building on these insights, scholars have also explored how the larger societal context shapes women's reproductive options. Kalindi Vora (2015) has interrogated Indian surrogacy through the prism of colonial history, arguing that this history offers the conditions of possibility for the present international division of reproductive labour, that is, why some bodies and not others are seen as possible sources of commodification. Gondouin and Thapar-Bjorkert (forthcoming, 2022) analyse policies and practices regulating native women's claim to motherhood of children fathered by European men, during British India, as a legacy of contemporary Indian surrogacy. Some scholars have used a reproductive labour approach, through which ovulation, gestation, pregnancy, child birth and mothering are analysed as value-producing practices within the extractive and exploitative regimes of global capitalism (Cooper and Waldby, 2014; Newman and Nahman 2020; Sunder Rajan, 2007; Vertommen and Barbagallo, 2021; Vertommen et al., 2021; Vora 2015; Waldy and Cooper, 2008; Weinbaum, 2019). Addressing the Indian context more specifically, Amrita Pande (2014a, 2014b) and Sharmila Rudrappa (2015) include India's history of population control and coercive reproductive policies targeted against marginalised communities. Pande interprets the narratives of surrogate mothers through the paradox of an aggressively anti-natalist state becoming a global hub for ART procedures. Rudrappa explicitly rejects the relevance of a reproductive rights approach to investigate the distinct stratifications of Indian society. Instead, she argues for a reproductive justice framework that accounts for 'the endemic social, political and economic inequalities among different communities which shape individual's abilities to access a good life. (Rudrappa, 2015: 170)

The intersectionality of Dalit feminism

The assertions by Dalit feminists in the 1990s have been part of a discourse of dissent in both mainstream women's movements and the male dominated Dalit movement. Sharmila Rege (2018) argues that middle-class, upper-caste women's experience, or alternatively Dalit male experience, became universalised, resulting in 'a masculinisation of dalithood and a savarnisation of womanhood' (Rege, 2018: 1–2;

see also Rege, 1998). Akin to these articulations, one of our research participants, an activist from Bangalore, stated: 'One of the things that I have been doing a lot is critiquing Indian feminists: there is a lack of connect[ion] with real life issues of marginalized women. But the fact is that they are the ones who set the agenda and basically define the issues which feminists talk about in India'.

Dalit feminism implies an interrogation of privilege and discrimination embedded within the Ambedkarian notion of 'Brahminical patriarchy', 'a specific modality of patriarchy' governed by 'a set of discriminatory levels constituting a hierarchical organization of society based on caste, which is quite unique to the Indian subcontinent' (Arya and Rathore, 2020: 8). This "graded inequality" determines the location of all individuals according to caste and gender, with upper-caste men and lower-caste women at the beginning and end of the spectrum. The Ambedkarian understanding of caste positions endogamy as its grounding principle, which makes the control of women central to caste ideology (Rege, 1998: 165; Velayudhan, 2018).

While both Dalit women and caste Hindu women are disempowered by patriarchal practices, Dalit and lower-caste women are more prone to violence as they face oppression at three levels: 1) caste, 2) class and 3) gender (Dutt, 2019; Malik, 1999; Moon, 2000), that is, the triple burden of economic marginalisation (low-wage labourers working for upper-caste landowners as most of the land is owned by upper-caste or upwardly mobile castes), caste discrimination and gender subordination. Our research participants would commonly refer to this 'intersectionality of oppression'. Thus, engaging with a Dalit feminist perspective demonstrates the importance of intersectionality for grasping gender inequality in India, However, prominent feminists such as Nivedita Menon oppose its relevance to Indian feminism (Menon, 2020), which Dalit feminists have perceived as a reluctance on the part of mainstream feminists to acknowledge and address their own caste privilege.

Towards a Dalit feminist standpoint theory

A Dalit feminist standpoint, as elaborated by Rege (2018) and Kanchana Mahadevan (2020), has significant parallels to other feminist standpoint theories (Collins, 2009; Haraway, 1988; Harding, 2004).

Standpoint theory designates the epistemological shift that occurs when marginalised communities gain public voice, and foregrounds the concept of experience. The location of the subject affects the experience and thus the knowledge that it generates. From a Dalit feminist perspective, experience is the origin of knowledge and, like standpoint theories, power is seen as integral to epistemology. The failure of dominant groups to critically interrogate their advantaged situation makes their social position a disadvantaged one for generating knowledge. As stated by one of our research participants, a Dalit journalist: 'we need to articulate women's experience and theory from the perspective of the marginalised sections, which mainstream feminists clearly are not doing. Indian feminists lack an insight or an experience […] the entire perspective that we would bring to the table'. On a similar tack, a social activist among our research participants describes the importance of having worked in the slums: 'my feminist theory sprung from there you know, and my understanding of caste, class, gender came from the slums that I work [in]'. What is emphasised in these narratives is the importance of *lived experience*, a kind of knowledge that has been omitted from traditional epistemologies, which spans over a register that includes feelings and more elusive elements, what Linda Martín Alcoff describes as 'textures' (Alcoff, 1996, 2008: 294).

Grounding knowledge in experience is democratic and provides an alternative to normative understandings. However, this does not imply a belief in unmediated 'authentic' experience. Rather than a subject merely registering the imprint of reality, which then qualifies as knowledge, experience is regarded as a dialectical process of collective articulation by persons belonging to conflicting social locations. As Alcoff elaborates: 'the oppressed do not have an epistemic privilege over understanding oppression generally; they are not more likely, for example, to know the causes of their oppression. However they are more likely to know the lived reality of the oppression, its emotional costs, its subtler manifestations, what it is like to live it' (Alcoff, 2008: 294).

Claiming one's experience as the foundation of knowledge and theory is particularly audacious in the Indian context, where a divide has been instituted between theory ('theoretical Brahmins') and experience ('empirical shudras') (Guru, 2020; Mahadevan, 2020:

229–3). As Cynthia Stephens (2009) suggests, Dalit feminist theoretical claims 'is a conscious effort to break the existing stereotype of Dalit women as mainly activists (doers) who have little to contribute (as thinkers) to ideological discourses in society, politics, governance, ethics, economics, and development'.

There is a risk of subsuming Dalit feminism within dominant feminist discourse through a mere acknowledgement of difference, and making room for 'different voices' from non-hegemonic locations within mainstream feminism (Harding, 2008: 158). If that was sufficient, caste discrimination would be a concern only for Dalit and other lower-caste women, just as feminists of colour reject seeing race as something only they should attend to. Instead, seriously engaging with Dalit feminist perspectives entails challenging the dominant paradigm of thought. The goal is not difference in itself, but the relations of power that it legitimates. In Rege's words, the aim is 'to address the social relations that convert difference into oppression' (Rege, 1998: 157). Here there are significant parallels to Black feminist standpoint theory, which challenges what counts as knowledge. Constructing new knowledge is crucial for empowerment because it provides alternatives to the way things are supposed to be (Collins, 2009: 286). Rege's idea of 'oppositional Dalit feminist pedagogies' resonates with Black feminist thought when she describes that the importance of Dalit women's narratives lies in the potential to destabilise received truths and locate debates in the complexities and contradictions of historical life (Rege, 1998: 133).

Importantly, standpoint theory's rethinking of experience is not an excluding gesture. The 'we' designated by Dalit feminism is an acquired community. Although it may not be possible to 'speak as' or 'for' Dalit women, it is possible to 'reinvent' oneself as a Dalit feminist, which entails rejecting the Brahmanical, middle-class outlook that structures mainstream Indian feminism, and become sensitive to the specific disempowerment created by the intersection of caste, class and gender. Furthermore, as Gopal Guru (2020) points out, the subject of a Dalit feminist standpoint is not homogenous but multiple, heterogeneous, and sometimes even contradictory. While the Dalit feminists in our study offered a different perspective on reproductive labour, our interviews also revealed a significant variety of standpoints within this perspective.

The aim of our study was to understand the respondents' social world through their own perspectives and words. Mohan Rao conducted semi-structured interviews with eleven respondents, which allowed for flexibility to pursue issues brought up by the respondents and sensitivity to their ideas and experiences. All respondents were women who had worked on areas of reproductive health in various capacities – as activists, journalists or academics – who were from the Dalit castes, and were based in the cities of Bangalore and Chennai in Karnataka and Tamil Nadu respectively. These two states share a history of strong Dalit movements and, more importantly, Dalit women's movements, with which all the women interviewed had been involved. It must be mentioned that not all the women identified as Dalit women primarily, some of them, especially the academic, were clear that they were feminists who were also Dalits. The interviews were conducted at locations suggested by our respondents – at their offices, at their homes and in cafés– and all interviews were recorded with their permission. The respondents were recruited through snowballing. The first respondent was aware of the interviewer's work over many years and suggested other respondents, mainly from NGOs and Dalit journalists. Another respondent had worked with the interviewer on a sub-Committee of the National Population Commission a long time back, and suggested other prospective respondents from the Dalit women's movement. The lone academic was an old friend of the interviewer, who had worked on Dalit women's issues with reproduction. In accessing these different networks, we were able to assemble a more heterogeneous sample.

The 'intersectionalit[ies] of oppression': reproductive labour and beyond

The intersections between gender, class and caste, in both their material and cultural dimensions, emerged as decisive – throughout our interviews – for the choices Dalit women make in relation to livelihoods, including reproductive labour. The triple burden of class (economic deprivation and lack of access to income-earning assets), caste (discrimination and threat of caste-related atrocities) and gender (patriarchal subordination), framed the responses of Dalit feminists.

Intersections of caste and class

One of the formative manifestations of caste is its coexistence with class as a system of stratification and social differentiation whereby 'Within a single caste, class identity may influence the use of caste as a strategic resource, just as within a single class, caste identity will affect the way people accumulate and deploy class assets and express their dominance spatially' (Jeffrey, 2001: 232; Chakravarti, 2018). The intertwining of caste and class often leads to a dominance of higher castes in white collar professional occupations while Dalits, and in our specific context, Dalit women, are confined to the least attractive jobs, including manual scavenging and sanitation, which one of our respondents described as a 'huge human rights violation'. As Gopal Guru reiterates, 'The Indian state ... could not offer more dignified alternative vocations for the Dalits. They (Dalits) found themselves limited to sanitary work, scavenging, tanning and lately rag picking, occupations that are considered defiling and socially inferior by civil society with a "Hindu mindset"' (Guru, 2000: 125; also see Mendelsohn and Vicziany, 1998). Since many rural women do not get economic independence through the inequitable labour market, and their absorption in the non-agricultural sector is confined to specific occupations, the agricultural sector offers an 'economically gainful occupation [...] not in terms of adding assets, but to just ensure survival' (Louis, 2001: 4) through manual and unskilled work. Nonetheless, cuts in agricultural work have further contributed to the unsustainable livelihoods of Dalit women and caused them turn to surrogacy and egg donation as a mode of survival. In combating commercial surrogacy and sex work – 'modern kinds of slavery' – the rejuvenation of the agricultural sector is key, a respondent argues. Lack of property also means that women seek livelihood options through viewing their own bodies as an 'asset' – undertaking tasks that contribute to the sustenance of society but with little value attached to their labour (see Madge, 2015: 49).

Social protection and anti-poverty programmes such as the Mahatma Gandhi National Rural Employment Guarantee Act

(MNREGA), implemented and enacted through a decentralised governance model, aim to aid the empowerment of marginalised communities, especially women, Scheduled Castes and Scheduled Tribes. Of specific significance is that NREGA recognises women's work as wage labour and now 'with some cash in their hands, women have greater degree of economic independence and self-confidence, [together with having] control rights to their wages in bank deposits' (Kelkar, 2009: 8; also see Kelkar, 2011). Just recently, in 2020, during the coronavirus pandemic, the Modi government allocated forty-thousand crores to the MGNREGA scheme, to enhance the 'livelihood security of the household' (GoI, 2005, MNREGA Act; *India Today*, 2020; MoRD, 2012). Nonetheless these government measures are perceived as not always sufficient. As one respondent stated:

> they are getting very poor wages, now this uh … hundred days work … NREGA work. It also comes once in a while, and then one job for one family, not all the family members are … and uh how do you expect Dalit women to depend on this … Dalit women forever landless.

Several respondents also spoke of cuts in educational budgets, which makes unaffordable private schooling the only remaining option – which government schemes are unable to bridge.

The vulnerability of Dalit livelihood was also connected to the non-accessibility to land. This is compounded by slum evictions. One of our Chennai-based respondent spoke of slum evictions as something that had led women to enter into surrogacy arrangements:

> There is this Semmanjeri (outside Chennai), there is this where people uh slum dweller in Chennai are dislocated and sent into ghettos kind of. So because they are dislocated from the city they have lost their jobs, and they can't make the commute to Chennai easily. So … options for getting work in that area was less so the women … the women were like 40 plus, they were not young women so they were surrogate mothers and their husbands … the whole community knows. There was like a bunch, at least ten women in that Semmanjeri housing board were pregnant at any given time until this regulation came.

During the monsoon flooding in Tamil Nadu in November–December 2015, the Chennai district was among the worst affected, with devastating consequences for the urban poor living on the banks of the affected rivers. In early January 2016, the Government of Tamil Nadu issued an order to relocate river bank families. A report published by the Information and Resource Centre for the Deprived Urban Communities and Housing and Land Rights Network, suggests that the state government took advantage of the flood disaster to clear valuable land under the guise of providing 'safety housing' (Peter, 2017). The report also indicates that between 60% and 71% of the resettled flood-affected families were Dalit, the rest belonging to Other Backward Castes, all of which lived below the poverty line. In addition, it states that 85% of informal settlements did not have legal land titles, which allowed the state to see these communities as 'illegal occupants' and 'squatters'. Numerous human rights violations were committed by the government during the process of relocation, including the rights to land and property of the urban poor, motivated by the growing demand for the land on which they live. 'It further stated that the deliberate denial of provision of security of tenure has been the root cause of forced evictions, wherein the people are coerced by the State government to move to ghettos under the guise of "post-disaster rehabilitation" and "affordable housing"' (Peter, 2017: 9; Aditi, 2017).

As mentioned by our respondent as well as the report, the remote location of these sites meant the majority of the community – which relied on livelihoods in the informal sector close to their homes – lost their jobs, while being offered no alternative occupations due to the remote location. Schools and other facilities such as public healthcare are also reported to be lacking in such sites. Although a place to which flood-affected families have been relocated, Semmanjeri is flooded every year. A news report (PARI, 2020) showed streets turned into rivers. While the 2015 disaster has led to adjustments regarding street drainage in some parts of the district, no such considerations have been taken in Semmanjeri, where the construction of high-rises cut off already insufficient avenues of water drainage. Thus state-projected gains only result in nclaves of prosperity for some at the cost of exclusion of the poor. As a result of the combined forces of caste and class – in particular regarding caste right or lack therof to land – the case of Semmanjeri shows the extreme vulnerability of Dalit communities. For the socially marginalised, economic development and social (in)justice are deeply intertwined since dislocating these communities, and diminishing their economic resource base and their ways of living, is one of the fallouts of development.

Intersections of class, caste and gender

In addition to aforementioned economic vulnerabilities, the bodies of low-caste women are seen as impure and sexually available (Aloysius, Mangubai and Lee, 2020). As one respondent puts it:

> The most exploited women are the Dalit women, 61% more than that in our area […] and the … whole economic conditions forces them into […] selling their wombs for surrogacy. And I blame the society which has the purity-impurity concept in everyone's mind which is also the sexual purity. Where they don't bother about the purity-impurity and they have the sexuality aspect.

As noted by Thapar-Björkert (2006: 481) 'While control over the labour and sexuality of upper caste women is legitimized through the purity/pollution concept, the economic and sexual labour of lower caste women is made available for the consumption by upper castes'. The idea of the impurity nexus in caste was also manifested in the kinds of reproductive labour that Dalit women were recruited for. One of the journalists shared the following account: 'the doctors I have discussed with at that time have told me […] they want fair looking babies, they want intelligent babies so they openly ask for Brahmin eggs. Some doctors have told me that people openly ask for some Brahmin eggs, or Brahmin sperm. So for uterus they are hiring lower caste people … women … They won't opt [for] their eggs […] but for eggs and sperm they only seek upper caste [donors]'. 'Brahmin eggs' and 'Brahmin sperm' are juxtaposed with the womb of the lower-caste woman, whose defiled and impure sexuality makes her own eggs undesirable. As earlier studies suggest, intended parents would ideally prefer a higher caste or Brahmin surrogate, with the expectation that they would produce 'healthy and good-looking babies' (Dhar, 2012).

Many of our participants referred to the historical exploitation of Dalit women's sexuality, and the practices of Dalit devadasis and joginis[2] as contributing to the coercive forces surrounding Dalit womens' labour. As stated by one of the journalists: 'We have experienced sexual slavery for … simply centuries, whereas mainstream feminists haven't had this experience'. Our respondents also spoke of ongoing religious practices of bonded sexual labour involving young girls. The journalist respondent emphasised the economic reality underlying these practices: 'dedications do still happen. The reason is that locally the economy pushes them into it because they don't … the labour … farm labour wage doesn't give them enough to live on. Another respondent shared her thoughts on her work in getting girls 'dedicated to Matama' into school: 'Last month one particular village stopped bringing the girl, and most of the girls dedicated to the Goddess we send them to schools. They are getting education, we are vigilant, we are watching … they should not be brought back to the practices. But how long?'

While it may be said that the bodies of women have always been a kind of capital, the bodies of Dalit women – who lack land and other property – have been an asset in a more concrete way. Sabala and Gopal argue that women with 'stigmatised' bodies have challenged feminist conversations on the body by suggesting that resistance against using the body as a resource is an expression of privilege. As an example, the voices of sex workers and bar dancers have 'made feminists rethink the use of the body as a resource for livelihood in a context of diminished options for survival' (Sabala and Gopal, 2010: 49, see also Kotiswaran, 2011; Makhija, 2010; Tambe, 2008). Such conversations have also addressed surrogacy.

Many of our participants approached commercial surrogacy through the lens of sex work. All our respondents emphasised the socio-economic reality in which surrogacy or sex work becomes a livelihood option. Some participants clearly opposed the idea of a commerce in sex or pregnancy, stating that anything that commercialises […] the body […] has to be seriously questioned'. One of our respondents, a Dalit academic and social activist with experience of working with women in sex work, explained:

> rural women like X, sex work, forced by the husband, by the family and also absence of work at the agricultural sector. All this made them … it is not their choice. I feel no women will get into this kind of selling sex, also selling their wombs for surrogacy. And the … whole economic conditions forces them to get into this. The most exploited women are the Dalit women […]. Surrogacy is another thing that we cannot accept.

Others regarded it as one kind of (relatively lucrative) work among others within a restricted spectrum of livelihood options. One of our respondents said:

> as long as in this political game, this economical game – as long as the poor can get a good share and she is paid part of it. So if I am able to produce the eggs and if I am able to get pregnant maybe I would have become a surrogate. I would have definitely, for a big lump of money you know.

This perspective made the conditions under which reproductive labour was performed a key concern. She elaborates by arguing that rather than prohibiting commercial surrogacy, a clear regulation would protect women from undue exploitation: 'If I am a surrogate and I am ... I've told I'll be paid 5 lakhs, and then I am left with 5000 after giving birth it's ... It's unfair. For that laws should be made not to ban it at all you know.'

An aspect of significant importance that emerged in our interviews was caste as 'social capital'. In fact, in these narratives, class and caste (dis)privileges were seen as reinforcing each other. As one of our respondents argued:

> it's an extremely uh embedded kind of conditions in which, and the huge uh caste social capital that other feminist, upper caste feminist, have that will not let them you know ... I don't think caste as a social capital uhh will allow them to go into sex work. Because she probably has far more part of the social capital available to her which is not there for Dalit woman.

Two interrelated ideas emerge from this narrative. First, caste-capital can enable access and mobilisation of resources, which facilitates class-based mobility and a better bargaining stance. As the same respondent stated:

> somewhere all kind of external conditions that sort of force Dalit women to take surrogacy, may uh also tell us the story of again another form of bondedness with which surrogacy may thrive by, for instance this thirty thousand paid to a Dalit woman may not be the case for uh the non-Dalit woman who may bargain better [...] She may bargain, she may have a choice of going in to surrogacy and bargaining for better you know sort of allowance, better kind of conditions of uh gestation etc. That may not exist for the Dalit.

On a similar tack, Madge (2015) in her research on surrogates at a clinic in Anand, Gujarat, suggests that surrogates from the schedule castes were paid less generally, and even less if they were Muslims. The second idea is that caste capital confers benefits comparable to those accrued from social capital. As 'embodied in relations among persons' (Coleman, 1988: 118), social capital is productive and enables the achievement of certain ends while conferring power and profit to its holders (Skeggs, 1998). Through membership of a caste, a person is able to access social networks and information channels on economic opportunities, and to develop and transmit skills which strengthen human and economic capital (Coleman, 1988). But since social capital accrued through caste-based networks is relational and embodies both the processes of inclusion and exclusion, it can further entrench existing systemic and structural inequalities. In explicating the interdependent relationship between various forms of capital and the social reproduction of inequalities, Bourdieu (1997), points out that economic capital is at the 'root' of all other types of capital, and in the context of our research, the landed castes (upper castes and upwardly mobile backward castes) are able to use their economic assets for accruing social and cultural capital; to reinforce structures of stratification and to transmit hegemony intergenerationally.

Conclusion

The central aim of this chapter has been to explore the salience of caste for reproductive labour and reproductive choices within the context of commercial surrogacy and egg donation in India. Placing the argument that gender, class and caste identities are inseparable, and locating Dalit women's sexuality at the core of caste, illuminates conflicting views regarding a number of issues involving women's sexuality, not least in the area of sexual labour. Dalit feminists consistently highlight the continuum of gendered caste-based reproductive labour, which includes not only surrogacy and egg donation but also sex work within its ambit. All our respondents highlighted how wider socio-economic realities were decisive for women's reproductive lives, a perspective that we understand through the lens of reproductive justice.

Our findings suggest that Dalit women entered surrogacy and egg donation when alternative sustainable livelihoods were lacking, and that caste identity was decisive in shaping not only their positionality but also their working conditions, once they found themselves within the industry. Our interviews suggest a caste-based stratification of ART-related reproductive labour. An intersectionality of oppression is explicated by: historical legacies of gendered caste exploitation and lack of mobility; slum evictions due to caste-related lack of access to land and deprivation (caste and class); privatisation and cuts in social services; cutbacks in the agricultural sector; and unsustainable welfare oriented poverty eradication schemes (such as MNREGA), since they claim the same resources of land and other natural assets that are the only source of livelihood for a majority of urban and rural poor populations. While Dalit feminist perspectives have been marginalised in mainstream debates, our chapter demonstrates how bringing caste and social justice centre stage may be fruitful for forging new conversations on 'global fertility chains' (Vertommen et al., 2021). Our chapter elucidates how, on the one hand, economic development is crucial for the poor and socially marginalised, while, on the other hand, this trajectory of development may deepen social injustice for those lacking caste and class capital – Dalit women in particular.

Notes

This research has been funded by the Swedish Research Council (2016–01644).

1 The Surrogacy (Regulation) Bill, 2016. Ministry of Health and Welfare, Government of India, New Delhi, Bill No. 257, https://dhr.gov.in/document/acts-circulars/surrogacy-regulation-bill-2016. Accessed 1 January 2019.
2 Devadasi means 'servant of the deity' and refers to women who were married to deities. An elaborate initiation ceremony was performed before the girl reached puberty (Ramberg, 2011). The devadasi tradition was not confined to any specific caste, though, arguably, the girls recruited belong to the Scheduled Castes (see Jeevanandam and Pande, 2017). Jogini is a regional and local variant of the devadasi tradition.

References

Aditi, R (2017). Slum dwellers to get homes within city, *The Hindu*, 11 September. www.thehindu.com/news/cities/chennai/slum-dwellers-to-get-homes-within-city/article19656980.ece. Accessed 25 August 2021.

Alcoff, L. M. (1996). *Real Knowing: New Versions of the Coherence Theory*, Ithaca, NY: Cornell University Press.

Alcoff, L. M. (2008). Real knowing: a response to my critics, *Social Epistemology* 12:3, 289–305. DOI:10.1080/02691729808578885.

Aloysius, S. J., Mangubai, J. P. and. Lee, J. G. (2020). Why intersectionality is necessary. In Arya Sunaina and Aakash Singh Rathore (eds), *Dalit Feminist Theory: A Reader*, 173–82. London: Routledge.

Anandhi S. (1998). Reproductive bodies and regulated sexuality: birth control debates in early twentieth-century Tamilnadu. In Mary E. John and Janaki Nair (eds), *A Question of Silence? The Sexual Economies of Modern India*. Delhi: Kali for Women.

Arya, S. and Rathore, A. S. (2020). Introduction. In Arya Sunaina and Aakash Singh Rathore (eds), *Dalit Feminist Theory: A Reader*, 1–23. London: Routledge.

Bailey, A. (2011). Reconceiving surrogacy: toward a reproductive justice account of Indian surrogacy, *Hypatia* 26:4, 715–41.

Bharadwaj, A. (2008). Biosociality and bio- crossings: encounters with assisted conception and embryonic stem cells in India. In S. Gibbons and C. Novak (eds), *Biosocialities, Genetics and the Social Sciences: Making Biologies and Identities*, 98–116. London: Routledge.

Bhatia, S. (2012). Revealed: how more and more Britons are paying Indian women to become surrogate mothers. *Telegraph*, 26 May. www. telegraph.co.uk/news/health/news/9292343/Revealed-how-more-and-more-Britons-are-paying-Indian-women-to-become-surrogate-mothers.html. Accessed 24 June 2021.

Bourdieu, P. (1997). The forms of capital. In A. H. Halsey, H. Lauder, P. Brown, and A. S. Wells (eds), *Education: Culture, Economy, Society*, 46–58. Oxford: Oxford University Press.

Briggs, L. (2002). *Reproducing Empire: Race, Sex, Science, and U.S. Imperialism in Puerto Rico*. Berkeley, CA: University of California Press.

Briggs, L. (2012). *Somebody's Children: The Politics of Transracial and Transnational Adoption*. Durham, NC: Duke University Press.

Chakravarti, U. (2018). *Gendering Caste: Through a Feminist Lens*. New Delhi: Sage.

Coleman, J. S. (1988). Social capital in the creation of human capital, *American Journal of Sociology* 94: 95–120.

Colen, S. (1995). 'Like a mother to them': stratified reproduction and West Indian childcare workers and employers in New York. In F. D. Ginsburg and R. Rapp (eds), *Conceiving the New World Order: The Global Politics of Reproduction*. Berkeley, CA: University of California Press.

Collins, P. H. (2009 [2000]). *Black Feminist Thought: Knowledge, Consciousness and the Politics of Empowerment.* London: Routledge.

Connelly, M. (2008). *Fatal Misconception: The Struggle to Control World Population.* Cambridge, MA: Harvard University Press.

Cooper, M. and Waldby, C. (2014). *Clinical Labour: Tissue Donors and Research Subjects in the Global Bioeconomy.* Durham, NC: Duke University Press.

Corea, G. (1985). *The Mother Machine: Reproductive Technologies from Artificial Insemination to Artificial Wombs.* New York: Harper and Row.

Deomampo, D. (2016). *Transnational Reproduction: Race, Kinship and Commercial Surrogacy in India,* New York: New York University Press.

Dhar, A. (2012) 'Beautiful and fair' preferred among surrogate mothers too, *The Hindu,* 25 October. www.thehindu.com/sci-tech/health/policy-and-issues/beautiful-and-fair-preferred-among-surrogate-mothers-too/article4028640.ece. Accessed 13 February 2021.

Dutt, Y. (2019). *Coming Out As Dalit: A Memoir.* New Delhi: Aleph Book Company.

Ghose D. (2018) Chhattisgarh sterilisation tragedy: two and a half years, deaths of 13 mothers later. *The Indian Express,* 25 June. https://indianexpress.com/article/india/chhattisgarh-sterilisation-tragedy-two-and-a-half-years-deaths-of-13-mothers-later-4605460/. Accessed 15 October 2019.

GoI (2005). National Rural Employment Guarantee Act. *The Gazette of India.* New Delhi: Government of India.

Gondouin, J. and Thapar-Bjorkert, S. (forthcoming, 2022). Indian native companions and Korean camptown women: unpacking coloniality in transnational surrogacy and adoption. In S. Vertommen, M. Nahman and B. Parry (eds), *Spring.* Catalyst: Feminism, Theory, Technoscience, Special Issue Colonial Lineages of Global Fertility Chains.

Gupta, J. A. (2006). Towards transnational feminisms: some reflections and concerns in relation to the globalization of reproductive technologies, *European Journal of Women's Studies* 13:1, 23–38.

Guru, G. (2000). Dalits in pursuit of modernity. In Romila Thapar (ed.), *India: Another Millennium.* London: Viking Penguin.

Guru, G. (2020). Dalit women talk differently. In Arya Sunaina and Aakash Singh Rathore (eds), *Dalit Feminist Theory: A Reader,* 150–4. London: Routledge.

Haraway, D. (1998) Situated knowledges: the science question in feminism and the privilege of partial perspective, *Feminist Studies* 14:3, 575–99.

Harding, S. (2004). Rethinking standpoint epistemology: what is strong objectivity? In L. Alcoff and E. Potter (eds), *Feminist Epistemologies.* New York/London: Routledge, 1993.

Harding, S. (2008). *Sciences from Below: Feminisms, Postcolonialities and Modernities*. Durham, NC: Duke University Press.

The Hindu (2016). Surrogacy bill gets the Cabinet nod. 24 August. www.thehindu.com/news/national/Surrogacy-bill-gets-the-Cabinet-nod/article14591267.ece. Accessed 12 January 2021.

India Today (2020). Rs 40,000 crore increase in allocation for MGNREGA to provide employment boost: Nirmala Sitharaman. 17 May. www.indiatoday.in/business/story/increase-mgnrega-provide-employment-boost-finance-minister-nirmala-sitharaman-coronavirus-economic-package-5th-tranche-1678920-2020-05-17. Accessed 13 December 2021.

Jeevanandam S. and Pande, R. (2017), *Devdasis in South India – a Journey from Sacred to Profane Spaces*. New Delhi: Gyan Books.

Jeffrey, C. (2001). A fist is stronger than five fingers: caste and dominance in rural north India, *Transactions of the Institute of British Geographers* 25:2, 1–30.

Kamin, D. 2015. Israel evacuates surrogate babies from Nepal but leaves mothers behind. *Time*. https://time.com/3838319/israel-nepal-surrogates/. Accessed 13 September 2020.

Kelkar, G. (2009) Gender and productive assets: implications of national rural employment guarantee for women's agency and productivity. Paper presented at the FAO-IFAD-ILO Workshop on gaps, trends and current research in gender dimensions of agricultural and rural employment: differentiated pathways out of poverty. Rome, 31 March–2 April.

Kelkar, G. (2011) Gender and productive assets: implications for women's economic security and productivity, *Economic & Political Weekly* 46:23, 59–68.

Kotiswaran, P. (2011). *Dangerous Sex, Invisible Labour: Sex Work and the Law in India*. Princeton, NJ: Princeton University Press.

ICMR (Indian Council of Medical Research) (2005). National Guidelines for Accreditation, Supervision and Regulation of ART Clinics in India, National Academy of Medical Sciences (India), New Delhi-110029.

Louis, P. (2001). 'Regaining our lost faith', *Seminar* 508, 'Exclusion: A Symposium on Caste, Race and the Dalit Question', New Delhi, December. www.indiaseminar.com/2001/508/508%20prakash%20louis.htm. Accessed 12 June 2021.

Madge, V. (2015). *Surrogacy in India: A Case Study of a Clinic in Anand, Gujarat*. Unpublished doctoral dissertation, Centre of Social Medicine and Community Health, School of Social Sciences, Jawaharlal Nehru University.

Mahadevan, K. (2020). Dalit women's experience: toward a Dalit feminist theory. In Arya Sunaina and Aakash Singh Rathore (eds), *Dalit Feminist Theory: A Reader*, 223–37. London: Routledge.

Makhija, S. (2010) Bar dancers, morality and the Indian law, *Economic &* *Political Weekly*, September–October, 45:39, 19–23.

Malik, B. (1999). Untouchability and Dalit women's oppression, *Economic* *& Political Weekly*, 34: 6, 323–4.

Mendelsohn, O. and Vicziany, M. (1998). *The Untouchables: Subordination, Poverty and the State in Modern India*. Cambridge: Cambridge University Press.

Menon, N. (2020). A critical view on intersectionality. In Sunaina Arya and Singh Aakash Rathore (eds), *Dalit Feminist Theory: A Reader*, 25–39. Routledge: London.

Moon, V. (2000). *Growing up Untouchable in India: A Dalit Autobiography*. Lanham, MD: Rowman and Littlefield.

MoRD (2012). *MGNREGA Sameeksha*. New Delhi: Ministry of Rural Development.

Nayak, P. (2014). The three ms of commercial surrogacy in India: mother, money, and medical market. In Sayantani Das Gupta and Shamita Das Dasgupta (eds), *Globalization and Transnational Surrogacy in India: Outsourcing Life*, 1–22. Lanham: Lexington Books.

Newman S. and Nahman, M. (2020). Nurture commodified? An investigation into commercial human milk supply chains, *Review of International Political Economy*, DOI:10.1080/09692290.2020.1864757.

Pande, A. (2011). Transnational commercial surrogacy in India: gifts for global sisters? *Reproductive Biomedicine Online* 23, 618–25.

Pande A. (2014a). *Wombs in Labour: Transnational Commercial Surrogacy in India*, New York: Colombia University Press.

Pande, A. (2014b). This birth and that: surrogacy and stratified motherhood in India. *philoSOPHIA: A Journal of Continental Feminism* 4:1, 50–64.

Peter, V. (2017). From deluge to displacement: the impact of post-flood evictions and resettlement in Chennai. New Delhi: Information and Resource Centre for the Deprived Urban Communities, and Housing and Land Rights Network.

PARI (People's Archive of Rural India) (2020). In Semmanjeri: 'We get a tsunami every year'. https://ruralindiaonline.org/en/articles/in-semmanjeri-we-get-a-tsunami-every-year/. Accessed 15 October 2019.

Ramberg, L. (2011). When the devi is your husband: sacred marriage and sexual economy in South India, *Feminist Studies* 37:1, 28–60.

Rao, M. (ed.) (2004a). *The Unheard Scream: Reproductive Health and Women's Lives in India*. New Delhi: Zubaan.

Rao, M. (2004b). Abiding appeal of Neo-Malthusianism: explaining the inexplicable, *Economic & Political Weekly*, 7–13August, 39:32, 3599–604.

Rao, M. and Sexton, S. (2010). *Markets and Malthus: Population, Gender, and Health in Neo-liberal Times*. New Delhi: Sage.

Rege, S. (1998). Dalit women talk differently: a critique of 'difference' and towards a Dalit feminist standpoint position, *Economic & Political Weekly*, 31 October, WS39–WS46.

Rege, S. (2018). A Dalit feminist standpoint, *Seminar* (No. 710), October.

Roberts, D. (1996). Race and the new reproduction, *Hastings Law Journal* 47, 935–49.

Ross, L. and Solinger, R. (2017). *Reproductive Justice: An Introduction*. Oakland, CA: California University Press.

Ross, L. J., Roberts, L., Derkas, E., Peoples, W. and Bridgewater Toure, P. (eds) (2017). *Radical Reproductive Justice: Foundations, Theory, Practice, Critique*. New York: Feminist Press.

Rudrappa, S. (2014). Mother India: outsourcing labour to Indian surrogate mothers. In *Globalization and Transnational Surrogacy in India: Outsourcing Life*, ed. Sayantani DasGupta and Shamita Das Dasgupta, 125–46. Lanham, MD: Lexington Books.

Rudrappa, S. (2015). *Discounted Life: The Price of Global Surrogacy in India*. New York: New York University Press.

Sabala and Gopal, M. (2010) Body, gender and sexuality: politics of being and belonging, *Economic & Political Weekly*, April 24–30, 45:17, 43–51.

Sama (2012). *Birthing a Market: A Study of Commercial Surrogacy*. New Delhi: Sama, Resource Group for Women and Health.

Sangari, K. (2015). *Solid:Liquid: A (Trans)national Reproductive Formation*. New Delhi: Tulika Books.

Saravanan, S. (2018). *A Transnational Feminist View of Surrogacy Biomarkets in India*. Singapore: Springer.

Shalev, C., Eyal, H. and Samama, E. (2017). Transnational surrogacy and the earthquake in Nepal: a case study. In M. Davies (ed.), *Babies for Sale? Transnational Surrogacy, Human Rights and the Politics of Reproduction*. London: Zed Books

Skeggs, B. (1998). *Formations of Class and Gender: Becoming Respectable*. London: Sage.

Stephens, C. (2009). Feminism and Dalit Women in India. www.countercurrents.org/stephen161109.htm. Accessed 20 May 2019.

Sunder Rajan, K. (2007). Experimental values: Indian clinical trials and surplus health, *New Left Review* 45, May–June 2007, 66–88.

Tambe, A. (2008). Different issues/different voices: organization of women in prostitution in India. In R. Sahni, V. K. Shankar and H. Apte, *Prostitution and Beyond: An Analysis of Sex Work in India*. New Delhi: Sage Publications India.

Thapar-Björkert, S. (2006). Women as arm-bearers: gendered caste-violence and the Indian state, *Women's Studies International Forum* 29:5, 474–88.

Twine, F. W. (2015). *Outsourcing the Womb: Race, Class and Gestational Surrogacy in a Global Market*. London: Routledge.

Velayudhan, M. (2018). Linking radical traditions and the contemporary Dalit women's movement: an intergenerational lens, *Feminist Review* 119, 106–25.

Vertommen, S. and Barbagallo, C. (2021). The in/visible wombs of the market: the dialectics of waged and unwaged reproductive labour in the global surrogacy industry, *Review of International Political Economy*. DOI:10.1080/09692290.2020.1866642.

Vertommen, S., Pavone, V and Nahman, M. (2021). Global fertility chains: an integrative political economy approach to understanding the reproductive bioeconomy, *Science, Technology, and Human Values* 1–34.

Vora, K. (2008). Others' organs: South Asian domestic labour and the kidney trade, *Postmodern Culture* 19:1. DOI:10.1353/pmc.0.0036.

Vora, K. (2012). Limits of 'Labour': accounting for affect and the biological in transnational surrogacy and service work, *South Atlantic Quarterly* 111:4, 681–700. DOI:10.1215/00382876-1724138.

Vora, K. (2015). *Life Support: Biocapital and the New History of Outsourced Labour*. Minneapolis, MN: University of Minnesota Press.

Waldby, C. and M. Cooper (2008). The biopolitics of reproduction: post-Fordist biotechnology and women's clinical labour, *Australian Feminist Studies* 23:55, 57–73.

Weinbaum, A. E. (2019). *The Afterlife of Reproductive Slavery: Biocapitalism and Black Feminism's Philosophy of History*. Durham, NC: Duke University Press.

Wilson, K., Loh, J. U. and Purewal, N. (2018). Gender, violence and the neoliberal state in India, *Feminist Review* 119:1, 1–6.

11

Hamstrung by hardship: protecting egg donors' reproductive labour in Kolkata, India

Meghna Mukherjee

India is one of the world's fastest growing egg donation industries, contributing to a global in-vitro fertilisation (IVF) market worth US$15 billion and growing at a rate of 10% annually (Grand View Research, 2018). Although India's 2016 Assisted Reproductive Technology (ART) Bill aims to stringently police laws on third-party reproduction through surrogacy, the same legal framework does not exist for egg donation. The Indian Council of Medical Research has established guidelines under which egg donation should be practised; however, without laws in place, these guidelines are not regulated across clinics and rarely legally enforced (Reddy and Patel, 2015; Shah, 2009; Vora, 2013). Within an unregulated legal space, the experience of egg donors in India relies on the discretion of the clinic at which they are donating (Bailey, 2011). Interrogating the extent to which in Kolkata, India's egg donors relinquish ownership over their reproductive labour, thus enabling fertility clinics to instrumentalise their bodies, this chapter culturally contextualises agency bound by poverty. It moves beyond discourses that negate bodily commodification to question the parameters required to safeguard donors' bodily ownership in third-party reproduction.

Kolkata is a major city in West Bengal, India, serving as a centre for medical, including fertility, services within West Bengal and neighbouring countries like Bangladesh. Its streets are teeming with fertility clinics perched on every corner, ranging from small dilapidated building facades to much larger, contemporarily designed spaces. Yet West Bengal remains one of India's least economically developed states, with a third of Kolkata's population living in slums below the poverty line – here, we find the women who fulfil the fertility industry's donation and surrogacy demands (Kundu, 2003; Mitra, 2016; World Bank, 2017). The typical egg donor in India has not completed middle school, works as a housemaid for less than US$150 per month, and often bears the brunt of an absent or abusive husband (Reddy and Patel, 2015; Rudrappa, 2015). While there is no credible data on the number of donors in Kolkata (due to lack of formal regulation), current estimates suggest that over 3000 women are impregnated using donor eggs each year in Kolkata, with donors earning Rs. 10,000 (US$145) to Rs. 20,000 (US$289) per donation (Niyogi, 2012).

This chapter examines commercial egg donation – a term representing arrangements in which clinics pay women to provide their oocytes for use in fertility treatments – in Kolkata, India. It teases out the interactions between institutions, their individual intermediaries, and low-income women providing eggs, in order to unpack the agentic complexity that lies between individual struggle and institutional demand. The politics of ownership over one's bodily labour has been analysed through discourses studying third-party fertility medicine (Dickenson, 2007; Pande, 2011; Rudrappa, 2015), human organ trading (Cohen, 2003; Scheper-Hughes, 2000), and sex work (Hoang, 2015; Kempadoo, 1998). This existing scholarship on commodifying women's bodies ranges from considering women as passive objects to recognising legitimate autonomy (Dickenson, 2017; Waldby, 2008; West, 2000). The implications of these discourses are meaningful. In this case, the degree of bodily ownership afforded to egg donors determines the extent to which we can consider their 'donation' to be legitimate labour, which frames moral, policy, and legal decisions around justifying and protecting third-party roles in the ART industry. Acknowledging that most women donating eggs in the global south are impoverished (Deomampo, 2013; Reddy and Patel, 2015), the chapter negotiates existing literature on bodily agency with the personal and financial constraints placed on the Indian egg donor. How is commercial egg donation organised in unregulated fertility markets, such as Kolkata, India, and what are the implications for the wellbeing of vulnerable donors? Moreover, given that low-income, uneducated women often decide to sell their eggs, to what extent can they be positioned to better 'own' their bodily labour in this transaction? Analysing the narratives and interactions that take place between meso-level clinic institutions and micro-level networks of low-income women, I unpack the theoretical potentiality of agency constrained by financial desperation, unequal gendered positions, and institutional imposition. The chapter argues that greater institutional accountability for clinics goes hand in hand with recentring donors' agency, which is both undeniable and necessary within Kolkata's third-party fertility exchanges. In doing so, it emphasises the need for greater contextual specificity to develop meaningful discourses about bodily labour, agency, and altruistic moralisation in the global south's fertility industries.

The chapter harnesses data about donors' networks, decision making, and clinical institutional power through interviews and participant observation. In doing so, it shows how clinics structure a financially incentivised donor market targeted at low-income women while also strategically distancing themselves from these networks of women. This neglect from the clinic – the most resourced institutional actor in the egg donation exchange – has severe consequences on the wellbeing and safety of donors, which in turn compromises their ownership over their bodily labour. The findings are organised into three sections: (i) the clinic's role in structuring the occupational market structure around egg donation; (ii) the consequences of the clinic's institutional neglect for donors; and (iii) the networks of nurture and support among low-income women who participate in Kolkata's egg donation market. Throughout, the discussion reinforces the need for better alignment between the meso-level institutions and micro-level individual networks driving currently unregulated fertility markets. Guided by national regulations that protect donors' bodily labour, clinics must engage and inform donors more thoroughly and take accountability for their intermediary actors.

Does poverty allow for agency?

To analyse the transaction of bodily material from one person to another, this chapter draws on the concept of 'bioavailability'. Conceived as a framework through which to analyse kidney donation (read: selling) between impoverished sellers and wealthier recipients, bioavailability defines 'the extent to which a person's body is available to be reincorporated into something or someone else given the relation between (surgical) techniques [...] and market structures' (Cohen, 2003: 685). Amrita Pande (2010, 2011), Sharmila Rudrappa (2015), and Sayantani DasGupta and Shamita Das DasGupta (2014) allow us to extend the bioavailability framework to third-party reproductive services, such as gestational surrogacy and egg donation (read: selling), as they examine how the deep-seated class inequality between low-income Indian surrogates and wealthier, often foreign, commissioning parents compromises surrogates' voice in biomedical processes and commercial transactions related to their bodily labour. Unpacking the ethics around bioavailability, these authors lead us to question, 'are those living under conditions of social insecurity and economic abandonment on the periphery of the new world order really the 'owners' of their bodies?' (Scheper-Hughes, 2000: 197).

Many authors studying third-party reproduction in India recognise the crippling effects of poverty when contending with women's ownership over their reproductive or bodily labour. For instance, Rudrappa (2012) affords surrogates some extent of choice, illustrating how these women actively pursue surrogacy as a source of material income; however, she recognises that the liberal westernised concept of 'autonomous reproductive rights' presents an empty rhetoric for these women who must resort to bodily commodification to subsist (Rudrappa, 2012). Conversely, Jyotsna Gupta and Annemiek Richters (2008) argue that reproductive labour negates agency because financial coercion, social pressure, and lack of information on health risks always violate the dignity required for autonomous choice. However, Cohen (2003) disentangles autonomous choice from agency. While arguing that financial compulsion negates voluntary donation of biological material, he still presents donors as 'informed agents making rational choices under unenviable but real conditions' (Cohen, 2003: 665). Finally, Pande (2010) problematises the concept of choice itself: although women choose to perform reproductive or bodily labour, this arises as an obligation toward supporting their families (Pande, 2010: 302). Pande (2020) urges us to move beyond the stalemate of impossible agency in commodified bodily work, toward understanding donors' desires foremost when evaluating global fertility markets. These authors urge us to situate agency under poverty in the global south, where 'choice' is necessarily contoured by the circumstances of financial duress, and where reproductive labour presents a tantalising, though transient, escape (Reddy and Patel, 2015; Rudrappa, 2012).

This complexity of bioavailability highlights the often-circular debates around whether to prohibit based on bioethical violations or regulate based on individual autonomy (Dickenson, 2017; Gupta and Richters, 2008; Pande, 2010; Rudrappa, 2012; Scheper-Hughes, 2000; Waldby, 2008). Along these lines, we must critique the normative understanding of agency – untainted freedom to make a choice – as a neoliberal concept that cannot translate to the lives of most marginalised women. West (2000) discusses that untainted decision making does not exist in most women's social environments. Rather, women often enter into precarious circumstances as a result of social crises and accordingly redefine their agentic identity to comport with their decisions (Almeling, 2006; Pande, 2010; Rudrappa and Collins, 2015; West, 2000). Studying non-trafficked sex workers in Vietnam, Hoang (2015) presents an empirical account of this agentic theory: these sex workers describe themselves as strategic agents, harnessing their positions within a patriarchal global economy to their financial and social advantage. Hoang (2015) suggests that choice is always constrained by power structures, and yet this does not discount the legitimacy of one's ownership over one's decisions. Translating this re-defined agentic theory to reproductive labour, scholars like Allison Bailey (2011), Anindita Majumdar (2014), Michal Nahman (2008) and Amrita Pande (2010) encourage a revisioning of donors' agency. Pande states: 'even though women may feel obliged to perform reproductive work to support their families, it is a decision they have ownership over' (Pande, 2010: 302). While the 'stolen rhetoric' of women's 'reproductive rights' would inappropriately impose empowerment on impoverished donors, their reproductive labour nonetheless warrants dignity and ownership, however constrained their options may have been (Majumdar, 2014; Nahman, 2008).

Recognising that third-party fertility markets are a global phenomenon, especially in India, this chapter launches from bioavailability – whether legalised, illegalised, or somewhere in between – being a stark reality for low-income women in the global south (DasGupta and DasGupta, 2014; Dickenson, 2017; Pande, 2010; Rudrappa, 2015). While westernised liberal debates often condemn bodily labour as immoral, for Kolkata's low-income women, earnings from egg donation are non-negligible and their effort to improve life circumstances cannot be minimised. Negating the agency of a marginalised woman in this way would risk imposing a false consciousness on her, discounting her personhood overall (Hoang, 2015). Therefore, this chapter understands agency being necessarily constrained, but nevertheless present and attainable. Rather than positioning donors as victims, safeguarding their involvement in a well-established fertility industry provides more concrete relief from the perils of commercialised reproductive work (Bailey, 2011). Accordingly, this chapter contributes to a pressing need for discourses that reconcile, rather than polarise, the conventional ban versus regulation debates, exploring conditions that can protect vulnerable and bioavailable women in owning their decision to donate eggs.

Poor, bioavailable, *and* altruistic?

While egg donors often justify their bodily labour on moral grounds, drawing on altruistic narratives of helping someone, research has questioned whether these moral narratives are after-thoughts or impositions that are complicit in coercing bioavailability (Pande, 2011; Rudrappa and Collins, 2015). Rene Almeling (2006, 2011) locates narratives of altruism within egg donation agencies, illustrating how agency staff guide donors to purport altruistic narratives that align with the traditional presentation of feminine, selfless mother-hood. While the altruism narrative may be institutionally controlled, research in the global south has shown that moral framing is also critical on the individual level, as altruism helps women justify reproductive labour and shroud their stark bodily commodification (Hochschild, 2011; Pande, 2020; Rudrappa and Collins, 2015). Moralisation mitigates the personal and social effects of stigmatised bodily work, which is particularly important in India where reproduc-tive labour is often conflated with 'dirty' sex work (Pande, 2010).

Although moral frames may provide low-income women a means to legitimise their reproductive labour, the institutional imposition of such narratives can disguise coercion (Reddy and Patel, 2015; Rudrappa and Collins, 2015). The medical institute stands as an independent locus of power, coercion, and regulation over the management of the human body and societal norms (Foucault, 1978;

Gupta and Richters, 2008; Scheper-Hughes, 2000). In countries like India where body markets remain unregulated, these institutions are legitimate sources of authority, and their discretion to perform ethically determines the protections and bodily ownership a donor is granted (Bailey, 2011; Gupta and Richters, 2008; Shah, 2009; Vora, 2013).

Furthermore, Pande (2011) argues that the drastic socio-economic rift between low-income surrogate and wealthier patient precludes conditions for genuine altruism, based on both parties' awareness of an irreconcilable class difference. The 'gift of motherhood' remains a financially coerced act. Although Pande (2011) treads the line of imposing a false consciousness on surrogates, her emphasis on the stark class inequality between surrogate and patient is important to the conditions surrounding bioavailability in the global south. Considering that donors in Kolkata are motivated by financial desperation, it is difficult to imagine how the transaction of eggs for money can be fundamentally altruistic. This does not deny room for moral motivation within bioavailability, but urges us to reconsider whether altruism is an impetus, ex post facto justification, or an all-together coercive narrative that has been imposed by the clinic and its actors.

Where is agency found within the bioavailability process?

The exchange of biological material includes several milestones at which agency may be derived. For Catherine Waldby and Melinda Cooper (2008), the defining moment lies in discussing egg donors as workers, not romanticised givers: 'the assumption of passivity seems to be a particular danger when analysing women's bodily work' (Waldby and Cooper, 2008: 66–7). Rather than positioning donors as empowered clinical labourers, reproductive labour contracts establish terms to give the clinic control over donors' bodies (Waldby and Cooper, 2008; Waldby et al., 2013). Supporting this need for a fair labour contract, Pande (2010) asserts that legitimation of reproductive labour as work would provide women ownership over their roles and diminish stigma. Further, Rudrappa (2010) urges a transition from seeing reproductive bioavailability as a 'reproductive right' to a decision that is better situated within women's 'workers' rights' (Rudrappa, 2012). However, while these authors locate donors' agency in fair, protective labour terms, Scheper-Hughes' (2000) notes that starkly unequal power dynamics in the global south preclude the conditions needed for an equitable reproductive labour contract (Scheper-Hughes, 2000). When faced with a doctor's medical authority and a patient's looming class status, impoverished donors in Kolkata are often too intimidated to question a contract, simply signing where they are told to. A fair contract cannot be realised without ameliorating the nodes of power and coercion that medical institutions hold over individual donors.

Charis Thompson (2005) identifies the clinical procedure as a key site in which to interrogate female agency and personhood. Thompson makes an important distinction between the medical status of patients and donors: unlike donors, 'patients willingly accept the role of being the object of the medical gaze and in fact actively participate in it' (Thompson, 2005: 191). Both patients and donors accept the objectifying medical gaze in exchange for treatments and income, respectively. Yet, since she is not the clinic's patient-of-interest, the donor is relegated to a secondary status and her trade-off for medical objectification is higher. 'Patients are better able to participate in their own care because they have been initiated into the *epistemic environment* of the clinic. Producing informed citizens also produces epistemic standards. Certain facts about bodies [...] and about treatment options are learned or are expected to be known' (Thompson, 2005: 201; emphasis added). Here, Thompson describes the 'epistemic orientation' as patients being initiated into the clinic's epistemic environment. Further, Mukherjee (2020) argues that because donors and intended parents receive varying types and qualities of epistemic orientations, they face discrepant medical experiences and outcomes during egg donation. Unlike donors, patients are central actors within the clinic: they are well-informed of treatment processes, risks, and rewards, and are entitled to consult doctors with questions and concerns. For donors in an unregulated fertility industry, these are benefits of working with a clinic that chooses to perform ethically, rather than entitlements for an individual undergoing medical procedures. These systemic shortcomings in care afforded to donors underscore issues of information dearth and medical treatment inequality, which compromise donors' owner-ship over their bodies. In order to uphold the legitimacy of a labour contract, the rift between donor and patient status within medical sites must be bridged.

The subordination of donors in medical settings raises Donna L. Dickenson's (2007, 2017) concept of the 'vanishing lady'. While the donor's gametes become the subject of medical consideration, the donor herself is bereft of rights and protections concerning her labour (Dickenson, 2017). Dickenson (2007) draws on Marx and Locke's theories of property rights and body ownership to re-centre the donor's agency in bioavailability. Per the logic of owning the products of one's labour, the egg donor who has undergone medical stimulation to produce an unnatural number of mature oocytes should own her resulting eggs. However, Dickenson's (2007) framework raises functional questions in the clinical setting. If a donor is to own her resulting eggs, should she also be financially responsible for the medical treatment that is required to stimulate these follicles? Further, what risks does the clinic assume if a donor is to exercise discriminatory judgement in choosing recipients or renege on a commitment? While some suggest that the answer lies in leaving the clinic out of donor-patient relationships altogether, greater issues arise from not holding the clinic accountable for *all* aspects of facilitating treatments. Dickenson suggests that the solution to financial coercion and exploitation of bioavailable bodies is de-commercialisation (Dickenson, 2007).

In contrast, those like Hoang (2015) would argue that denying low-income women the choice of compensated bioavailability is more damaging to selfhood and consciousness than protecting constrained agency. Waldby (2008: 28–9), too, aptly critiques the de-commercialisation perspective:

> The well-established, highly mobile, clandestine and transnational nature of both recruitment clinics and vendor (donor) populations suggests that attempts to ban oocyte markets will simply push trade underground, into black markets with more likelihood of criminal involvement and further possibilities of harm to the women.

This is particularly concerning for low-income women in India's unsupervised oocyte industry. Rather than de-commercialisation, some researchers urge a 'uniform oversight of these clinic's operations [...] (combining) issues of safety, consent and clinical conditions with those of workers' rights, organized representation for vendors, and regulated negotiation of conditions' (Waldby, 2008: 28). Rather than withdraw payment, women should be positioned as central voices in policies governing their reproductive labour, addressing medical and social risk, procedural transparency, and ownership over one's bodily work (Thompson, 2007).

It is from this solutions-oriented perspective that the chapter launches. If bioavailability can be responsibly regulated without needing to ban commercialisation, where do interventions begin? This chapter proposes a two-fold starting point: require greater accountability for clinics with regard to protecting all bodies in the fertility treatment; and relatedly, re-centre the donor as the owner of her bodily labour, which entitles dedicated support and thorough, accurate information on the medical interventions and risks she will undertake. Recognising deeply rooted global economies centred on bioavailable bodies, we can begin a productive discourse on safeguarding, rather than diminishing, the tenuous ownership that low-income women have over their bodily labour.

Methods

The data presented here is drawn from 225 hours of participant observation and 21 in-depth interviews conducted at Progya Fertility Clinic (pseudonym) in Kolkata. After two months of preliminary observations during December 2014 and January 2015, a targeted study on egg donation was carried out between June and July 2018. In 2018, Progya's main location shifted to a central, luxury building, and it operated numerous branches throughout Kolkata and neighbouring cities. The main facility employs eight fertility doctors, eight nurses, three embryologists, one lab technician, two fertility coordinators, and five administrative staff who attended to around seventy to eighty fertility patients a day.

Data was obtained through shadowing clinical staff and attending doctor-patient consultations. Interviews were conducted with twelve egg donors, Progya's two main recruiters, and ten clinical staff, including fertility doctors, nurses, and coordinators. The interviews focused on understanding the treatment of egg donors: the recruitment process; donors' education about medical processes; clinic's management of donors; maintenance of donor-patient anonymity; and women's psychological and physical navigation through the donation process. The narratives reveal how women are taught to rationalise their donations and moralise stigmatised bodily labour, highlighting the class inequalities and institutional forces that compromise donors' informed ownership over their bioavailability.

Discussion

Occupational market structure

Without enough education or income, donors in Kolkata are typically unemployed or part of the unskilled workforce of domestic workers or day labourers, with a household income of less than US$130 a month (DasGupta and DasGupta, 2014; Pande, 2010; Rudrappa, 2015). In Kolkata, donating eggs does not require education qualifications or formal training, making it a tangible income opportunity for impoverished women. As such, most women in Kolkata enter the egg donation market (and donate several times) to relieve financial burdens. A donor named Rabeya describes her motivations:

> I first took up this job to make some money. My husband had so many loans. I needed to pay them back. [...]. [My friend] told me that I would be able to give back at least 3 or 4 months' worth of his loans at once. His loans are for an entire year, so it'll take time. I just wonder what will happen to me, to my body, after doing all this. But what can I do? I have to do this job. It's the only way I can make enough money. (Rabeya Khatun, 2018, Interview)

Like so many other donors, Rabeya's choice to provide eggs is motivated by financial constraint and a lack of better alternatives. She feels the pressure to repay her late husband's loans and sees egg donation as her only opportunity to make consistent large sums of money. Similarly, other egg donors described using their income to relieve debts or meet short-term life expenses. Many provided for emergency medical care for relatives or supported daily household and child rearing expenses. In many donors' narratives, there was a sense of helplessness. Even though many, like Rabeya, are fearful for their health and wellbeing, their financial need is overwhelming enough to compel their bioavailability. For impoverished women in

Kolkata, donating eggs is often a result of having one's back against the wall.

The overwhelming need for money cripples one's ability to freely choose reproductive labour (Cohen, 2003; Gupta and Richters, 2008; Majumdar, 2014). However, the fact remains that these women require substantial financial support that cannot be achieved through their regular means of income (Bailey, 2011; Pande, 2010; Rudrappa, 2012). For many women, performing reproductive bodily work through egg donation or surrogacy is often the only feasible and morally justifiable (in terms of donors' perception of chastity) route to earning money. As a result, there is a robust referral network among low-income women in Kolkata, who help connect each other to recruiters who operate as fertility clinic liaisons.

Women in Kolkata learn about egg donation through a close friend or family member who has previously donated her eggs, and who then relays willing candidates to recruiters. Recruiters are low-income women who have also donated their eggs. They are familiar with the procedures and closely support donors. Moreover, since women must go through recruiters to donate their eggs at fertility clinics, recruiters occupy a crucial node of the referral networks (Deomampo, 2013). Puja, a second-time donor who learned about egg donation through her cousin, explains, 'We all know at least one recruiter. Everyone has the recruiters' numbers. So, if you want to donate, you can call the recruiter when you get your period and tell them you want to donate that month' (Puja Debjyoti, 2018, Interview). The ubiquity of donating eggs within Kolkata's low-income communities, as well as recruiters' embeddedness within donor referral networks, allows recruiters convenient regular access to women who are willing to donate their eggs. At Progya, recruiters bring two or three willing donors into the clinic each day to undergo a transvaginal scan examining their ovaries. If the scan goes well, the candidate is 'selected' and proceeds for a blood test and serology report to verify her overall health. Finally, each month, clinicians match approved donors to recipients who are on the docket based on their biophysical features.

This recruitment process also creates a dense word-of-mouth referral network, which not only connects low-income women but also creates a support system through which they can rely on one another while undergoing unfamiliar medical processes. Thus, the recruiter functions as a gatekeeper for who can donate as well as a key figure to liaise between donors and fertility clinics. Recruiters are responsible for explaining the egg donation process to willing candidates, guiding them through the medical procedures, and addressing their concerns. As donors often share the same recruiter, it is not uncommon for women to have similar recruitment experiences (Deomampo, 2013).

Subsequently, poor women are not only entering egg donation due to financial compulsion, but the systemic nature of poverty in Kolkata is contributing to a structured and self-perpetuating referral system between bioavailable women, recruiters, and the clinic. While it may seem like the occupational market structure is contingent on individual women who comprise these donor networks, it is imperative to underscore the clinic's institutional role in driving the financial incentives that sustain this market and incoming flow of donors.

Using strategic compensation practices, clinics sustain the occupational market structure around donating. They provide recruiters with regular deposits into their bank accounts, which are calculated in ways to allow for tiered financial incentivisation. Although recruiters establish the specifics of their payment schemes themselves, each trying to present more competitively to potential donors, the institutional force driving this market structure comes from the clinic. Rajeshri, a former donor and recruiter with 10 years' experience, explains:

> If a donor has a positive result, the clinic tells me to bring her back again after six months. [...] So, in that case, I just give her some money to keep her loyal to me, and I tell her to come back to me when enough time has passed if she wants to (donate) again. [...] We get direct deposits to our bank accounts every two weeks. I make about Rs. 25,000 (approximately US$362) per donor I secure. From there, I give a new donor maybe Rs.15,000 (approximately US$217), or if it's someone who has worked with me before I give her Rs.18,000 (approximately US$260) for loyalty. Then there are also our sub-agents, who were donors with us before, but who now also connect us with new donors. So, sometimes I have to pay the sub-agent and the donor. In this case, I give the sub-agent around Rs.3,000 (approximately US$43) and the donor around Rs.12,000 (approximately US$173).
> (Rajeshri Rai, 2018, Interview)

In Kolkata, low-income women are institutionally encouraged (by the clinic) to urge one another into bodily labour. Fertility clinics ensure that recruiters are consistently paid and that their compensation depends upon the number of successful donors they enlist. In turn, recruiters are motivated to pay donors for loyalty, that is repeat donations. Moreover, every time a woman refers someone to a recruiter, she receives a commission from the recruiter and becomes her 'sub-recruiter'. This payment structure, underwritten by the fertility clinic, not only compels financially desperate women into bodily labour but also inclines impoverished women to 'target' one another's bioavailability as a solution to financial urgency. Further, though women may be helping one another with financial opportunity, the motivation for doing so lies primarily in compensation over commiseration. Much like Hoang's (2015) analysis of power dynamics between sex workers and their 'mommies' (managers), there is a degree of top-down emotional care but this is primarily directed toward incentivising women's profitable bodily work. Parallel to the mommy's relation to her sex workers, recruiters are important sources of care and support for donors but their objective in cultivating the relationship is to secure additional income through donors' bioavailability. As such, the decision to donate belongs less to the donor, and more to the institutional actors, like recruiters and clinics, who manipulate her financial desperation (Towghi and Vora, 2014).

The systematic use of money to secure donor loyalty and donor-to-donor referral is also central to incentivising repeat donations and broadening the market of willing 'career donors'. Egg donors are able to donate several times, and often do, as the amount they earn from egg donation is rarely ever an all-encompassing solution to their financial needs (Rudrappa and Collins, 2015). Together, donors' continuous need for money and the financially incentivised payment structure rewarding 'loyalty' creates an alarming cycle of bioavailability, where egg donation becomes a profession. Arpita does not know how many times she has donated her eggs, but has done so regularly over the last four years:

> They say not to do it frequently like every month. I'm not doing that. I do it like every six months or one time three months. This type of work is convenient for me to do. [...] I will do this work for as long as I can. Right now, I am around 28 years old. For as long they will

take me, I will try to continue donating. I have heard that they don't take donors above the age of 30, so, I have about 2 years left. Then, when I am 30, I will do a surrogate job. The amount for surrogacy is much bigger. (Arpita Chandra, 2018, Interview)

Arpita, a career donor, insists that she will provide reproductive labour for as long as possible, even considering surrogacy after she has aged-out of donation. Egg donation is seen as convenient because it does not require formal training, can be performed somewhat regularly, and is available to all women who are healthy enough. Many donors shared Arpita's sentiment of wanting to donate as many times as possible, indicating reliance on egg donation for consistent income (Reddy and Patel, 2015). Women see donation as a core part of their household earnings, which likens their bioavail-ability to a scheduled job rather than a one-time occurrence.

Although the Indian Council of Medical Research guidelines state that women should not donate their eggs more than six times, in this study neither the donors nor the recruiters responsible for conveying such information were aware of this limitation, placing donors in potential harm (Niyogi, 2012; Shah, 2009). As Kolkata's impoverished women gravitate toward bioavailability as an occupa-tion, and given that fertility institutions structure medical markets to compel their continued bioavailability, it is important to examine (and resolve) how coercive financial motives alongside undeniable financial need perpetuate harm for donors.

The consequences of institutional neglect

As discussed, recruiters come from similar impoverished communities as donors and have often faced similar life challenges. Although clinics entrust them with explaining egg donation to potential donors, recruiters lack the education and medical literacy to do so. Conse-quently, they do not present an accurate overview of the donation process to women and thus many donors do not thoroughly understand, if at all, what is happening to their bodies while donating. However, the clinic is ultimately responsible for any harm caused to donors as it wilfully neglects the oversight and professionalisation of recruiters it relies on. Fundamentally, this institutional neglect calls into question donors' informed consent and thereby their ownership over their bodily labour.

Given that recruiters supply donors for the clinic's profit, these women should be considered and professionally trained as clinic representatives. However, the clinic strategically keeps them at arm's length, so as to not take responsibility for recruitment strategies. Several doctors told me that they 'did not get involved' with the recruiters and 'their business', that they did not want to deal with 'all these women asking for more money'. However, recruiters were also given the impression that they were linked to the clinic, so that the clinic could maintain donor supplies. During their daily interactions, Progya's IVF coordinators would often subtly mention that they had to 'manage' the recruiters skilfully, to make them feel important so they would continue supplying the clinic with donors. In turn, recruiters spoke highly of their 'clinic jobs', saying working for the medical field was the most prestigious occupation they had. Still, Progya did not supervise or hold recruiters accountable for *how* they brought donors into the clinic. Rather than formal clinic representatives, Progya intentionally kept recruiters as intermediaries that they did not professionalise. As a result, we see the spread of problematic recruitment narratives that include financial coercion or lack of medical information:

> There is a recruiter who lives near me. [...] She told me, 'Just come and try to do it once. You have so many expenses and debts, you can take care of those with this money.' I am of course scared about what will happen, but I am here because I need money. [...] The recruiter just told me that they would give me injections to take out an egg and that after 10–12 days I would get my money. (Pratima Sen, 2018, Interview)

Like Pratima, almost all donors indicated that the women who recruited them relied on expedient monetary benefit as the primary rationale to persuade them into donation. Financial compulsion is also overwhelmingly what women focus on during their donation. As Pratima says, she continues to be scared but is centred on the income she will receive. She, like so many other donors, does not understand the exact medical procedures and risks she is undertaking, viewing donation pragmatically as a series of injections leading to a final payment. This is a sentiment many recruiters and donors in Kolkata share, as they come to see their bodies as a tool for profit (Pande, 2010; Rudrappa, 2012, 2015).

However, there are significant consequences to donors being uninformed or misinformed actors in their bioavailability. One result of the medical misinformation among donors is the creation of pseudo-medical narratives that can become pernicious. For example, two such narratives among donors are that of the 'wasted egg' and 'gift of motherhood' – eggs are being wasted each month through menstruation, in which case not donating squanders both an opportunity to earn and help a family (Kroløkke, 2015; Pande, 2020). Recruiters intertwine the wasted egg rationalisation with emotional pleas to share motherhood, as they urge women to realise that their 'wasted egg' could help another woman become a mother. Rajeshri explains:

> I tell the women, 'Look, this egg, this thing we have inside our stomach, it's getting wasted every month with our periods. It leaves your body in any case. [...] [The doctors] take it out and put it in another woman's womb. This woman is someone who cannot have children naturally the way we can. She needs the egg. So, you're also helping someone become a mother. You are a mother, you understand how beautiful this motherhood is. If you can help someone also feel the emotion of being a mother, what is wrong in that? That's so amazing' After I explain it like this, the women usually understand. (Rajeshri Rai, 2018, Interview)

Cohen (2003: 663) captures these moralisation logics as 'flexible ethics' and 'ethical publicity'. By emphasising the morality of enabling someone's motherhood, recruiters teach donors a 'win-win' logic to justify income through contentious bodily labour (Cohen, 2003). Similarly, the logic of 'excess', that is having eggs that go unused, becomes a source of guilt, engendering a skewed sense of obliged altruism (Scheper-Hughes, 2000). This coaxing toward bioavailability is emotionally manipulative, as donors are presented with incomplete truths and made to feel responsible for not providing their unused eggs to a couple in need (Gupta and Richters, 2008; Reddy and Patel, 2015). Although one egg may be 'wasted' each month through menstruation, this does not account for the risks associated with stimulating and extracting twenty to thirty eggs when a woman agrees to donate. Peter Digeser (1992), in his analysis of Michel Foucault's theories of ubiquitous power, outlines manipulation as inculcating a false consciousness: actor A (recruiter) persuades actor

B (donor) to do something (donate eggs) that is fundamentally against B's interest by convincing B (employing narratives of wastage, financial gain, and moral obligation) that the action is indeed in B's best interest. There is no overt force – power lies in coercing self-interest. The institutionally imposed gift and wasted egg narratives mask evident bioethical concerns regarding the donor, taking precedence over discussing her risks and wellbeing (Reddy and Patel, 2015; Rudrappa and Collins, 2015; Scheper-Hughes, 2000; Tober and Kroløkke, 2021). However, in allowing the free reign of misinformed and coercive narratives, it is the clinic who benefits most, as it receives a steady source of donors to profit from.

Another consequence of the clinic's neglect toward formalising its recruiters and recruitment strategies is the substantial emotional and psychological harm caused to donors. Without adequate medical understanding, donors harbour a host of fears and anxieties about the donation procedures. Many donors expressed fears about what the doctor would *really* do after administering anaesthesia during the egg retrieval. It was not until women had donated their eggs multiple times that they came to understand, or rather became accustomed to, the medical processes. Lalita has donated her eggs twice and is now working as a surrogate mother because, at age thirty-two, her eggs are no longer desirable. Her first donation was not with Progya, but she still remembers the overwhelming fear:

> I was so afraid of the operation. Fear, like how can I explain to you? My heart was beating so hard. I just worried what the doctors would do to be when they would make me unconscious. [...] They told me there was nothing to be afraid of and that I wouldn't feel anything. Then, they gave me the saline. They tied my hands and feet down. I was even more scared then. There were two people standing beside me, two by my head, two by my feet. They were all talking to me, just trying to distract me until I became unconscious. [...] I never talked about these things with anyone else. Even though I was scared and nervous and all that, I didn't want to discuss it with anyone. At that point in my life the only concern I had was for my money. (Lalita Biswas, 2018, Interview)

Lalita agreed to be an egg donor without fully understanding what the medical process would entail, illuminating how financial pressure induces bioavailability regardless of informed consent. Despite her fears, Lalita, like so many other donors, forged ahead in her donations in order to receive money. As she describes, many donors do not openly discuss their concerns at the time of donation, fearing that this will disqualify them from being able to complete the procedure and receive income. Although Lalita goes on to discuss that donating was ultimately manageable, and her fears subsided the second time around, it remains problematic that women feel that they must endure major surgical procedures that they do not understand.

Although the clinic creates the financially incentivised market structure for egg donation, it neglects to adequately train its inter-mediaries and protect the individuals it relies on for continued bioavailability. Without professionalised recruiters, donors can be enlisted by any means necessary, including financial compulsion, ultimately benefiting the clinic's productivity in a for-profit fertility industry. As a result of clinics intentionally retaining recruiters as informal intermediaries in this way, donors are emotionally and psychologically harmed, which compromises their consent and autonomy in their bodily labour. Donors lack an appropriate epistemic orientation into the clinic, as they do not meet with doctors or other medical professionals before enlisting as donors (Mukherjee, 2020; Thompson, 2005). They are unable to ask the clinicians questions or express concerns, and are often hesitant about doing so as they fear losing donation as a source of income. All of this combines to put donors in a position where they can be coerced and harmed, as they don't have the tools or accurate information to guide their choices.

While becoming bioavailable is compelled by financial duress, it is arguably the donor's lack of knowledge about the medical process and the resulting emotional stress that compromise her ability to provide informed consent. Without the appropriate professional resources and thorough counselling prior to enlisting as a donor, the psychological trade-off for income through bodily labour is untenable (Gupta and Richters, 2008; Thompson, 2007; Vora, 2013; Waldby, 2008).

Moralisation and camaraderie among low-income women

Although I have shown how women of low socio-economic status in Kolkata are often incentivised to target one another's bioavailability, it is also important to note that there is a network of trust and care among them (Deomampo, 2013). Donors must overcome significant hurdles if they are to continue being bioavailable, including intense fears about the medical procedures and judgement from friends and family who stigmatise egg donation as immoral bodily work (Pande, 2010; Rudrappa and Collins, 2015). Through this, donors become important sources of support for one another, especially when it comes to managing the stigma around performing bodily work. In addition, recruiters provide care and comfort for donors; they host an informal epistemic space (though misinformed) for donors to make sense of bioavailability, a responsibility the clinic absolves itself of. Accordingly, donors describe recruiters as their confidantes:

> I really trust [my recruiter]. We have a good relationship. She takes care of me like I am her own family. I know I can trust her to be good to me. She takes care of my health, she looks after me, she never lies to me, she is really good to me. The recruiters explain everything to us for the most part. [...] If I have any questions or worries, I will refer to my recruiter. They help us with everything. (Puja Debjyoti, 2018, Interview)

Donors like Puja who have good relationships with their recruiters describe positive experiences, illustrating the crucial support found in these networks. In some cases, donors who were close to their recruiters were able to find out whether their eggs resulted in successful pregnancies, information that donors often desired but were denied access to. Still, the issue remains that recruiters are not formally trained or professionally bound to the clinic. They are freelance middle-women who, through donating their own eggs, have met fertility doctors and harnessed this relationship to get paid for providing donors to clinics. Despite well-intentioned efforts, recruiters often perpetuate medical misinformation (i.e. pseudo-medical narratives) when trying to comfort donors. Menaka, a former donor and recruiter with thirteen years' experience, explains how she placates donors' fear of injections:

> If they are really worried, I just tell them that the injections are good for them. These are poor people, they don't have that much to eat, so taking these injections adds so much strength to their bodies, right? I think so. I tell them all this stuff to make them ready and convince them to come here. (Menaka Raj, 2018, Interview)

Menaka describes being unsure about the purpose or effects of these injections, but she says what she needs to in order to reduce women's fears and 'convince' them to donate. In reality, these injections do not add strength or nutrients to donors' bodies. They solely contain hormones intended to increase follicle stimulation and prevent premature ovulation. Without adequate clinical guidance or oversight, recruiters are at liberty to say what is needed to comfort and recruit women, even if their narratives are wholly inaccurate or coercive (and thereby harmful to donors). As such, for donors to genuinely benefit from trusting networks with recruiters, it is important to recognise that recruiters have become the donor's primary resource for medical information and emotional support, and should thus functionally occupy a role likened to formal clinical staff.

Donors also crucially support one another in their bioavailability. A traditional Bengali society, Kolkata deeply values female chastity with engrained traditions around sex, motherhood, and family. Here, reproductive labour is stigmatised, often conflated with sex work or 'baby selling'. Although donors primarily seek this bodily work for financial gain, their motivations are more complex and can parallel Scheper-Hughes' (2000: 193) account of kidney sellers – a 'blend of altruism and commerce, of science and magic, of gifting, barter, and theft, of choice and coercion'. As such, to cope with stigma, donors moralise their bioavailability. They look to experienced donors to reinforce the notion that egg donation will not compromise their chastity. Darshana, a first-time donor, explains:

> I am doing this work because what I am doing is helping someone and I am also getting money that I need. Doing this is not a bad or immoral job – my friend [former donor] made sure to make me understand this. For someone who is not able to be a mother, what I am doing is helping her be a mother. What I am giving her is going to help her see the face of a child. What I am doing is helpful. Also, at the same time I am making money. (Darshana Kayal, 2018, Interview)

Moral framing enables women to see egg provision as a noble act of sharing motherhood. Coming from communities with little formal knowledge about egg donation, interviewees describe suspicions that arises when a poor woman suddenly makes a large income, wherein the woman's sexual character is called into question. Accordingly, moralising donation enables women to overcome the stigmatisation around their reproductive labour and continue pursuing bioavailability (Pande, 2010, 2020; Rudrappa and Collins, 2015). Here, it is important to recognise that donors are undertaking substantial emotional and psychological labour for one another, none of which constitutes professional resources. In order to respond to their cultural contexts around bioavailability, clinics should be accountable for providing these resources – such as, professional mental health counselling – to donors. Further, the professionalisation of recruiters as clinic actors would allow for more reliable networks of support that are built on medical accuracy and therefore donor wellbeing.

Conclusion

As third-party reproductive technologies continue to shape family production, the demand for bioavailable bodies increases. Moreover, as global patterns have suggested, these bodies will be those of impoverished women in the global south (Cohen, 2003; Pande, 2011; Rudrappa, 2015; Scheper-Hughes, 2000,). While many have urged de-commercialisation and prohibition, the growing ubiquity of third-party reproduction, as well as precarious black markets in countries where it is illegal, suggests a need to protect bioavailable bodies without imposing blanket bans or negating individual autonomy (Dickenson, 2007; Gupta and Richters, 2008; Nahman, 2008; Thompson, 2007; Vora, 2013; Waldby, 2008). Egg donors, like many others who regularly resort to risky bodily labour for financial need (e.g. coal miners, commercial fishermen, sex workers) deserve the industries that they embed themselves in to protect their involvement.

Poverty underscores each of the hazardous circumstances that donors face: financial compulsion, lack of education and access to medical information, marginalised treatment within the clinic, and ever-present vulnerability due to inferior class status (Bailey, 2011; Gupta and Richters, 2008; Pande, 2011; Shah, 2009). Although resolving India's poverty is a large and important task, the pressing need to assure ethical bioavailability demands immediate and realistic regulatory interventions. Drawing on narratives from Kolkata's donation industry, I suggest that regulations prioritising increased meso-level overview can create a more equitable clinic environment, addressing class-based power imbalances and holding all clinic representatives accountable for donor support. Most importantly, these regulations must be aimed at re-centring donors' bodily ownership through access to accurate and thorough medical information, and legitimation of reproductive labour as an integral component of the ART industry worth safeguarding (Pande, 2010; Thompson, 2007; Vora, 2013; Waldby, 2008). While Foucault's (1978) framework of power ubiquity posits that egg donors (like all actors) can never be free from compulsion, it is worth discussing approaches to even *limited* ownership over one's bodily labour, where coercive mechanisms are minimised as much as possible (Digeser, 1992).

The stakeholder with the most power in the egg donation transaction is the clinic. It manages each of the medical processes and interactions involved in the transfer of biological material, dictating the terms around who is provided with what extent of access to resources and care from medical professionals. When the clinic fails to recognise its responsibility toward donors as patients undergoing medical procedures, for example by not encouraging donors to voice concerns, ask questions, and access accurate medical information, donors fall at the whim of pseudo-narratives and cannot be genuinely informed, consenting actors. Further, because India's egg donation norms remain un-legislated, clinics effectively self-monitor ethical standards. With so much left to the discretion of fertility clinics, it is imperative that these institutions be held to greater account in providing fair treatment to donors (Bailey, 2011). This brings us to the 'epistemic orientation' that is afforded to patients, but rarely to donors (Mukherjee, 2020; Thompson, 2005). If clinics are to rely on egg donors to complete fertility treatments, they must entitle donors to equal access of space and resources, allowing for sufficient medical education and emotional counselling, knowledge of short- and long-term risks, and a space to seek basic information on the resulting use of their biological material. The epistemic orientation, then, requires an established and equitable partnership between clinic and donor, where the donation is protected as clinical labour and the donor is afforded the same standards of safety and consideration afforded to patients undergoing IVF. These provisions pave a foundation for women to own their decision to donate eggs as one that is thoroughly informed.

Even though recruiters have emerged as the central and often only resource for donors to receive medical information, they are not recognised as formal, clinic representatives. Since clinics rely on recruiters to identify and guide women through the donation process, clinics must assume responsibility over these recruiters as staff bound to the same ethical standards as clinicians. This would require a professionalisation of the recruiter's role as a clinic representative, standardisation of the recruitment strategies and narratives, and regulation of payment schemes incentivising repeat donations. Still, the issue remains, can we trust clinics to regulate themselves? The straightforward answer is 'no' (Bailey, 2011; Towghi and Vora, 2014). As India contemplates its national laws and regulations around third-party regulation, a key component must be developing an independent regulatory body to monitor bioethical practices within fertility clinics.

Greater accountability for the clinic and its representatives can lay the groundwork for more adequate donor education and genuine informed consent. Although a donor may continue to face financial compulsion, ensuring that she has accurate information about the medical processes her body will undergo provides her with tools to consider whether the trade-off for bioavailability is worth temporarily alleviating financial duress. Poverty may constrain her options, but information and resources begin to transform her into an agent who is able to make an informed decision regarding whether to donate eggs.

As the global machine commercialising reproduction proliferates, the option to make oneself bioavailable becomes more tangible and conscionable for low-income women. When women express a desire to continue donating their eggs for as long as possible, it is difficult to imagine implementing a ban that would not drive them into a far more perilous black market. Considering the gamut of empirical cases that illustrate low-income women's reliance on reproductive labour as a source of income, research should consider how best to protect women in this machine that is already deeply entrenched worldwide. While this article has focused on on-the-ground solutions at the clinic level, Scheper-Hughes (2000: 210) provides a framework for the broader picture: a country must have 'national laws and international guidelines outlining and protecting the rights of ... donors', a 'reasonably fair and equitable health care system', and a 'reasonably democratic state in which basic human rights are guaranteed'. It is important that future research looks into the international contexts in which third-party ART operates, questioning how legislation can safeguard bioavailability across various global markets. With interdisciplinary contributions from the social sciences, law, and medicine, we can inform equitable systems that reinforce the wellbeing of bioavailable bodies as a shared commitment among medical institutions leading ART advancements.

References

Almeling, R. (2006). 'Why do you want to be a donor?' Gender and the production of altruism in egg and sperm donation. *New Genetics and Society* 25:2, 143–57.

Almeling, R. (2011). *Sex Cells: The Medical Market for Eggs and Sperm.* Berkeley, CA: University of California Press.

Bailey, A. (2011). Reconceiving surrogacy: toward a reproductive justice account of Indian surrogacy. *Hypatia* 26:4, 715–41.

Cohen, L. (2003). Where it hurts: Indian material for an ethics of organ transplantation. *Zygon* 38:3, 663–88.

DasGupta, S. and Das Dasgupta, S. (2014). *Globalization and Transnational Surrogacy in India: Outsourcing Life.* Lanham: Lexington Books.

Deomampo, D. (2013). Transnational surrogacy in India: interrogating power and women's agency. *Frontiers: A Journal of Women Studies* 34:3, 167–88.

Dickenson, D. L. (2007). *Property in the Body: Feminist Perspectives.* Cambridge: Cambridge University Press.

Dickenson, D. L. (2017). Disappearing women, vanishing ladies and property in embryos, *Journal of Law and the Biosciences* 4:1, 175–80.

Digeser, P. (1992). The fourth face of power, *The Journal of Politics* 54:4, 977–1007.

Foucault, M. (1978). *History of Sexuality, Volume 1: An Introduction.* New York: Random House.

Grand View Research (2018). *In-Vitro Fertilization (IVF) market size, share and trends analysis report by instruments (culture media, capital equipment, IVF disposable devices), by end use (hospitals, clinics), by type, and segment forecasts, 2018–2025.* www.grandviewresearch.com/industry-analysis/in-vitro-fertilization-market. Accessed 28 October 2018.

Gupta, J. and Richters, A. (2008). Embodied subjects and fragmented objects: women's bodies, assisted reproduction technologies and the right to self-determination, *Journal of Bioethical Inquiry* 5:4, 239–49.

Hoang, K. (2015). *Dealing in Desire: Asian Ascendancy, Western Decline, and the Hidden Currencies of Global Sex Work*. Berkeley, CA: University of California Press.

Hochschild, A. (2011). Emotional life on the market frontier. *Annual Review of Sociology* 37:1, 21–33.

Kempadoo, K. (1998). Globalizing sex workers' rights, *Canadian Woman Studies* 23:3/4, 143–50.

Krøløkke, C. (2015). The golden egg: the business of making mothers through egg donation. In A. T. Demo, J. L. Borda and C. Krøløkke (eds), *The Motherhood Business: Consumption, Communication, and Privilege*, 28–51. Tuscaloosa: University of Alabama Press.

Kundu, N. (2003). The case of Kolkata, India. The global report on human settlements. www.ucl.ac.uk/dpu-projects/Global_Report/pdfs/Kolkata.pdf. Accessed 1 September 2018.

Majumdar, A. (2014). The rhetoric of choice: the feminist debates on reproductive choice in the commercial surrogacy arrangement in India, *Gender, Technology and Development* 18:2, 275–301.

Mitra, P. (2016). Egg donation on the rise in Kolkata. *The Times of India*, 28 August. www.timesofindia.indiatimes.com/city/kolkata/Egg-donation-on-the-rise-in-Kolkata/articleshow/53898364.cms. Accessed 10 December 2017.

Mukherjee, M. (2020). The management of unequal patient status in fertility medicine: donors' and intended parents' experiences of participatory and imposed enrolment, *Social Science and Medicine* 247, 112807.

Nahman, M. (2008). Nodes of desire, *European Journal of Women's Studies* 15:2, 65–82.

Niyogi, S. (2012). Kolkata's poor poorer than the rest. *The Times of India*, 12 September. https://timesofindia.indiatimes.com/city/kolkata/Kolkatas-poor-poorer-than-the-rest/articleshow/16367595.cms. Accessed 1 September 2018.

Pande, A. (2010). 'At least I am not sleeping with anyone': resisting the stigma of commercial surrogacy in India, *Feminist Studies* 36:2, 292–312.

Pande, A. (2011). Transnational commercial surrogacy in India: gifts for global sisters? *Reproductive Biomedicine Online* 23:5, 618–25.

Pande, A. (2020). Visa stamps for injections: traveling bio-labour and South African egg provision, *Gender and Society* 34:4, 573–96.

Reddy, S. and Patel, T. (2015). 'There are many eggs in my body': medical markets and commodified bodies in India, *Global Bioethics* 26:3–4, 218–31.

Rudrappa, S. (2012). Working India's reproduction assembly line: surrogacy and reproductive rights? *Western Humanities Review* 66:3, 77–101.

Rudrappa, S. (2015). *Discounted Life: The Price of Global Surrogacy in India*. New York: NYU Press.

Rudrappa, S. and Collins, C. (2015). Altruistic agencies and compassionate consumers, *Gender and Society* 296, 937–59.

Scheper-Hughes, N. (2000). The global traffic in human organs, *Current Anthropology* 41:2, 191–224.

Shah, C. (2009). Regulate technology, not lives: a critique of The Draft ART (Regulation) Bill, *Indian Journal of Medical Ethics* 6:1, 32–5.

Thompson, C. (2005). *Making Parents: The Ontological Choreography of Reproductive Technologies*. Cambridge, MA: MIT Press.

Thompson, C. (2007). Why we should, in fact, pay for egg donation, *Regenerative Medicine* 2:2, 203–9.

Tober, D. and Kroløkke, C. (2021). Emotion, embodiment, and reproductive colonialism in the global human egg trade, *Gender, Work and Organization* 28: 5, 1766–86.

Towghi, F. and Vora, K. (2014). Bodies, markets, and the experimental in South Asia, *Ethnos* 79:1, 1–18.

Vora, K. (2013). Potential, risk, and return in transnational Indian gestational surrogacy, *Current Anthropology* 54:S7, S97–S106.

Waldby, C. (2008). Oocyte markets: women's reproductive work in embryonic stem cell research. *New Genetics and Society* 27:1, 19–31.

Waldby, C. and Cooper, M. (2008). The biopolitics of reproduction, *Australian Feminist Studies* 23:55, 57–73.

Waldby, C., Kerridge, I., Boulos, M. and Carroll, K. (2013). From altruism to monetisation: Australian women's ideas about money, ethics and research eggs, *Social Science and Medicine* 94, 34–42.

West, R. (2000). The difference in women's hedonic lives: a phenomenological critique of feminist legal theory, *Wisconsin Women's Law Journal* 15:1, 149–215.

World Bank (2017). *West Bengal: Poverty, Growth, and Inequality.* http://documents.worldbank.org/curated/en/315791504252302097/pdf/119344-BRI-P157572-West-Bengal-Poverty.pdf. Accessed 28 October 2018.

12

The egg donation economy in South Africa: different levels of biopolitics

Verena Namberger

Over the last fifteen years South Africa has developed into one of the top destinations for so-called reproductive tourism (Bergmann, 2011; Nahman, 2016)[1] and into an important hub in the transnational market for donor eggs in the context of in vitro fertilisation (IVF) and commercial surrogacy. Part and parcel of the country's flourishing egg donor market is its 'large pool of racially diverse donors' in combination with 'first world' medical standards and clinics, English-language proficiency, favourable exchange rates and tourist attractions. Overall, the South African egg donation economy is a paradigmatic example of the reshaping of global politics of reproduction through the normalisation and marketisation of assisted reproductive technology (ART) (Lie and Lykke, 2017). This chapter explores the biopolitical dimension of this particular local market for reproductive tissue, which is closely entwined with the global fertility industry. It revolves around the following twofold question. In which ways do Foucauldian biopolitics play out in the economy of egg donation in South Africa; and how are they possibly reshaped and altered?

The chapter shows that in the context of commercialised egg donation, biopolitical efforts to exercise the power to 'make live and to let die' (Foucault, [1976] 2002: 241) operate on different levels: on the molecular level of embryo selection in the laboratory; on the level of the body proper with regard to the (medical, psychological, genetic) screening and pre-selection of suitable oocyte donors and the possibility for recipients to choose the 'perfect donor'; on a national level in terms of regulatory efforts to manage the national gene pool and prevent interbreeding; and on a global level insofar as it is only a particular, privileged group that can afford expensive fertility treatment and the outsourcing of reproductive services to the global south. While mapping these different dimensions of biopolitics I will argue that the South African fertility industry is a paradigmatic site to study the emergence of a new, subtle form of eugenics, which comes in the frame of choice – or 'positive eugenics', to use Amrita Pande's (2014: 34) term – and frames egg providers as rational, responsible biocitizens (Pande and Moll, 2018). In contrast to scholars like Nikolas Rose (2007), who considers the concept of eugenics inadequate in the context of genomics and reproductive choice, this chapter employs the term to highlight both continuities and changes regarding the reproduction of existing hierarchies. My analysis is based on an extensive corpus of ethnographic data collected during two research stays in South Africa (November/December 2014 and January/February 2016), which I analysed through 'situational analysis' (Clarke, 2005) in combination with text and metaphor analysis in the tradition of cultural studies.[2]

Biopolitics and reproduction

Michel Foucault (1978, [1976] 2002) describes biopolitics as a new governmental rationality that emerged in the eighteenth-century political economy and that is concerned with phenomena relating to a group of living beings who constitute a population. Biopower, or the modern governmental rationality of making live and letting die, seeks to discipline and regulate birth and mortality rates, health, hygiene and the quality of the population's gene pool. It 'deals with the population, with the population as a political problem, as a problem that is at once scientific and political, as a biological problem and as power's problem' (Foucault, [1976] 2002: 245). Foucault did not pay much attention to the gendered and racialised dimension of biopolitics. This is a major point of criticism from a (Black) feminist perspective. Silvia Federici (2004: preface) for instance, points out that 'Foucault's analysis of tile power techniques and disciplines to which the body has been subjected has ignored the process of reproduction, has collapsed female and male histories into an undifferentiated whole'. It is important to realise that the biopolitics of reproduction are furthermore played out differently on white women's bodies than on the bodies of Black women or women of colour, and again differently according to women's socio-economic status, class and sexual orientation (Hill Collins, 2000; Barbagallo, 2015). One just has to recall the early days of European colonialism when Black female slaves working on planta- tions were forbidden to have children of their own as 'it was cheaper to purchase than to breed' (Mies, 1986: 92), to use the language of slave owners, while the natural role and destiny that was ascribed to white bourgeois women was being mothers and housewives. Such a historically grounded sensitivity to intersectional power relations is crucial in the South African context. It stresses that population control and pro-natal policies, as diametrically opposed dimensions of reproductive politics, are two sides of the same biopolitical coin. This complex interrelationship is at the core of the thematic frame of this book.

Interestingly, those two poles of reproductive politics have common technological roots, which further underlines their entanglement. One aspect of this genealogical link is the history of so-called sex hormones and especially the hormones oestrogen and progesterone, which are commonly associated with femininity (Fausto-Sterling, 2000; Oudshoorn, 1990).[3] Beatriz Preciado (2013) describes the genealogy of the manufacturing and trafficking of sex hormones as beginning in the 1920s and involving both human research subjects and research material derived from dead animals. It is intriguing how largely unheard of the historical trajectories are that led to today's mass industrial production of synthetic hormones. This is even more astonishing as oestrogen and progesterone are 'the most manufactured synthetic substances in all the pharmaceutical industries of the world' (Preciado, 2013: 167). They are also key actants in every IVF treatment. In other words, the South African fertility industry and egg donation market would not exist without them. From the outset there has been a distinct gendered bias in hormonal research, as Preciado stresses. While testosterone, the 'male' sexual hormone is associated with sexual desire, health, youth and vitality, the 'female' counterparts are seen as useful only within the biopolitical frame of controlling reproduction and women's sexuality – or, to frame it in pharmaceutical bestsellers, Viagra on the one side and the birth control pill on the other side.

The history of the pill, and with it the history of the synthetic production of oestrogen and progesterone, is deeply rooted in disciplinary policy regimes and postcolonial power relations. The pill can be seen as the scientific outcome of US policy efforts of the 1950s and 1960s to restrict the reproductive power of non-white or deviant women; and as such it is closely linked with other techniques of 'public hygiene' (Preciado, 2013: 176) in a Foucauldian sense. When clinical trials in prisons and psychiatric institutions in the US did not provide enough data for the US Food and Drug Administration (USFDA) to allow the commercialisation of the pill, the pharmacological industry had to look for alternatives. In Puerto Rico it eventually found the perfect pseudo-colonial setting and a live laboratory for a large-scale pill trial outside medical institutions. Embedded in a state-controlled birth control programme the pill was tested on uneducated and low-income Puerto Rican women. This marked a new era for clinical trials as it moved both from animal to humans and from controlled clinical settings to the larger population. The feminist activist Katherine McCormick, who heavily funded research on the contraceptive pill through the 1960s, infamously compared the involved challenges to finding and getting access to a 'cage of ovulating females' (cited in Preciado, 2013: 180). Puerto Rico came quite close to such laboratory settings. As an island it resembled a hermetically sealed cage full of docile, low-income women who had no choice but to follow the instructions, which were enforced by close monitoring through social workers. This historical example shows that the by now normalised administration of hormones, be it in the form of the pill or in the context of IVF treatment and the procurement of donor oocytes, does come with a heavy biopolitical burden. Synthetically produced hormones are paradigmatic examples of how the bodies of egg donors in South Africa are connected with US foreign policy and postcolonial dependencies, with pharmaceutical companies' pursuit of profit and politically motivated research funding, with population control and biopolitics. Those entanglements remain hidden behind the glossy picture of ARTs and the possibilities they yield for infertile heterosexual women and couples or gay intended parents to realise the dream of a child of their own. Against this backdrop, I will now turn towards the empirical case study of this chapter, namely the egg donation market in South Africa.

The biopolitics of egg donation: consumer choice, genetics and geopolitics

As already mentioned in the introduction, South Africa is the site of a thriving economy that revolves around donor oocytes as sought-after reproductive matter. While egg donation was practised very rarely in the early 2000s, it is now a routine medical procedure and a professionalised market. A growing number of private fertility clinics and egg donor agencies are offering their services, the number of recipients (predominantly from overseas) is constantly rising and yet there are no waiting lists for donor eggs (in stark contrast to many other countries, especially in Europe). South Africa is renowned for high medical standards, a wide choice of donors and comparatively low treatment costs (especially in combination with favourable exchange rates for patients coming from Europe, the US or Australia). Catalysts of this remarkable development have been egg donor agencies, which constitute key intermediary actors in the field and have significantly professionalised the commercial procurement and brokering of donor oocytes in South Africa. Part and parcel of the professionalisation of the industry are, furthermore, the ethical guidelines established by the Southern African Society of Reproductive Medicine and Gynaecological Endoscopy (SASREG).[4] The guidelines work as a code of conduct that is not mandatory but intends to provide a normatively binding set of rules in addition to the legal framework of the National Health Act (National Department of Health, 2003). They pertain to the age of egg donors (between eighteen and thirty-six), context sensitive advertisements and recruiting (i.e. avoiding statements about financial gains), the practice of informed consent, the requirement of physiological and psychological screening of donors and the maximal number of donations (six times). Besides this, the guidelines make a recommendation regarding the payment of egg donors, which is framed as monetary compensation for the donor's time, inconvenience and financial costs. SASREG proposes a sum of R7000 (US$525), which should be received via the fertility clinic after the procedure.

All in all, the South African egg donation economy is an emblematic case of the increasing normalisation of reproductive technologies and outsourcing of reproductive services to third parties and countries in the global south. ARTs have strengthened the desire for one's own biological children (either genetically or epigenetically related) and have turned procreation into a seemingly manageable project – with the aim of minimising risks while maximising control and predictability. This development is linked to a depoliticised perspective on infertility, 'insofar as the new technologies locate the problem of infertility within individuals' (Sawicki, 1999: 194). The following section discusses to what extent Foucauldian biopolitics play a role in the South African industry around donor eggs. In doing so, it shows how they are partly reshaped in this specific setting. It thereby pays particular attention to the close relationship between biopolitics and the pseudo-scientific discourse of eugenics, the link between the 'degeneracy' of individuals and the hygiene and vitality of the population at large (Foucault, [1976] 2002).

Choosing the perfect donor

At the heart of the egg donation economy are the online databases of egg donor agencies that offer a wide choice of available donors just a click away. Thanks to agencies and their online presence, intended parents all over the world have access to detailed profiles of South African women enrolled as potential donors. These profiles transform the vague desires and traits that recipients are seeking into a standardised form and into neat categories. Donor profiles include photos of the donor as a child and allow searching for specific physical features and genetic traits (race, hair and eye colour, complexion, height) or more personal characteristics (religion, education, special talents). Recipients especially appreciate the wide choice of donors of all races and ethnicities that South Africa offers. The colonial and apartheid history of the country is thereby turned into an asset in the global fertility business. The option for recipients to base their choice of a donor on extensive medical and personal information gives South Africa a competitive advantage on the international market, as in countries like Spain, where recipients are assigned a phenotypically matching donor. An agency owner put it aptly when she said: 'South Africa is all about offering choice' (Interview with agency owner, 2014). The possibility to choose the perfect donor goes hand in hand with the logic of consumerism and the desire for healthy babies with specific genetic traits (Becker, 2000; Strathern, 1995). It fits into a cultural setting marked by freedom of choice, the privatisation of risks and the desire for perfect bodies.

Accordingly, donors are pre-selected during the application process. There are a number of conditions that exclude women from becoming donors from the outset, for example: HIV positive women, women with a high BMI (above 28), or diagnosed schizophrenia. In addition, the application process involves a detailed medical and psychological screening to rule out further genetic disorders, family dispositions for diseases or mental illness and pre-existing medical problems. With the prospect of genetic panel tests soon becoming commercially available and affordable, the importance of genetic testing is likely to increase even more, as one of the leading IVF specialists of the country explained to me:

> That opens a door to a whole lot of other genetic testing that can be done. And these new genetic panels that are being introduced now may be a massive factor in egg donation in the future because it could be that they become commercially available for a small fee. So you can check 200 genes on a donor and get this whole panel of results and then decide whether you want the donor. (Interview with physician, 13 November 2014)

In other words, only a specific group of healthy, 'defect-free' women passes the barrier to be added to one of the agencies' databases. In addition to those screening processes I found another, more subtle and indirect mechanism of donor pre-selection based on class, a category that heavily intersects with race in the South African context. It is an (unintended) effect of the situation that the South African egg donation industry mainly takes place online and is moreover a predominantly white and English- or Afrikaans-speaking world. The application process and the way agencies are run in South Africa make it quite hard for socio-economically deprived women, who are often Black women, to be accepted as donors. Seemingly banal but not to be underestimated obstacles are the lack of a computer with internet access (many of the well-known agencies require having an email address and/or applying online) and childhood photos (cute toddler pictures are part of a donor's human capital). Besides, all donor application forms are in English; not one agency offers an additional form in isiXhosa or another vernacular language. Also, in the clinic donors are mostly expected to master the English language well enough to understand the medical details and instructions they are given. For Black women from rural areas or poorer backgrounds who did not go to an English-speaking school this poses a major challenge. Moreover, some Black donors told me off the record that they would not feel comfortable in the white, English-speaking world of egg donation; for others the fact that agencies are predominately run by white women had been a reason to refrain from applying altogether. Hence, racialised structures and requirements tend to subliminally impede women from poor socio-economic backgrounds, predominantly Black women, from enrolling in a donor programme.

In the combination of recipients choosing the 'perfect donor' and the upfront screening of women applying as donors there is a danger of a clandestine arrival of a new form of eugenics. It is a form of 'positive eugenics' (Pande, 2014: 34) or 'flexible eugenics' (Taussig et al., 2003), which is embedded in the rhetoric of personal choice and driven by the desire for perfection, individual preferences and health. The application of the term eugenics in this context is not uncontested. Nikolas Rose (2007) for instance, rejects the reference to eugenics in the context of selective reproductive technologies because of the term's association with particular Nazi practices, such as ethnic cleansing and insectification. What Rose (2007) sees at work in today's fertility-related services is not eugenics as part of national interests and governmental strategies but a new form of self-government based on individual choice and the desire for self-fulfilment. I agree that it is important to differentiate clearly between state eugenics and racism, like in Nazi Germany, and new possibilities to choose the desired traits of offspring or rule out genetic diseases. Unlike Rose, however, I suggest using the term with the necessary caution to precisely make visible both differences and continuities between 'old' and 'new' forms of eugenics. I favour a critical rethinking of the term that takes into account the changed context, as Amrita Pande (2014) suggests. She speaks of 'positive eugenics' to stress the positive appeal of a language of selection and individual choice: 'While the concepts of "waste" and "burden" are intrinsic to negative eugenics, the concept of "consumer choice" is intrinsic to positive eugenics and the promotion of new reproductive technologies' (Pande, 2014: 34).

This characterisation applies, to a great extent, to the South African egg donation market where the positively framed notion of consumer choice is pivotal – starting with the choice of the donor profile representing the perfect (genetic) traits from the database. Yet it is important to note that the trend towards individual choice in markets for reproductive tissue is not completely generalisable. During my field research, I learned that not all recipients attach the same value to detailed information about donors and the vast possibilities of choice. My data suggests that there is a difference between women or couples coming from overseas (predominantly from Australia and New Zealand, but also from Europe and the US) and the increasing number of Black recipients from South Africa or other African countries. Whereas for the former, choosing a donor tends to be a difficult and complex decision the latter are mostly not interested in detailed profiles and genetics. As a physician told me: 'it is like they will choose anyone as long as she is Black. She does not have to look like a movie star and be this and that, they just want a baby' (Interview with IVF specialist, 24 November 2014).

Selecting 'beautiful embryos'

The possibility of choosing and selecting the (genetic) traits of the desired baby continues on a molecular level, and hence in the laboratory space. This empirical observation from my research supports Rose's (2007) claim that in the age of biomedicine biopolitics move from whole bodies to the molecular level. Once donor oocytes have been fertilised and cultured in the lab for three to six days, the 'best' embryos are selected for transfer. In most South African clinics this is done through a visual assessment of the embryos in the petri dish by the embryologist. Even though practitioners stressed that it is not a 'beauty contest' (Interview with physician, 12 November 2015) staged under the microscope, the grading systems are based on norms of beauty and aesthetics. Symmetry, especially, is highly rated in the lab, along with clear lines and boundaries and evenly shaped cells. The criteria are always already co-constituted by the embryologist's eye in seeing beauty in embryos. In addition, pre-implantation genetic diagnosis (PGD) is routinely used to detect gene defects in embryos prior to transfer.

A significant innovation in the context of visual embryo grading is the use of technological devices like the EmbryoScope™ or Primo Vision™, which are currently finding their way into the laboratories of South African fertility clinics. Due to their high cost and effortful handling they are not yet used in standard IVF procedures in South Africa but can be booked for an additional fee in some of the bigger clinics. Those clinics mostly work with the EmbryoScope™, 'a system that is an incubator, a microscope with an integrated camera and advanced software at the same time' (Cape Fertility Clinic). It allows the embryologist to assess the development of embryos through automated imaging without removing them from the incubator. The integrated time-lapse technology furthermore enables a dynamic image of cell growth and cleavage, in contrast to the snapshot the embryologist gets through a once-a-day peek. Additionally, it comes with integrated computer software that scores embryos according to set parameters and selects the ones with the highest implantation potential. Thereby, the software partly substitutes the experienced eye of the embryologist. This means a qualitative change with regard to the selection of embryonic cells and ultimately bodies that deserve to live. With the automated and standardised embryo selection based on a population-derived norm of embryonic development, Foucauldian biopolitics are updated and raised to a new level. The population of embryonic cells replaces the population of a nation as the target and norm-setting collective of biopolitics. Biopolitics then also move from 'wet DNA' (physical tissue) into 'dry DNA' (information and data): the 'survival of the fittest' is written into algorithms that are designed to calculate deviances from the norm. Overall, time-lapse technology leads to an 'increased digitization and standardization of selection' (van de Wiel, 2017: 290) while reiterating existing ideas of able-bodiedness, health and lives worth living.

The selection of 'beautiful embryos' – be it through the trained embryologist's eye or through time-lapse technology and computer software – adds another, molecular level to the 'positive eugenics' that are at play in the egg donation economy. While there is a qualitative difference between the state-led eugenics that Foucault described, the biopolitical link between the 'degeneracy' of individuals and the hygiene and vitality of the population at large is also discernible in the laboratories of IVF clinics. For the ideal of the perfect child is embedded in a socio-cultural context in which dis-abled or sick bodies tend to be seen as burdens for health systems and societies. For that reason I disagree with Rose, as already stated above, who writes that PGD and selective reproductive technologies have nothing to do with 'Nazi insectification' and are not 'remotely similar to the view that those who are born afflicted by any of these conditions are of less worth than others' (2007: 69). The routine use of PGD in the context of IVF treatment in general, and hence also in the case of IVF using donor eggs, normalises a 'geneticisation of conception' (Bock von Wülfingen, 2007) based on the linking of pro-natal and anti-natal technologies. This normalisation establishes the basis for a new form of 'positive eugenics' that is embedded in the rhetoric of personal (consumer) choice. For the normalisation and routinisation of embryo selection might in the long run foster a social climate and health policies in which disabilities and genetic defects are considered preventable and the lives of affected people less worth living.

Managing the 'gene pool'

The idea of the body as an expression and bearer of individual genetic information is also relevant for biopolitics on a macro level. The South African state is an important, or at least a potentially important, actor with regard to the legislation of gamete donation. As mentioned earlier, the respective South African legislation is published in the National Health Act (Chapter 8), supplemented by SASREG's ethical guidelines. With the limit of six donations resulting in live births, both South African law and SASREG guidelines address a key biopolitical concern, namely the danger of interbreeding and the health of the nation's gene pool. It is also a central concern for professionals working in the field, as my research revealed. The head of the fertility unit in a private clinic shared his memories with me about the old days of egg donation, when the clinic had not cooperated with egg donor agencies but had relied on a group of local donors.

> We had our own pool of donors, they didn't cost anything. We did the screening for free, the blood test for free, we did everything for free for the donors. The patients could actually come and choose but the pool was only ten to fifteen donors. As time went on we saw that we were using the same donors over and over. And then I said 'Whoa,

what is going on here? Is this the genetic pool you are going to choose from? Shouldn't we just change this formed dam to the ocean?' (Interview with IVF specialist, 24 November 2014)

The ocean stands here for the vast choice of donors that only agencies can offer. Despite initial reservations against the agency business, the clinic started cooperating with agencies that were operating nationwide. The main reason for that step was the described concern about genetic interbreeding.

The management of the biology of a population with regard to its reproduction, including the regulation of the population's gene pool, is at the core of what Foucault termed biopolitics. Regulatory efforts in the context of egg donation exceed medical ethics in a narrow sense as they pertain not only to the individual body but simultaneously address the social body as an object of biopolitical governance. A widely discussed, yet not embarked on policy measure is a national registry of all South African donors. Physicians and most SASREG registered agencies advocate for such a central database in order to keep track of the number of donations per woman (including the number of live births). At the moment, clinics and agencies have no means to track and control how often a woman has donated in South African clinics. One argument that professionals in favour of this control tool put forward is medical concern about the long-term health and fertility of the donor. The other reason is the peril of genetic interbreeding:

> Say she has donated five times and she has produced five live births, which is rare, but it happens. Now she goes on and has her own family of three children. There are eight children that potentially are all living within a radius in South Africa. Maybe two or three in Australia, which is a good immigration business of South Africans and there they generally move to one or two cities. And you can have interbreeding happening. Therefore I think that the central registry is critical. (Interview with agency owner, 10 November 2014)

Both the individual body as a carrier of a specific set of genes and the national body are addressed here as a target of biopolitical measures. Due to the demand for ever more detailed information about donors, whereby genetics and the desire for 'good genes' play a pivotal role, the body in egg donation is not only a source of reproductive matter but also of valuable data. What is remarkable, in this regard, is the subtle 'reification of race' on a cellular level (Pande, 2021; see also Chapter 14, this volume) and the normalised framing of individual dispositions, personality traits and socio-cultural factors as genetically anchored and inheritable. Here, the South African egg donor market, as part of the global fertility industry, fosters the cultural power of genes as the 'script of life' and produces bodily configurations – donor bodies, embryos, imagined bodies of 'desired babies' – that are valued and enacted in relation to their genetic make-up.

Like in Foucauldian biopolitics, the state remains an important addressee in the biopolitical task of managing the 'genetics' of egg donation, as the demand for a central, state-run registry illustrates. Even though the South African government is at present not able or willing to perform this controlling function, it is primarily seen as being the actor in charge. This ascribed role fits Foucault's description of biopolitics as concerned with the regulation of reproduction in order to maximise the health and wellbeing of the national population. Apart from this continuity the management of South Africa's gene pool in times of IVF and egg donation differs significantly in terms of scale, as described above. Reproductive technologies add another level of intervention to biopolitics, namely the molecular level of genes and embryos as new objects of biopolitics. The 'nationally governed managerial effort to manage life [...] has "descended" and been refocused at the level of reproductive substance itself', as Franklin (2013: 50) notes. At the same time nation states like South Africa are quite restricted in their ability to regulate reproduction in the face of a globalising fertility industry. In other words, biopolitics are simultaneously moved to a global level, as outlined in the following final section.

Biopolitics meets geopolitics: the global fertility industry

The importance of the transnational dimension of the South African egg donation economy can hardly be overestimated. Between 60% and 80% of patients seeking IVF treatment with donor eggs come from abroad (figures vary from clinic to clinic). Additionally, a significant number of internationally operating agencies facilitate cross-border donor arrangements. In this case, South African women are flown to IVF clinics in, for example, India, Nepal,[5] Mexico,

Ukraine or Barbados to provide 'fresh' oocytes for IVF treatment or gestational surrogacy there (Kroløkke, 2015; Pande, 2021; Pande and Moll, 2018; Sama, 2010). Oocytes from South African women are a particularly sought-after resource in the context of transnational surrogacy arrangements in South Asia and South America where oocytes from 'European looking' donors are rare. Even though SASREG guidelines ethically disapprove of this practice, the phenomenon of 'travelling donors' seems to be widespread (and an issue of concern for most practitioners I spoke with). This means that the South African egg donation economy is in many ways interlinked with the international fertility industry and part of a global topography of reproductive politics in times of ART.

South Africa is a geopolitical place marked by histories of conquest and colonialism that have always been entwined with questions of mobility and geopolitical power relations. When European or US American citizens fly to Cape Town to purchase the reproductive capacities of South African women, they do so against the historical background of European colonialism and imperialism. This is not to claim an unbroken continuity. The commodification of enslaved Black women as 'breeders' and workers in colonial times is markedly different from the way South African women – in itself a highly variegated group in terms of race and class – are enrolled in the egg donor business today. Past and present forms of commodifying human reproductivity are incommensurable, yet they are not unrelated. On the one hand neo-colonial dependencies, networks and the symbolic value of the Cape, which goes back to its reputation as a health resort in colonial times (Deacon, 2000), have contributed to South Africa becoming a global player in the fertility sector. On the other hand, intended parents from the global north with a relatively high socio-economic status benefit from unequal structures of economic exchange rooted in postcolonial power relations. They share the privilege to move across national and geographical space on their journey towards fulfilling their procreative desires both from a legal perspective, that is, thanks to holding a valid passport and being a citizen of a nation that grants the right to travel, and regarding financial means. Moreover, the cross-border arrangements often serve an economic purpose in the most immediate sense: one of the main reasons for IVF patients seeking treatment in South Africa is the cost factor, the good price-performance ratio they find there. Clinic costs, agency fees and the compensation for donors are significantly lower than in their home country or continent. A historical perspective of today's landscape or rather multiple geographies of reproductive travels is hence indispensable.

Such a historically informed perspective needs to consider, as Charis Thompson (2011: 206) points out, that 'medical migrations tend to run down well-traveled pathways, even as they re-inscribe, reinvent, or subvert those pathways'. My data shows that egg donation in South Africa today does not in every aspect 'map [...] onto older histories of race and empire' (Cooper and Waldby, 2014: 88). There are also discontinuities. An important deviation from 'well-traveled pathways' is that South Africa is seeing more and more fertility patients from other African countries, as it is, at the moment, the only country on the continent that offers cutting-edge fertility treatment and facilities. This trend mirrors the findings of a recent study initiated by the Southern African Migration Project (SAMP), that by now a high number of patients seeking treatment on the African continent are coming from other African countries (Crush et al., 2012). My research supports the demand of the study's authors that the idea of medical tourism running north–south needs to be adjusted to account for the increasing numbers of south–south travels for treatment. I hence agree with Bronwyn Parry's (2015: 32) critique of the widespread assertion in the literature that cross-border reproductive services would be 'largely unidirectional and characterised by a dynamic of provision in which "the rest" services "the West"'. Even though historically grown power relations between the global north and the global south play a major role in the transnational organisation of reproductive tourism, those structures are, at points, also reshaped and changed. What is needed is an empirically grounded and differentiated mapping of the 'complex "reproscape"' (Inhorn, 2011: 89–90), which includes not only whole bodies that move from A to B but also the global circulation of technologies, bodily tissue, money, ideas and medication.

Such a mapping of reproscapes makes visible that the biopolitics of egg donation have acquired an additional global dimension. Nation states, and especially the relations between them, still play an important role for the organisation of commercial oocyte brokering. Despite the global spread of ART and donor agencies those technologies and services are only accessible for a specific group, predominantly located in the global north. The economy of choice within the transnational fertility industry moves national biopolitics to a global level. It creates a 'biopolitical sphere located beyond national containers' (Beck, 2012: 374). A new type of global biopolitics is emerging insofar as the technologically enabled possibilities to enhance and optimise the genetic make-up of bodies are distributed unequally according to class, race and geopolitical location. In other words, 'biopolitics has merged with geopolitics', as Bruce Braun (2007: 8) writes. Global regimes of reproduction, geopolitics and neo-colonial power relations are at the core of a new subtle form of eugenics that come in the frame of choice but reproduce, to a great extent, unequal global power relations and existing hierarchies. On top, the divide between those who can afford to procreate by any (technological) means and those who are deprived of reproductive rights is aggravated by the depoliticisation of infertility due to ART. Reproductive technologies foster the individualisation of infertility as a medical condition and draw attention away from structural risk factors for infertility, such as poor living conditions, environmental pollution and inadequate healthcare, which disparately affect the poor and women in the global south.

Conclusion

Based on data from ethnographic research, this chapter explored the biopolitical dimension of the egg donation economy in South Africa. It showed that biopolitical technologies and strategies of controlling and regulating reproduction play a role on four different levels: on the molecular level of embryos and genetics; on the individual level of donor screening and selection; on the national level of legal and ethical regulations; and on the level of geopolitics and global power relations. Foucauldian biopolitics are thereby re-actualised as they are at the same time scaled down and up. Notwithstanding those changes I argued that the logics of selective reproduction through ART need to be seen as a continuation of eugenics, understood as a set of interventions in order to maximise the health and wellbeing of the national body, under new premises. I hence share the concern of scholars like Amrita Pande (2014) over the emergence of a new form of subtle, 'positive eugenics' linked to individual choice, technologically managed procreation and norms of able-bodiedness and healthy genes. The picture I drew was partial and inevitably biased, not least due to my social positioning as a white woman from Europe, and only provided a rough sketch of the actors, structures, practices and norms that constitute the South African market for human oocytes. By drawing attention to the biopolitical dimension of the fertility industry in South Africa, I aimed to contribute to the overarching debate of this book on the interrelations between population control, reproductive injustices and pro-natal technologies.

Notes

1 'Reproductive tourism' or 'fertility tourism' describes the search for fertility treatment, human gametes and/or surrogates across national borders due to financial reasons, legal restrictions and shortage of gamete donors or surrogates in the home country. The term tourism is increasingly criticised because it neglects the emotional pain and distress of IVF patients (Inhorn, 2011). Alternatively, more neutral and wider terms like 'repro-migration' (Nahman, 2011), 'cross-border reproductive care' or 'reproductive travel' (Inhorn and Pasquale, 2009) are suggested.

2 The corpus consists of thirty-six semi-structured interviews with physicians, clinic staff, owners of egg donation agencies, psychologists, and donors, complemented by anonymous donor questionnaires, participatory observation in clinics as well as of a heterogeneous corpus of textual and visual material published in the field (e.g. websites, information brochures, advertisement, blog posts, online forums). The analysis of the chapter is based on a more comprehensive study of the South African bioeconomy of egg donation (Namberger, 2019).

3 The idea that there are 'female' and 'male' hormones is a result of the field of endocrinology as it emerged in the 1930s and 1940s. Even though research has since clearly disproven this binary classification it is still deeply ingrained in everyday understanding and language.

4 These include general guidelines for gamete donation (published in 2008) and special guidelines for egg donation agencies (published in 2012, updated in 2015). Both documents can be retrieved from the SASREG website: www.fertilitysa.org.za/EggDonation/index.asp (accessed 4 May 2017).

5 Both India and Nepal have officially banned commercial surrogacy for foreigners now. It remains an open question how effectively those laws

will be enforced and to which countries the surrogacy business will move instead. Some agencies that facilitated transnational surrogacy programmes in the past still list Nepal and India on their website. It is likely that some existing schemes will continue covertly.

References

Barbagallo, C. (2015). Leaving home: slavery and the politics of reproduction, *Viewpoint Magazine* 5. www.viewpointmag.com/2015/10/31/leaving-home-slavery-and-the-politics-of-reproduction/. Accessed 9 September 2020.

Beck, S. (2012). Biomedical mobilities: transnational lab-benches and other space-effects. In M. Knecht, M. Klotz and S. Beck (eds), *Reproductive Technologies as Global Form: Ethnographies of Knowledge, Practices, and Transnational Encounters*, 357–74. Frankfurt and New York: Campus.

Becker, G. (2000). *The Elusive Embryo: How Women and Men Approach New Reproductive Technologies*. Berkeley, CA: University of California Press.

Bergmann, S. (2011). Fertility tourism: circumventive routes that enable access to reproductive technologies and substances, *Signs* 36:2, 280–9.

Bock von Wülfingen, B. (2007). *Genetisierung der Zeugung: Eine Diskurs- und Metaphernanalyse reproduktionsgenetischer Zukünfte*. Bielefeld: transcript.

Braun, B. (2007). Biopolitics and the molecularization of life, *Cultural Georaphies* 1:1, 6–28.

Clarke, A. E. (2005). *Situational Analysis: Grounded Theory after the Postmodern Turn*. London: Sage.

Cooper, M. and Waldby, C. (2014). *Clinical Labor: Tissue Donors and Research Subjects in the Global Bioeconomy*. Durham, NC: Duke University Press.

Crush, J., Chikanda, A. and Maswikwa, B. (2012). Patients without borders: medical tourism and medical migration in southern Africa. In J. Crush (ed.), *Migration Policy Series*. Cape Town: Southern African Migration Programme.

Deacon, H. (2000). The politics of medical topography: seeking healthiness at the Cape during the nineteenth century. In R. Wrigley and G. Revill (eds), *Pathologies of Travel*, 279–98. Amsterdam: Rodopi.

Fausto-Sterling, A. (2000). *Sexing the Body: Gender Politics and the Construction of Sexuality*. New York: Basic Books.

Federici, S. (2004). *Caliban and the Witch: Women, the Body and Primitive Accumulation*. New York: Autonomedia.

Foucault, M. ([1976] 2002). *Society Must be Defended: Lectures at the Collège de France, 1975–76*. New York: Picador.

Foucault, M. (1978). *The History of Sexuality, Vol. 1. The Will to Knowledge.* London: Penguin.

Franklin, S. (2013). *Biological Relatives: IVF, Stem Cells and the Future of Kinship.* Durham, NC: Duke University Press.

Hill Collins, P. (2000). *Black Feminist Thought: Knowledge, Consciousness, and the Politics of Empowerment.* London: Routledge.

Inhorn, M. C. (2011). Globalization and gametes: reproductive 'tourism', Islamic bioethics, and Middle Eastern modernity, *Anthropology and Medicine* 18:1, 87–103.

Inhorn, M. C. and Pasquale, P. (2009). Rethinking reproductive 'tourism' as reproductive 'exile', *Fertility and Sterility* 92:3, 904–6.

Kroløkke, C. (2015). Have eggs, will travel: the experiences and ethics of global egg donation, *Somatechnics* 5:1, 12–31.

Lie, M. and Lykke, N. (eds) (2017). *Assisted Reproduction Across Borders: Feminist Perspectives on Normalizations, Disruptions and Transmissions.* New York and Milton Park: Routledge.

Mies, M. (1986). *Patriarchy and Accumulation on a World Scale: Women in the International Division of Labour.* New York: Zed Books.

Nahman, M. (2011). Reverse traffic: intersecting inequalities in human egg donation, *Reproductive Biomedicine Online* 23:5, 626–33.

Nahman, M. (2016). Reproductive tourism: through the anthropological 'Reproscope', *Annual Review of Anthropology* 45:1, 417–32.

Namberger, V. (2019). *The Reproductive Body at Work: The South African Bioeconomy of Egg Donation.* London: Routledge.

National Department of Health (2003). National Health Act No. 61. *Government Gazette No. 26595.* Pretoria: Government Printers.

Oudshoorn, N. (1990). Endocrinologists and the conceptualization of sex, *Journal of the History of Biology* 23:2, 163–87.

Pande, A. (2014). *Wombs in Labor: Transnational Commercial Surrogacy in India.* New York: Columbia University Press.

Pande, A. (2021). 'Mix or match?' Transnational fertility industry and white desirability, *Medical Anthropology.* DOI:10.1080/01459740.2021.1877289.

Pande, A. and Moll, T. (2018). Gendered bio-responsibilities and travelling egg providers from South Africa, *Reproductive BioMedicine & Society Online* 6, 23–33.

Parry, B. (2015). Narratives of neoliberalism: 'clinical labour' in context, *Medical Humanities* 41:1, 32–7.

Preciado, B. (2013). *Testo Junkie: Sex, Drugs, and Biopolitics in the Pharmacopornographic Era.* New York: Feminist Press.

Rose, N. (2007). *The Politics of Life Itself: Biomedicine, Power, and Subjectivity in the Twenty-First Century.* Princeton, NJ: Princeton University Press.

Sama Resource Group for Women and Health (2010). *Constructing Conceptions: The Mapping of Assisted Reproductive Technologies in India.* New Delhi.

Sawicki, J. (1999). Disciplining mothers: feminism and the new reproductive technologies. In J. Price and M. Shildrick (eds), *Feminist Theory and the Body. A Reader*, 190–202. New York: Routledge.

Strathern, M. (1995). Displacing knowledge: technology and the consequences for kinship. In F. D. Ginsburg and R. Rapp (eds), *Conceiving the New World Order*, 346–68. Berkeley, CA: University of California Press.

Taussig, K., Rapp, R. and Heath, D. (2003). Flexible eugenics: technologies of the self in the age of genetics. In R. V. Santos, S. Silverman, S. Franklin, R. Rapp, C. Royal, D. Haraway, H. Rose, K. S. Taussig, F. Kaestle, T. Duster and C. Heller (eds), *Genetic Nature/Culture: Anthropology and Science Beyond the Two-Culture Divide*, 8–76. Berkeley, CA: University of California Press.

Thompson, C. (2011). Medical migrations afterword: science as vacation? *Body and Society* 17:2/3, 205–13.

van de Wiel, L. (2017). Cellular origins: a visual analysis of time-lapse embryo imaging. In M. Lie and N. Lykke (eds), *Assisted Reproduction Across Borders: Feminist Perspectives on Normalizations, Disruptions and Transmissions*, 288–301. Abingdon: Routledge.

13

Subjects of scarcity: making white egg providers in the repro-hub of South Africa

Tessa Moll

I met Kelly in late 2015 at a coffee shop in Cape Town, alongside a representative of an egg provision[1] agency. Kelly had applied to provide her eggs anonymously, part of the maturing market in reproductive services and material in South Africa. When we first met, Kelly hadn't yet provided eggs, merely submitted an application. But just weeks later when we met a second time, Kelly had already gone through the whole procedure – medical examination, hormone stimulation, and egg retrieval in one of Cape Town's clinics. In fact, she was selected by intended parents within days of her application going 'live' onto the digital database of available providers. In our second meeting, I voiced surprise at how fast her movement from applicant to first-time provider had moved. She attributed this to her 'Celtic' looks – blue/green eyes, dark blonde hair, fair skin. Having never met or asked the intended parents, I could never be sure what it was about Kelly's profile that attracted immediate attention. But undoubtedly agency representatives sought providers like Kelly, that is, highly educated, employed, young, and, for the largest sector in the global market in reproductive material, white.

South Africa may seem a strange place to come for white egg providers. For one, white people are a distinct minority, roughly only 10% of the current population. Certain countries, like South Africa, are emerging as global hubs due to the availability of white egg providers (Bergmann, 2015; Homanen, 2018; Speier, 2016); and certain locales are becoming recruiting hubs for the global movement of egg providers (Nahman, 2018; Pande and Moll, 2018).

Why is it that South Africa, in particular, has emerged as a node in this ever-shifting global fertility market?

This chapter examines the case of white egg providers in South Africa, situating it within the particular histories of race and whiteness and the emergence of the local fertility industry to demonstrate how white biodesirability functions to produce a 'hub' for the global flow of services and tissues. Race is a defining and structuring feature of the global market in reproductive services and tissues (Deomampo, 2019; Moll, 2019; Pande 2021; Roberts, 2012; Thompson, 2009). Race structures the pathways, mobilities, and geographies between key actors, for instance, as brown women acting as surrogates for white reproductive travellers (Deomampo, 2016; Pande, 2014, 2015). The geography of reproductive markets, the mobilities of patients, medical professionals and those who provide gametes and surrogacy labour, and the circulation of fertility services and biological material are shaped by and within inequalities and global racial imaginaries. The force of racial imaginaries is especially acute when it comes to the way it shapes markets in egg 'donation', the colloquial descriptor for the process of ovarian stimulation and egg extraction to provide those eggs for a third party.

International demand for the oocytes from white women (particularly those mediating the line between 'acceptable whiteness' that makes them sought after, and economic disadvantage which may compel women to provide), and high local demand both from South African patients (as white patients seeking 'racial matches' make up the vast majority of those engaging in reproductive technologies – Moll, 2019) and international patients (as described further below), coupled with a relatively small white population in South Africa means that the eggs from white women are a hot commodity. I think of white providers as *subjects of scarcity*, their racial subjectivity enacted through recurrent donations and reinscribed as 'biological capital' (Cooper and Waldby, 2014) through ongoing engagement with globalising markets for tissues both racialised and commodified (Deomampo, 2019). As scarce subjects, white egg providers articulate their experiences as a form of cosmopolitan cool, enacting scarcity through their unique and particular participation in forms of high-tech reproduction. In this way, the commodity of whiteness is both seemingly globalising, connecting disparate corners through the logics of ancestry and colonial legacies, and, seemingly paradoxically, through particularity and scarcity of genetic material, limited participation, and a unique experience. That is, providers racialised as white in South Africa can substitute for genetic material from Australia, but not everyone can provide, not everyone is 'suitable'. I demonstrate these twinned characteristic of whiteness as both globalising, on one hand, and scarce and particular, on the other, and how they operate in the functioning of the South African market in egg provision.

'Super-ovulators' and 'egg safaris': regulations and industry machinations that make a market

In 1988, the first pregnancy in South Africa from a third-party egg provider resulted in the birth of triplets at Groote Schuur Hospital in Cape Town, one of the three public facilities that initiated in-vitro fertilisation (IVF) programmes in South Africa (Vrou word ma ..., 1988). The provider in that case was another woman undergoing treatment, who also fell pregnant during the cycle. These so-called 'super-ovulators' – women undergoing their own IVF treatment who produced 'excess' eggs – provided the bulk resource for third-party egg provision in the first fifteen years of the South African industry. Any eggs over a certain threshold, often fifteen, became framed as 'excess'. Doctors approached such women to ask if they would donate those 'extra' eggs to other couples. Alternatively, known donation also occurred, with patients bringing in friends, cousins, or sisters. The patchwork system between known donors and 'super-ovulators' facilitated limited egg provision, largely for the local market.

This all changed in the early 2000s, when an American woman temporarily living in South Africa started a medical tourism business bringing patients from the global north (mostly the US) to South Africa for private healthcare. The idea, she explained to me in an interview, was conceived as part of a larger facilitation agency for medical tourism, for treatments such as plastic surgery, and where patients could enjoy a holiday, get treatment at a reduced cost of what they would pay at home, and enjoy the high-quality care in South Africa's booming private medical sector.[2] As a former patient of IVF herself, she understood the need for egg donors for an American market, and that South African providers and fertility services would be a much cheaper option. She began working with a fertility specialist in Cape Town, and her agency for third-party egg provision launched in 2002. Her agency would recruit young local women, largely for international clientele. The agency paid egg providers ZAR10,000 (~ US$1000 in 2002).

The agency came under fire from media, the local fertility industry, and regulators. The media labelled it 'egg safaris' and made references to surrogacy as a form of slavery (Brits, 2004). The South African Society for Reproductive Medicine and Gynaecological Endoscopy (SASREG), a professional society for fertility specialists, felt ZAR10,000 was too much money for compensation, driving the price up to unaffordable levels for locals and constituting coercion for egg providers. The Ministry of Health temporarily shut down the agency. It soon reopened, albeit following new regulations set out by SASREG that limited compensation to, at that time, a ZAR5000 (~ US$750 in 2004) flat rate per egg provision (it has now gone up to ZAR7000). Numerous other agencies opened subsequently; at one point in my research there were seven SASREG-accredited agencies, but the number of agencies fluctuate. In addition to compensation, patients using agencies must also pay additional fees (reportedly around ZAR15,000 – ~ US$970), which the companies say covers recruitment and pre-screening of egg providers, management of provider databases, follow-up care, and support and curated matching between recipients and providers. Verena Namberger (2016; see also chapter 12 above) describes this shifting landscape as the growing normalisation and professionalisation of procurement and the surrounding local industry and infrastructure, which set out the conditions necessary to create a growing hub in the global movement of services and reproductive materials.

South Africa receives numerous 'reproductive travelers' (Inhorn, 2015) from areas both in the global south and global north within this global bioeconomy. This is not entirely a new phenomenon. Ironically, the first IVF baby born in South Africa was conceived overseas. In 1982, Dominique was born in South Africa, conceived as a result of IVF in the UK (Tuit, 1982). Magdelene and Joe Darvas had their IVF cycle carried out in the UK, then travelled back to South Africa, their home country, to deliver their baby in Pretoria. Thus, the first IVF baby born in South Africa in 1982 was the product of reproductive travel in the early 1980s. By the late 1980s, the local press reported that women were coming from multiple countries to South Africa for IVF treatment (Vorster, 1988). While not entirely new, infrastructure, such as the previously described agency system, and, as I shall describe in more detail below, the ways that white egg providers enter into market circulation, have certainty shaped and intensified the market and flows both in and out of South Africa. However, without quantitative, standardised, and regular data[3] on where patients in South African clinics travel from, evidence at this point comes from ethnographic research. During my own fieldwork in three private South African clinics, I observed patients from the following countries: Angola, Australia, Botswana, Cameroon, China, Germany, Namibia, Nigeria, Swaziland, Uganda, the UK, the US, Zambia and Zimbabwe. Some of the staff at the clinics I worked with estimated that as many as a third of their patients came from abroad for treatment; others estimated a quarter of their patients were from abroad. In my research, the reasons for reproductive travel to South Africa varied and often depended on the country of origin. Some patients came from countries that lacked IVF clinics, or had clinics that some patients regarded as sub-par and thus they preferred a well-reputed South African clinic. Others stated they wanted to go abroad for treatment to avoid gossip and slander in their home countries, or to avoid the perceived poor treatment in clinics in their home countries, staffed with local medical professionals that also harboured stigmatising views. A large percentage came to South Africa for IVF with third-party eggs, what is also one the greatest drivers of cross border reproductive care in Europe (Shenfield et al., 2010), because of the availability in South Africa (in contrast to their home countries). Australians undoubtedly make up the largest single country contributing to the influx to South Africa of global repro-travelers, largely attributed to long waiting lists for gamete donors at home (Goedeke et al., 2020).[4] One agency, one of the largest in South Africa, estimated that half their intended parents were from abroad, and 75% of these were from Australia.

Today, egg procurement in South Africa is legislated under the National Health Act (No 61 of 2003) and the subsequent 2012 regulations (Regulations Relating to Artificial Fertilisation of Persons, Department of Health, 2012). SASREG also issues industry guidelines on egg procurement (SASRSS, 2008). SASREG enforce this through a process of accreditation, whereby fertility clinics, to receive accreditation, may only work with accredited agencies, which must in turn abide by the egg provision guidelines. The latter include age restrictions, a prohibition on international egg provision (Pande and Moll, 2019), and setting the amount of money given to anonymous egg providers. According to these regulations, anonymous egg provision is only done for altruistic reasons. Payment for anonymous providers is explicitly glossed as 'compensation', not for oocytes or tissues, but for 'time, inconvenience, financial costs to the donor – eg. travel, loss of income and childcare costs, physical and emotional demands and risks associated with oocyte donation' (SASRSS, 2008).

The growth and stabilisation of the market in egg providers also benefits from the local hesitancy and discomfort over known egg providers. Providers are categorised as 'known donors', meaning they have a previous relationship with the intended parents, or are anonymous. Doctors and other clinic staff I worked with during my fieldwork overwhelming recommended that patients use anonymous providers. Fertility professionals feared that known donor scenarios, whereby a friend, sibling, or cousin would provide ovas for the intended parent, became complicated by questions of kinship, potential involvement of the 'genetic parent', and questions around secrets and disclosure to the resultant child. In sum, they worried it could strain social relations between known donors and recipients (who are oftentimes family members). Known donors, both egg and sperm, and the recipient couples have to undergo psychological evaluations to ensure that social roles were delineated in advance, to the satisfaction of the screening psychologist or social worker, in accordance with regulations. I saw a mere handful of known-donor scenarios during my fieldwork, several of them against the advice of fertility professionals who always treated them as a weary project of relationship management.

Thus, anonymous providers supply the bulk of third-party oocytes in South Africa. Under the anonymous system, clinics themselves or the egg provision agencies recruit providers, who must fill in applications detailing their social, medical, and familial profile, and undergo a medical examination and psychological screening. The South African law does not stipulate that providers also submit baby photos,[5] but they are common practice in both sperm and egg donation. Other information that must be provided to recipient patients include: identity particulars; family history, both medical and professional; educational attainments and occupation; hobbies and interests; information about looks, such as hair and eye colour, and complexion; 'population group', which is apartheid-linked parlance for racial categories; national identity; religion; and any wishes the egg provider may have for recipients of her gametes. The latter may refer to racial, religious, or sexuality stipulations for gamete recipients, such as requiring that the recipients be a married heterosexual couple or of a certain racial or religious group. Agencies and clinics may request more information or documents, and many do. Profiles often include information on what celebrity the provider thinks she looks like or favourite movies. Many agencies encourage applicants to try and get their 'personality' in their profiles. Agencies and clinics I worked with also requested that providers have a high school certificate and often asked for a copy.

When egg provider applicants are recruited or apply of their own accord, they go through agency 'pre-screening'. Clinics or agencies may refuse to allow someone to provide for numerous reasons. These include: medical criteria (such as problems with one's reproductive system); family genetic criteria (such as a family history of schizophrenia or bipolar disorder); or failure to meet certain social criteria (such as lacking a high school completion certificate, or appearing as 'irresponsible' during their clinic visits and psychological screening). Such egg screening suggests removing potential providers that are at risk for sexually transmitted diseases, including those engaging in 'casual sexual relations frequently with different partners' (SASRSS, 2008). Some criteria is not delineated in regulations but is common practice and sometimes debated. During my fieldwork, one such debate emerged among screening psychologists and social workers about whether to reject young women who admitted to smoking *dagga* (marijuana). Some argued that it was an extremely common habit among young women and not a significant reason to bar a potential egg provider. Others said it could affect the egg quality, similarly to smoking cigarettes. Yet others argued that if applicants admitted to *dagga* smoking, it was likely they were also using other, and ostensibly 'worse', substances. The debate, which was never formally settled during my fieldwork, also reflects how screening procedures, seemingly objective and fixed, are instead debated, fluid, and made from an assemblage of various elements

– medical criteria, ideas of anticipated markets for intended parents, egg provider 'sellability', and moral valuations – that delineate who is and who isn't 'suitable' to provide.

'Sellability' is important. Even those applicants who make it through pre-screening and onto databases of available providers may not ultimately provide eggs. An intended parent must select that provider for the process to ensue.[6] Thus, agencies are incentivised to recruit egg providers who they can ultimately 'sell', by which I mean those who are ultimately selected for provision and after which agencies can charge for their services. For instance, during my fieldwork I followed an agency representative, Ellen, to meet with potential providers.[7] During these meetings Ellen explained the procedure and follow-up care from the agency, asked questions about how the woman came to find out about egg provision, their motivation to provide, any reservations, and finally gain written consent for the woman to go onto databases and potentially be selected by intended parents. In this particular meeting with a potential provider, the applicant had been adopted. After the applicant left the meeting, Ellen mused aloud to me her weighing of the question of whether the agency should take her on to their database. As an adoptee, the potential provider knew little of her genetic family history (and thus could not answer questions related to familial schizophrenia or breast cancer, for instance). And most importantly, she didn't have any baby pictures. Baby photos are a key part of the profile package that recipients get to peruse. On the other hand, Ellen said, she was beautiful – white, slim, blonde hair, and big eyes. Ellen hoped the lack of baby photos would not prove a deterrent to her getting selected, and the applicant ultimately joined their database.

Ellen's interest in this provider, despite the limitations to her 'sellability' (her lack of baby photos and the lack of knowledge of her genetic family history), show the force of white desirability (Pande, 2021). The applicant's idealised presentation of white-ness – educated, slim, pretty, and blonde – made her a desirable provider, overcoming even the lack in other areas. Taken together, the system of regulations, pre-screening, medical restrictions, and profile-building creates an infrastructure to gate-keep egg provision. While some of the restrictions, such as age, are created in ensuring 'good quality' *eggs*, other restrictions, such as a high school diploma or assessments of provider 'responsibility', are created in ensuring 'good quality' egg *providers*. In the context of increasing demand for white egg providers, this system of gate-keeping, I argue, draws from a longer local history of '*policing the borders of whiteness among whites*' (Willoughby-Herard, 2007: 493, italics in original). The next section draws on this history of white racialisation and anxieties over those with questionable and insecure claim to the class status of whiteness.

Local histories and global whiteness

In South Africa, race has structured social, political, and economic life, and continues to do so. Unlike other settler colonial contexts, such as Canada, Australia, or New Zealand, whites in South Africa were always a distinct demographic minority. Never comprising more than 20% of the population during the height of apartheid, today whites comprise 9% of the population, yet have an overwhelming majority of the country's wealth (Orthofer, 2016; Steyn, 2001). As such, 'whiteness' in South Africa differs from many other western contexts in that it is more obvious in its potency and privilege: 'Self-conscious rather than deliberately obscured, and accepted rather than veiled as a sight of privilege' (Salusbury and Foster, 2004: 93). That is, unlike whiteness studies that seek to highlight invisible, unmarked whiteness[8] (Frankenberg, 1997), South African whiteness is in contrast 'hyper visible' (Willoughby-Herard, 2007).

Tiffany Willoughby-Herard (2007) argues that the historical hyper-visibility of whites arose, in part, from the legacy of the 1932 *Poor White Study*. Funded by the US-based Carnegie Corporation, the infamous study – that many consider foundational for apartheid policy just a decade later – sought to investigate different facets of the 'poor white problem' and provide recommendations for upliftment (Willoughby-Herard, 2015). The study consolidated anxieties over the potential vulnerability of white civilisation and whether those considered 'poor whites' were really white at all. The presence of 'poor whites' – those questionable in their access to acceptable whiteness – thus revealed the fallacy of a 'natural', inborn white supremacy (Willoughby-Herard, 2007: 485). White racialisation, Willoughby-Herard argues, was thus critical to the apartheid project:

'The *policing of the borders of whiteness among whites* was a critical terrain on which to map South Africa's racial hierarchy' (Willoughby-Herard, 2007: 493, italics in original). Thus, it was critical to ensure that those read as white maintained a certain social status and respectability. Willoughby-Herard (2015) contextualises the Carnegie study as part of a larger infrastructure in the sustenance of 'global whiteness', the border-crossing features that both help sustain national racial mythologies and supra-national investments in whiteness.

The transition to democracy in the 1990s has seen large parts of the minority white population maintaining and rearticulating its privilege in the 'New South Africa', while the formerly disenfranchised, dispossessed, and majority Black population has achieved political power (Steyn and Foster, 2008). Legacies of apartheid have meant that whiteness in South Africa almost always translates into economic privilege and middle- to upper-class social capital. On average, white people in the country have higher incomes, higher educational levels, and often live in the affluent, cloistered and well-serviced neighbourhoods formally delineated as 'white' under apartheid spatial planning (Burnett, 2018). Steyn's study of South African 'White Talk' (2004; Steyn and Foster, 2008) explores the discursive modes of asserting privilege in the 'New South Africa' through which 'White South Africans can reach out to their racial kin in the white mainlands through the ideological allegiances of whiteness, affiliations which are taking on new levels of importance as whites deal with loss of political dominance in the local context' (Steyn and Foster, 2008: 46).

While whites have become politically denuded, economically they remain advantaged. This in turn has shaped post-apartheid discourse that frames whiteness as 'naturally middle class' (Steyn, 2004: 100). Most significantly for this study, Salusbury and Foster link narratives from white, English-speaking South Africans (referred to in the academic literature as WESSAs) to contradictory forces within globalisation. Their interviewees navigate the paradoxes of globalisation; on one hand, they are sure to adhere to South African nationalism and justify their presence here, yet they also highlight their historical origins in Europe and Eurocentric ideals. This allows them to position themselves as 'civilising forces' from within. The authors conclude that 'WESSAs may 'tap into' a transnational culture of 'whiteness', allowing them to masquerade as cultureless, but also permitting the group to legitimise their ideological stance through the invocation of 'internationalism' (Steyn, 2004: 108). This choreography of insider and outsider allows them to remain politically concealed while socially hegemonic.

In this regard, I see the creation and imaginary of the South African market in provider oocytes as hinged on dual processes. In the first, it replicates projects of racialisation, sorting through prospective white providers in ensuring their qualifications, largely economic and moral. Secondly, it sustains the imaginaries of global whiteness, marketing local providers and their biogenetic 'assets' as transposable. This transposition offers white South Africans genes as mere substitutions for the genes from the UK, Germany, and Australia, forging links in the global whiteness imaginary. For providers, there is a third process at hand. While leveraging whiteness in a global market, providers also discursively present themselves as unique and particular. Their embodiment of whiteness not only stakes claims to global cache, but in providing eggs also makes them particular and scarce.

Both 'bioavailable' and 'biodesirable': situating white egg providers

Sara Ahmed (2007: 151), a critical race and feminist theorist, has argued whiteness shapes bodies and 'in turn what it is that bodies "can do"', meaning that comportment, orientation, and mobility in certain spaces becomes framed as a shared 'likeness' (Ahmed, 2007: 154). In very different contexts, accessing private reproductive medicine in Ecuador (Roberts, 2012), dancing to trance music in Goa (Saldanha, 2007), or transnational access via the 'visa whiteness machine' between South Africa and the UK (Andrucki, 2010) are among disparate, though interrelated projects of white racialisation.

Whiteness does not only shape bodies and space; 'whiteness has cash value' (Lipsitz, 2006: xxi). Lipsitz's argument details the political economic underpinnings of racism as whites in the US control land, wealth, and access to resources. This is undoubtedly true in South Africa, as Burnett (2018) has carefully tracked in the historical and contemporary debates over land. In the case of egg donation, whiteness most literally translates into cash value, as white egg providers leverage their acceptance in racial categories for compensation. The market value of racial distinctions has been tracked in egg donation (Daniels and Heidt-Forsythe, 2012; Deomampo, 2019), but also in other markets using biomedical technologies such as for-profit DNA testing, bio-banks, and precision medicine (Bliss, 2013; Daniels and Heidt-Forsythe, 2012; Lee, 2017; Reardon and TallBear 2012; Tupasela, 2017). Seeing how race operates, not only through individual desires and notions of kinship but through the market forces that leverage notions of difference, is an extension of the argument that ethnicity has been increasingly intertwined with market forces (Comaroff and Comaroff, 2009).

Lawrence Cohen (2005) reformulated the pharmaceutical term of 'bioavailability' to conceive of the ways that political economic forces render certain bodies 'available' for new bioeconomic markets in increasingly partible bodies. What forces shape the tendency for certain bodies to provide parts, tissues, and organs, and certain others to receive them? Economic geographies, argues Carolin Schurr (2018) underwrite the global flows of the fertility market, with its complicated intersections of transnational mobility, legacies of colonial exchange, and global racial imaginaries. Pricing and wage differentiation, payment to egg providers, and cost of medications, among other factors, contribute to mobilities and the creation of nodes in the global fertility market (Whittaker and Speier, 2010). In global surrogacy, for instance, poorer Indian women often serve as surrogates for white, wealthy women of the global north, replicating historical legacies of extractive labour from former colonial contexts to the metropole (Pande, 2011; 2015; Vora, 2015). Colonial, gendered, and racial relations are often pointed to as shaping the global imaginations of reproductive labourers and receivers of bodily commodities (Cooper and Waldby, 2014; Nahman, 2018; Pande, 2014; Vora, 2015).

Egg provision complicates the notion that 'donors' and 'receivers' have clear filiations through the legacies of unequal colonial exchange. Firstly, families seeking egg providers often search in terms of 'racial matching', what Amrita Pande describes as 'the desire for a single race family [that] is made natural and universal for intended parents who identify as white' (2021: 1). The notion that familial connection, affinity, and thus kinship take form through race undergirds matching practices (Moll, 2019). Rufaro Moyo (in chapter 14 below) unpacks the seeming 'obviousness' of this choice as an extension of the eugenic myth of racial purity. Egg provision and mediators continue to employ 'the look' (Erasmus, 2017) as the mode of determining race, fixing, naturalising and biologising race in the name of familial resemblance (Moyo, Chapter 14, this volume). Pande (2021) argues that ultimately these ideas of familial resemblance, intimacy and 'connection' serve to depoliticise questions of inequality and the privilege of whiteness in the transnational fertility industry.

Despite the fact that South Africa is a majority Black country, the logics of 'racial matching' propels the scarcity of white egg providers because those seeking egg providers are overwhelmingly white intended parents, both locally and internationally. In South Africa, the political economy of ART provisions means that despite the fact that Black couples may potentially have higher rates of infertility due to socio-economic marginalisation and environmental racisms (Hlatshwayo, 2004; Moll, 2021), white intended parents have, by far, greater access to high-tech reproductive technologies due to in part economic and geographical barriers. This, in part, drives the circuits of reproductive mobilities in the search for hubs of white egg providers. Beyond the economic and geographic barriers to access, there may be less material reasons at play. Philosopher Camisha Russell (2018) argues that to examine the way race works in ARTs, one must unpack for whom the technology was intended and for what problem. Infertility was overwhelmingly seen as a *problem* for white women (raced and gendered), contrasted with the imagination of Black women as hyper-fertile (Ikemoto, 1996). Russell writes that in unpacking ART and the work that race does within it, 'We begin to see that far from being an ideal solution for infertility at large, ARTs have arisen and developed with the concerns of a certain population in mind and bear many traces of that particular standpoint.' How that operates in South Africa is beyond the scope of this chapter, but it bears repeating that ART is not merely a 'treatment' for infertility but privileges the family-making of certain arrangements and populations over others.

The political economy of ART provision coupled with the logics of racial matching mean that white egg providers are sought after. Thus, white egg providers become valued – their genes sought after, their donations yielding higher compensation, or they are specifically targeted and recruited – along the lines of what Jenny Gunnarsson Payne (2015) calls 'biodesirability', which knot in particular and contextually specific constellations. Traits that render a provider desirable include phenotypic and historical relations between countries, ideas of social similarities, recruiters' ideas of what becomes 'sellable', scarcity of certain racial and ethnic groups (Deomampo, 2019), and recipients' imaginaries of their potential child (Hudson, 2019). Daisy Deomampo (2019: 622), studying the market in Asian-American providers, argues that racial preferences, either for 'sameness' or 'difference', 'influence[s] demand in the international market, making eggs a racialized commodity to be obtained and purchased'. Deomampo (2019) found that market forces of scarcity and demand, including valuations around ideas of racial 'purity' and notions of familial likeness, shaped recipients and matchers selection of providers. Whiteness, which in the ART industry is taken to be inheritable through the genetic contribution of egg providers, is particularly sought after, or what Pande (2021) refers to as 'white desirability'. So while economic precarity, for instance, may make some 'bioavailable' and pushed into egg provision, traits within hierarchies of race, class, education, and health make some women particularly desirable as egg providers. Fueled by a racial imaginary that whiteness is global in its reach and transposable, certain locales have become 'hot spots' in the global bioeconomy of third-party eggs. In addition to South Africa, Spain, Czech Republic, Romania, Greece, and Cyprus, among others, are places where growing neoliberal economic policies, high unemployment among young people, and lower incomes and purchasing power have been push factors for young women to provide eggs (Cooper and Waldby, 2014; Nahman, 2018). Yet these locales and the providers from them are also read as white, a form of 'biological capital' (Cooper and Waldby, 2014: 76). In South Africa, to put it pithily and to quote a colleague, 'We have cheap whites.'

Cosmopolitan aspirations, risky business?

As this chapter has thus traced, the demand for white egg providers, fuelled by the racial imagination of global whiteness, has led to South African agencies and clinics actively recruiting white egg providers to participate in the for-profit market for reproductive material. Thus, in receiving compensation for their donations, providers stand to benefit financially from their racial identities. However, the backgrounds and biographies of the white providers I interviewed complicated the clear filiations between white racial identity and upper-class cosmopolitan social standing. Here, I argue that more than cash is at stake; class, 'suitable' whiteness, and the active self-fashioning as cosmopolitan young women reflects the dual operations of whiteness – as both global racial imaginary and the unique, particular, and scarce.

The white providers I interviewed could broadly be classed into two groups. Either those who were active university students during their donation, or those with tenuous ties to middle-class life, an observation that echoes Amrita Pande's (2020) findings among egg providers that travel overseas. As university students, they may have middle-class access and networks, but are temporarily lacking monied resources. They are outside of their parents' daily financial assistance, yet in accessing higher education, they have access to social capital of middle-class life and the anticipated resources. University students make up a particularly desirable demographic of providers. For one, students are often young. They generally have more flexible schedules, allowing for medical appointments, interviews, and scans. They also have a reason for needing money that is viewed as 'respectable' – tuition fees. Thus, the age restrictions on who can provide is legitimated not only through medical reasoning (younger eggs are more likely to result in a child), but also market frameworks and historical ideas of respectability. With university students in particular, having completed high school education and with some tertiary education, they became more 'sellable' to the professional class of patients, according to matchers I interviewed.

The second group had semi-skilled urban work, but often at the lower socio-economic edges. These providers were bookkeepers, massage therapists, and receptionists. They may have moved to urban centres of South Africa, such as Cape Town or Johannesburg, but many grew up outside these national centres, in areas such as the suburbs of Port Elizabeth, Worcester, and Bloemfontein. While they are white, they may not have the same social capital as middle-class English speakers or wealthy Afrikaans-speakers, those who enact transnational mobilities as part of their claim to whiteness (Andrucki, 2010). Their biographies reflect much more nuanced expressions of the class politics of whiteness in South Africa.

Their precarious ties to middle-class life and the social capital of whiteness, I argue, led many providers to frame their experience as, simply put, 'cool'. Pande (2020) found similar narratives from egg providers who travelled outside of South Africa for their provision. In her interviews, egg provision similarly was an avenue toward cosmopolitanism and beyond the rural farms of South Africa where many of those she interviewed grew up. In my work, the discourses were similar. Egg provision was cool. It engaged young women in high-tech biomedical services, and rendered their biological and biographical profile as desirable. I read this as expressions of individuality and uniqueness; whiteness as not only global, and desirable, but particular, unique, and scarce.

Sophie, a young, urban professional with a university degree in her mid-twenties, had provided three times while studying. She first heard about egg provision through a friend at university.

> *Sophie*: I know this is going to sound very strange and a bit detached, but egg donating, the first time I did it, was kind of like getting a tattoo. It's kind of like one of these things, you want to do good, you want there to be some sort of positive outcome, and it's to kind of engage with something different. And to do something good.
>
> *Tessa*: Was it kind of a little ... I don't want to use the word rebellious because maybe that's a bit too strong, but kind of exciting or like ... ?
>
> *Sophie*: Definitely. There definitely was that element to it. But then the thing was, the morality issue of it was completely clear for me in that initial donation. 'I'm going to help someone have a child.' Whether they're gay or a single parent. And actually the person that I did donate to the first time was a single parent. There was a sperm donor and an egg donor. I don't know who she was or any of that. But that's what she did. So it was risky. It was like, in my head, rebellious, you know like getting an ear pierced or tattoo or going bungee jumping. I know that sounds completely strange ...

In addition to doing 'good', egg providers were able to do something 'different'. The ways that provisions allows for ways of enacting gendered forms of altruism and morality has been well covered by the literature (Almeling, 2006; Mohr, 2014). Less discussed has been how it makes providers 'different' – 'like getting an ear pierced', says Sophie.

Sophie was the most clearly spoken about the desire for difference through provision. Other providers often phrased this through allusions to 'disclosure' (my term) to family and friends. Crystal, a twenty-one-year-old provider in Cape Town, described telling her boyfriend about providing: 'He thinks I'm giving away my kids or something', said Crystal, in a joking manner that reflected to me she thought this was a naïve and silly notion. Discussing whether to disclose or not indicates that there is something that may need to be disclosed. Many providers chose not to tell family, particularly those members they thought would not agree with their decision, or, to use providers' common parlance, 'not understand'. This could mean family members or friends not understanding the process, the technology, the kinship meanings they were navigating, or understanding why they would want to donate. I read the providers' delineation of those who 'don't understand' in seeming contrast to themselves as reinforcing their status as modern subjects – knowledgable, participatory in high-tech modes of creating children, and engaging in niche biomedical realms. Like techno music in KwaZulu-Natal (Dolby, 1999), or the discursive differentiating between 'authentic' South Africa and 'bland' UK (Andrucki, 2013), the literature demonstrates that cosmopolitan aspirations and global imaginaries have become a significant avenue for post-apartheid enactments of whiteness. For some providers, particularly students and those without their own children, egg provision was an avenue for participation in an imagined cosmopolitanism.

However, whiteness, which contributes to their desirability as providers, also puts them at potentially greater bodily burden. The impetus to garner a greater number of eggs in a single egg extraction has led to accusations and fears of exploitation and putting young providers at risk of health complications, for instance ovarian hyper stimulation syndrome (OHSS) (Deveaux, 2016; Pande and Moll, 2019). The World Health Organization describes OHSS as an 'exaggerated response' to hormone stimulation, which may include, 'abdominal distention, ovarian enlargement, and respiratory, hemodynamic, and metabolic complications' (Zegers-Hochschild, 2009: 1523). In severe cases, OHSS can cause pulmonary conditions, infertility, and even fatality. While the published risks of OHSS put the incidence rate between 1% and 5% of all cases (Delvigne and Rozenberg, 2002), others research indicates that this is likely underreported (Jayaprakasan et al., 2009; Kenney and McGowan 2010; Kramer et al., 2009; Sarojini et al., 2011). There is a dearth of research on the long-term health effects of egg provision (Jain, 2013; Schneider et al., 2017). In my ethnographic research, most of the providers I interviewed had repeated procurements, an average of three and a half, at the time of our interviews. One woman provided eight times over a few years, and another said she felt pressured to donate a sixth time after the recipients from a previous provision wanted a sibling of the same genetic combination. Another provider I met, Almeda, ended up in hospital after her provision. Almeda had chest pains and difficulty breathing when she woke from the extraction, and was transferred to the hospital across the street from the clinic. The doctor later determined that she was not suffering from OHSS, although they had extracted a high yield of twenty-eight eggs. I visited her in the hospital, finding her in the maternity ward, where she was still suffering from chest pain and discomfort. The hospital physician intended to keep her overnight, but she did not yet have a diagnosis. Another one of the providers I interviewed was treated for OHSS and had to be hospitalised. That was the only case of diagnosed OHSS among providers that I encountered, but a few reported some complications, ranging from bloating to severe pain, discomfort, and swelling. Pressures to donate repeatedly, embodied health risks, and a lack of research on the long-term health implications reflect that the experiences of egg procurement an be at odds with the ways that the industry portrays 'donation'. The way that industry discourses reiterate that egg procurement is mere recycling of eggs that would go to 'waste', a gentle 'lighting the candle' of another woman, and the overwhelming use of the term 'donation' (both by industry figures and egg providers themselves) belies and minimises these real potential risks.

Several feminist scholars see the medical risk that comes with egg provision as part of the industry's exploitation of young women, who are enticed by compensation (Ballantyne, 2014; Heng, 2005; Pfeffer, 2011). Other scholars find egg provision and other reproductive services at the centre of emerging forms of neoliberal citizenship, medical markets, and technologies of the body (Kr;økke, 2012; Kr;økke and Pant, 2012). As Michal Nahman (2008) points out, the binary of agency/victim does little to elucidate the complicated intersections of reproductive desires, cosmopolitan aspirations, and fertility markets in which provisions take place. White egg providers are not merely supplying eggs; their engagement with reproductive markets is structured by complicated economic and racial geographies, desires, and imaginations that, in turn, shape their subjectivities.

Discussion: subjects of scarcity

Repro-hubs emerge for numerous reasons. South Africa's fertility industry specifications – that is 'altruistic' local regulations clamping egg provider payments, changing egg provision infrastructures such as the agency system, and the legacy of apartheid-era disparities in healthcare provision, coupled with neoliberal private and for-profit healthcare in the post-apartheid era – have contributed to a unique confluence of conditions that set the stage for an attractive market in reproductive material and services. But further to this, race, how racism shapes economic geographies (Schurr, 2018), and the biodesirability of whiteness structures the global fertility market (Pande, 2021), leading to a unique grouping of certain locales – South Africa, Spain, the Czech Republic – to emerge in the global bioeconomy.

Through the unpacking of local histories, processes to screening providers and through interviews with providers themselves, this chapter has also argued that while biodesirability may fuel a market, it in turn produces racialisation through engagement with egg provision. Reproductive markets reify racialisation and reinscribe a biogenetic notion of race. Further to that, the supply-and-demand logics of reproductive markets and the notions of kinship that underly these markets create eggs of white women as *scarce* and valuable. I think of this manner of racialisation I call 'subjects of scarcity' in the global bio-economy. This is drawing from Sunder Rajan's (2005) notion of 'subjects of speculation'. Sunder Rajan describes subjects of speculation as the populations that become enrolled in market speculations as consumers of postgenomic medicine and the populations of experimentation in the production of the research. In his analysis, life sciences and market frameworks in genomics configure particular subjects in their operation. In the global reproductive bioeconomy, white egg providers are configured through market arrangements, and racial imaginaries as subjects of scarcity. I think of scarcity as having two meanings. In the first, is its market connotations. The political economy of ARTs alongside the desirability of whiteness fuels a demand for white egg providers, and, aided further by gate-keeping processes that limit participation, create limited supply. In the second, it is a question of rarity, desirous in its infrequency and uncommonness. The enactments of whiteness through discourses of unique participation in a cosmopolitan industry reflect scarcity in this second meaning. In this case, the market for white egg providers produces a certain kind of whiteness. Simply put, white skin alone does not render one 'biodesirable' (Payne, 2015).

Historians and race scholars have noted the twinned anxieties of whiteness in South Africa: its hyper visibility and racist fears turned inward at being thought as not quite white enough (van der West-huizen, 2017; Willoughby-Herard, 2007). As egg providers participate in a market delineating 'whites' and the way in which participation becomes an avenue for imaginations of transnational cosmopolitanism, egg provision is an arena for the performance of a certain hegemonic vision of whiteness. Egg provision thus offers much more than 'compensation'; it allows for participation in spheres of mobility, cosmopolitanism, and high-tech biomedicine where one's racial subjectivity becomes a scarce object of capital.

Notes

Thanks to Amrita Pande for her editing of this volume, the opportunity to contribute, and her feedback on an earlier draft. Thanks to Emma Arogundade and anonymous reviewers who also provided enriching feedback. Also many thanks to Christopher Mayes who read an early version, and Fiona Ross who supervised the research from which this chapter emerged. The chapter came from my doctoral research in Social Anthropology at the University of Cape Town, which received financial support from the Mellon Foundation and the Oppenheimer Foundation.

1 Throughout this chapter, I refer to 'egg donors' as 'egg providers'. The language around egg provision and how to identify those who provide eggs is a lengthy and ongoing debate in the social science literature (Beeson et al., 2015). I myself have been inconsistent in my work on whether to refer to women as providers or donors. Actors within the industry overwhelmingly use the language of donation, which many have critiqued as glossing over the profit-making contexts and the exchange relations at its core (Jain, 2013; Roberts and Scheper-Hughes 2011). In response, some refer to 'egg vendors' (Pfeffer, 2011; Cooper and Waldby,

2014), 'egg transfer' (Leve, 2013), 'egg sellers' (Nahman, 2008), or 'egg providers' (Pande and Moll, 2018). However, I remain unconvinced of delineating this as an etic label in every instance, as the women providing eggs hold fast to the notion of donation. In this instance, I use provider in this chapter as a way to unsettle the industry's insistence on donation as I argue that part of the usage of this term is to render the process innocuous. Thanks to Christopher Mayes for raising this point.

2 Deregulation since the 1970s and 1980s has resulted in a thriving private sector healthcare system, which largely services about 16% of the population who have medical insurance (Mayosi et al., 2012).

3 None of the clinics I worked with registered the 'home countries' of patients in their intake papers.

4 There are reports of lengthy waiting lists for egg providers in Australia (Hope, 2020; Saunokonoko, 2017). Some attribute the cause to the legislation on non-anonymous egg provision, which means that providers are registered and may be contacted by potential adult offspring (Goedeke et al., 2020).

5 The regulations from SASREG delineate that 'baby photos' should only include photos of the provider from when they were ten or younger.

6 This is changing as egg banks become more common. In egg banking, donors will undergo the same hormone stimulation and egg extraction as with 'traditional' egg donation. Thereafter, eggs will be frozen and 'banked' for later use instead of being immediately fertilised.

7 Agencies by and large work 'online' and oftentimes the South African agencies had employees in different South African cities working remotely. Many agencies arranged to meet potential donors, either in person or through Skype, before bringing them on board to databases, where they would be potentially chosen.

8 The question is also, invisible to whom? This is Sara Ahmed's (2004) question of the refrain that whiteness studies seeks to highlight what is otherwise invisible as it 'only makes sense from the point of view of those for whom it is invisible' that is, white people. The question of invisibility re-instantiates the white gaze as the scholarly gaze.

References

Ahmed, S. (2004). Declarations of whiteness: the non-performativity of anti-racism. *borderlands*, 3:2. www.borderlandsejournal.adelaide.edu.au/vol3no2_2004/ahmed_declarations. Accessed 6 December 2021.

Ahmed, S. (2007). A phenomenology of whiteness, *Feminist Theory* 8:2, 149–68.

Almeling, R. (2006). 'Why do you want to be a donor?' Gender and the production of altruism in egg and sperm donation, *New Genetics and Society* 25:2, 143–57.

Andrucki, M. J. (2010). The visa whiteness machine: transnational motility in post-apartheid South Africa, *Ethnicities* 10:3, 358–70.

Andrucki, M. J. (2013). 'There's a drumbeat in Africa': embodying imaginary geographies of transnational whiteness in contemporary South Africa, *Geoforum* 49(C), 1–9.

Ballantyne, A. (2014). Exploitation in cross-border reproductive care, *International Journal of Feminist Approaches to Bioethics* 7:2, 75–99.

Beeson, D., Darnovsky, M., and Lippman, A. (2015). What's in a name? Variations in terminology of third-party reproduction, *Reproductive Biomedicine Online* 31:6, 805–14.

Bergmann, S. (2015). Assisted authenticity: naturalisation, regulation and the enactment of 'race' through donor matching. In V. Kantsa, G. Zanini and L. Papadopoulou (eds), *(In)fertile Citizens: Anthropological and Legal Challenges of ART Technologies*, 231–46. (In)FERCIT.

Bliss, C. (2013). The marketization of identity politics, *Sociology* 47:5, 1011–25.

Burnett, S. (2018). *Giving Back the Land: Whiteness and Belonging in Contemporary South Africa*. Doctoral Thesis. University of the Witswatersrand.

Brits, E. (2004). Eiersafari's in SA se doppie geklink. *Die Burger* (Cape Town). 24 April: p. 2.

Cohen, L. (2005). Operability, bioavailability and exception. In A. Ong and S. J. Collier (eds), *Global Assemblages: Technology, Politics and Ethics as Anthropological Problems*. Malden: Blackwell Publishing, 79–90.

Comaroff, J. and Comaroff, J. (2009). *Ethnicity, Inc.* Chicago: University of Chicago Press.

Cooper, M. and Waldby, C. (2014). *Clinical Labor: Tissue Donors and Research Subjects in the Global Bioeconomy*. Durham, NC: Duke University Press.

Daniels, C. R. and Heidt-Forsythe, E. (2012). Gendered eugenics and the problematic of free market reproductive technologies: sperm and egg donation in the United States, *Signs Journal of Women in Culture and Society* 37:3, 719–47.

Deomampo, D. (2016). Race, nation, and the production of intimacy: transnational ova donation in India, *positions* 24:1, 303–32.

Deomampo, D. (2019). Racialized commodities: race and value in human egg donation, *Medical Anthropology* 38:7, 620–33.

Delvigne, A. and Rozenberg, S. (2002). Epidemiology and prevention of ovarian hyperstimulation syndrome (OHSS): a review, *Human Reproduction Update* 8:6, 559–77.

Deveaux, M. (2016). Exploitation, structural injustice, and the cross-border trade in human ova, *Journal of Global Ethics* 12:1, 48–68.

Dolby, N. (1999). Youth and the global popular: the politics and practices of race in South Africa, *European Journal of Cultural Studies* 2:3, 291–309.

Erasmus, Z. (2017). *Race Otherwise: Forging a New Humanism for South Africa*. Johannesburg: Wits University Press.

Frankenberg, R. (1997). Introduction: local whiteness, localizing whiteness. In R. Frankenberg (ed.), *Displacing Whiteness: Essays in Social and Cultural Criticism*, 1–33. Durham, NC: Duke University Press.

Goedeke, S., Shepherd, D., and Rodino, I. (2020). Support for recognition and payment options for egg and sperm donation in New Zealand and Australia, *Human Reproduction* 35:1, 117–29.

Heng, B. C. (2005). Ethical issues in paying for long-distance travel and accommodation expenses of oocyte donors, *Reproductive BioMedicine Online* 11:5, 552–3.

Hlatshwayo, S. (2004). Infertility among Black South African Women, *Agenda* 60, 146–54.

Homanen, R. (2018). Reproducing whiteness and enacting kin in the Nordic context of transnational egg donation: matching donors with cross-border traveller recipients in Finland, *Social Science and Medicine* 203, 28–34.

Hope, E. (2020). Tasmanian couple forced to wait years in fertility queues due to donor egg shortage. *The Mercury* (Tasmania, Australia), 1 June. www.themercury.com.au/news/tasmania/tasmanian-couples-forced-to-wait-years-in-fertility-queues-due-to-donor-egg-shortage/news-story/859 6b8c83fcb087ca3b8b152f73bfe6c. Accessed 28 April 2021.

Hudson, N. (2019). Egg donation imaginaries: embodiment, ethics and future family formation, *Sociology* 54:2, 346–62.

Ikemoto, L. C. (1996). The in/fertile, the too fertile, and the dysfertile, *Hastings Law Journal* 47:4, 1007–61.

Inhorn, M. (2015). *Cosmopolitan Conceptions: IVF Sojourns in Global Dubai*. Durham, NC: Duke University Press.

Jain, S. L. (2013). *Malignant: How Cancer Becomes Us*. Berkeley, CA: University of California Press.

Jayaprakasan, K., Herbert, M., Moody, E., Stewart, J. A., and Murdoch, A. P. (2009). Estimating the risks of ovarian hyperstimulation syndrome (OHSS): implications for egg donation for research, *Human Fertility* 10:3, 183–7.

Kenney, N. J. and McGowan, M. L. (2010). Looking back: egg donors' retrospective evaluations of their motivations, expectations, and experiences during their first donation cycle, *Fertility and Sterility* 93:2, 455–66.

Kramer, W., Schneider, J., and Schultz, N. (2009). US oocyte donors: a retrospective study of medical and psychosocial issues, *Human Reproduction* 24:12, 3144–9.

Kroløkke, C. (2012). From India with love: troublesome citizens of fertility travel, *Cultural Politics* 8:2, 307–25.

Kroløkke, C. H. and Pant, S. (2012). 'I only need her uterus': neo-liberal discourses on transnational surrogacy, *NORA – Nordic Journal of Feminist and Gender Research* 20:4, 233–48.

Lee, S. S. J. (2017). Consuming DNA: the good citizen in the age of precision medicine, *Annual Review of Anthropology* 46:1, 33–48.

Leve, M. (2013). Reproductive bodies and bits: exploring dilemmas of egg donation under neoliberalism, *Studies in Gender and Sexuality* 14:4, 277–88.

Lipsitz, G. (2006). *The Possessive Investment in Whiteness: How White People Profit from Identity Politics*. Philadelphia, PA: Temple University Press.

Mayosi, B. M., Lawn, J. E., Niekerk, A. van, Bradshaw, D., Karim, S. S. A., and Coovadia, H. M. (2012). Health in South Africa: changes and challenges since 2009, *The Lancet* 380:9858, 2029–43.

Mohr, S. (2014). Beyond motivation: on what it means to be a sperm donor in Denmark, *Anthropology and Medicine* 21:2, 162–73.

Moll, T. (2019). Making a match: curating race in South African gamete donation, *Medical Anthropology* 38:7, 588–602.

Moll, T. (2021). Reproduction, sacrificial life, and the logics of attrition in the afterlife of apartheid. In R. Davis-Floyd (ed.), *Birthing Techno-Sapiens: Human-Technology Co-Evolution and the Future of* Reproduction, 90–102. London: Routledge.

Nahman, M. (2008). Nodes of desire: Romanian Egg sellers, 'dignity' and feminist alliances in transnational ova exchanges, *European Journal of Women's Studies* 15:2, 65–82.

Nahman, M. (2018). Migrant extractability: centring the voices of egg providers in cross-border reproduction, *Reproductive BioMedicine & Society Online* 7, 82–90.

Namberger, V. (2016). The South African economy of egg donation: looking at the bioeconomic side of normalization. In M. Lie and N. Lykke (eds), *Assisted Reproduction Across Borders: Feminist Perspectives on Normalizations, Disruptions and* Transmissions, 72–83. New York: Routledge.

National Health Act (No. 61 of 2003). Regulation (2012). *Government Gazette.* 35099. 1 March. Government notice no. R181. Pretoria: Government Printer.

Orthofer, A. (2016). Wealth Inequality in South Africa: Insights from Survey and Tax Data. REDI3x3 Working Paper 15, University of Cape Town. www.redi3x3.org/sites/default/files/Orthofer%202016%20REDI3x3%20

Working%20Paper%2015%20-%20Wealth%20inequality.pdf. Accessed 24 November 2021.

Pande, A. (2011). Transnational commercial surrogacy in India: gifts for global sisters? *Reproductive Biomedicine Online*, 23:5, 618–25.

Pande, A. (2014). *Wombs in Labor: Transactional Commercial Surrogacy in India*. New York: Columbia University Press.

Pande, A. (2015). Global reproductive inequalities, neo-eugenics and commercial surrogacy in India, *Current Sociology* 64:2, 1–15.

Pande A. (2020). Visa stamps for injections: traveling biolabor and South African egg provision, *Gender and Society* 34:4, 573–96.

Pande, A. (2021). 'Mix or match?' Transnational Fertility industry and white desirability, *Medical Anthropology*. DOI:10.1080/01459740.2021.1877289.

Pande, A. and Moll, T. (2018). Gendered bio-responsibilities and travelling egg providers from South Africa, *Reproductive Biomedicine & Society Online* 6, 23–33.

Payne, J. G. (2015). Reproduction in transition: cross-border egg donation, biodesirability and new reproductive subjectivities on the European fertility market, *Gender, Place and Culture* 22:1, 107–22.

Pfeffer, N. (2011). Eggs-ploiting women: a critical feminist analysis of the different principles in transplant and fertility tourism, *Reproductive Biomedicine Online* 23:5, 634–41.

Rajan, K. S. (2005). Subjects of speculation: emergent life sciences and market logics in the United States and India, *American Anthropologist* 107:1, 19–30.

Reardon, J. and TallBear, K. (2012). 'Your DNA is our history': genomics, anthropology, and the construction of whiteness as property, *Current Anthropology*, 53:S5, S233–S245.

Roberts, E. F. S. (2012). *God's Laboratory: Assisted Reproduction in the Andes*, Berkeley, CA: University of California Press.

Roberts, E. F. S. and Scheper-Hughes, N. (2011). Introduction: medical migrations, *Body and Society* 17:2–3, 1–30.

Russell, C. (2018). *The Assisted Reproduction of Race*. Bloomington, IN: Indiana University Press.

Saldanha, A. (2007). *Psychedelic White: Goa Trance and the Viscosity of Race*. Minneapolis, MN: University of Minnesota Press.

Salusbury, T. and Foster, D. (2004). Rewriting WESSA identity. In N. Distiller and M. Steyn (eds), *Under* Construction, 93–109. Sandton, SA: Heinemann.

Sarojini, N., Marwah, V., and Shenoi, A. (2011). Globalisation of birth markets: a case study of assisted reproductive technologies in India, *Globalization and Health* 7:27, 1–9.

Saunokonoko, M. (2017). 'Begging for eggs' inside Australia's altruistic donor system. 9News (Australia). 3 November. www.9news.com.au/health/australian-women-forced-to-beg-for-eggs-shortage-of-altruistic-donors-ivf/bc399ab4-c7cc-4435-ad99-05a4a5f9eda9. Accessed 28 April 2021.

Schneider J., Lahl J., and Kramer, W. (2017). Long-term breast cancer risk following ovarian stimulation in young egg donors: a call for follow-up, research and informed consent. *Reproducive BioMedicine Online* 34:5, 480–5.

Schurr, C. (2018). The baby business booms: economic geographies of assisted reproduction, *Geography Compass* 12:8, 1–15.

Shenfield, F., Mouzon, J. de, Pennings, G., Ferraretti, A.P., Andersen, A. N., Wert, G. de, ESHRE Taskforce on Cross Border Reproductive Care Goossens, V., and 2010. Cross border reproductive care in six European countries, *Human Reproduction* 25:6, 1361–8.

SASRSS (South African Society of Reproductive Science and Surgery) (2008). Guidelines for gamete donation.

Speier, A. 2016. *Fertility Holidays: IVF Tourism and the Reproduction of Whiteness*. New York: New York University Press.

Steyn, M. (2001). *Whiteness Just Isn't What it Used To Be: White Identity in a Changing South Africa*. Albany, NY: SUNY Press.

Steyn, M. (2004). Rehabilitating a whiteness disgraced: Afrikaner white talk in post-apartheid South Africa, *Communication Quarterly* 52:2, 143–69.

Steyn, M. and Foster, D. (2008). Repertoires for talking white: resistant whiteness in post-apartheid South Africa, *Ethnic and Racial Studies* 31:1, 25–51.

Tuit, M. (1982). Salute to test tube father. *Rand Daily Mail* (Johannesburg, SA). 8 February: p. 1.

Tupasela, A. (2017). Populations as brands in medical research: placing genes on the global genetic atlas, *BioSocieties* 12, 47–65.

van der Westhuizen, C. (2017). *Sitting Pretty: White Afrikaans Women in Postapartheid South Africa*. Durban, SA: University of KwaZulu-Natal Press.

Vora, K. (2015). Re-imagining reproduction: unsettling metaphors in the history of imperial science and commercial surrogacy in India, *Somatechnics* 5:1, 88–103.

Vorster, R. (1988). Vroue stroom na SA vir bevrugtning. *Rapport* (Johannesburg, SA), 20 November: p. 4.

Vrou word ma na skenker-eierselle (1988). *Die Burger*. 15 July, p. 1.

Whittaker, A. and Speier, A. (2010). 'Cycling overseas': care, commodification, and stratification in cross-border reproductive travel, *Medical Anthropology* 29:4, 363–83.

Willoughby-Herard, T. (2007). South Africa's poor whites and whiteness studies: Afrikaner ethnicity, scientific racism, and white misery, *New Political Science* 29:4, 479–500.

Willoughby-Herard, T. (2015). *Waste of a White Skin: The Carnegie Corporation and the Racial Logic of White Vulnerability*. Berkeley, CA: University of California Press.

Zegers-Hochschild, F., Adamson, G. D., de Mouzon, J., Ishihara, O., Mansour, R., Nygren, K., Sullivan, E., and Van der Poel, S. (2009). International Committee for Monitoring Assisted Reproductive Technology (ICMART) and the World Health Organization (WHO) revised glossary of ART terminology, 2009, *Fertility and Sterility*, 92:5, 1520–4.

14

The resurgence of eugenics through egg donation in South Africa: race as a central and 'obvious' choice

Rufaro Moyo

This routinized reinscription of race at the genetic and cellular level in donation programmes, which as medicalized organizations offer a veneer of scientific credibility to such claims, is worrisome given our eugenic history. (Almeling, 2007: 338)

Well, I think the problem is um, race is obviously an artificial construct ... I think racial profiling is different because certainly in South Africa it was more of a legal, arbitrary definition that people made. That's why it became so problematic because they couldn't fit some people in the boxes, in the terms of what the heck race is this person (Laughs). And they tried all these ridiculous ways of trying to figure it out (Laughs). (Participant 9)

The social science literature on infertility treatments or Assisted Reproductive Technologies (ARTs) has been growing since the 1980s after the first baby was conceived using assisted reproduction in 1978 in the UK (Dow, 2017). Although much of Africa and Sub-Saharan Africa is seen to be resource poor in terms of reproductive technologies, the first in vitro fertilisation (IVF) procedure took place in South Africa in 1983, merely five years after the first procedure (Dyer and Kruger, 2012). ARTs in South Africa have been expanding since then, with a market of reproductive technologies that attracts both locals and foreigners alike in the private sector (Dyer and Kruger, 2012).Given the specific apartheid and colonial history of South Africa, this makes it an exceptional case for social science study in reproductive technologies and race (Norling, 2015).

Existing social science scholarship in the field of reproductive technologies and race has focused on three phenomenon. First are the disparities that exist around access to ARTs according to one's racial group (Chin et al., 2015; Elster, 2005; Guendelman, 2011; Jain, 2006; Quinn and Fujimoto, 2016; Roberts, 2009). Second, is the reproduction of whiteness that is made possible by these technologies (Nahman, 2016; Pande, 2021: Quiroga, 2007; Roberts, 2012; Schuur, 2017). Third, scholars examine how race affects the choices of recipients when choosing donors, indicating that there is often a phenomenon of 'racial matching' or 'racial passing' taking place, leading to a resurgence of a biological conception of race (Valdez and Deomampo, 2019). This chapter examines the role that race plays in the process of recipients choosing a desirable donor. The findings are based on interviews I conducted with fertility staff (staff working in the field of reproductive technologies in fertility clinics and donor agencies) in Cape Town, South Africa. The purpose of choosing fertility staff was that, given the numerous cases of IVF that have occurred in South Africa, a more general and reliable assesment of the role race plays could be made by staff who have worked with a variety of patient cases. The insights of staff were not only pivotal, but consulting with them became a practical way of accessing the field of reproductive technologies for study.

In this chapter, I use the literature on racial matching and neo-eugenics as theoretical frameworks to make the argument that race is central to the egg donation process and this naturalisation of race in the process is a form of neo-eugenics. The repercussions of this resemble nineteenth- and twentieth-century eugenics and a desire to maintain the myth of racial purity, which would thereby indicate a possible resurgence of eugenics by reproductive technologies. Explorations such as this are relevant to understanding the ways in which race still asserts itself in our post-apartheid dispensation and how it is being recreated by reproductive technologies as a biological phenomenon. This biological conception of race is one that social scientists have disputed in the interests of racial justice.

For the purpose of this research, I conceptualised race using its modern definition, a means of classifying people based on their skin colour and other physical features as well as culture and geography (Erasmus, 2017: xxii). While I understand race to be a social construction, with no biological significance (and that is part of this chapter's argument), this modern conception of race, which influenced the apartheid racial categories, continues to reinscribe itself as apartheid racial categories persist in post-apartheid South Africa, not simply as markers for redress, but increasingly in the field of ARTs as biological or inheritable. Apartheid categories of race continue to be a means by which people are identified and identify themselves (racial identity). These processes, of identification and applying race are known as racialisation (Erasmus, 2017: 53). What subjects understand by race differs significantly outside and within South Africa, but the modes of racialisation, across South African society remain somewhat universal. One epistemology of racialisation that is of particular importance is what Erasmus terms 'the look' (Erasmus, 2017: 53). It is this understanding of race as being inscribed in a 'look' that persists and is reproduced as seemingly biological in the world of fertility in Cape Town, South Africa and it is this reinforcement of a biological understanding of race in the egg donation process that this chapter interrogates.

Setting the scene: the role of race in ART

Numerous scholars have examined the role of race in ARTs. The scholarship indicates arguments around the disparities of access based on race and the reproduction of whiteness within these technologies (Chin et al., 2015; Elster, 2005; Guendelman and Stachel, 2011; Jain, 2006; and Quinn and Fujimoto, 2016), the phenomenon of race matching when choosing donors, and the search for resemblance when choosing donors, which leads to the possible resurgence of a biological conception of race (Ikemoto, 1995; Krølokke, 2014; Quiroga, 2007; Russell, 2015). Of particular interest to this study was the scholarship on the phenomenon of race matching. This section explores some of the beginnings of scholarship on race and reproductive technologies, followed by attention to scholarship on race matching and emergent scholarship emphasising the need to use race as an analytic in examining reproduction. These arguments are critical to understanding the role race plays in ART.

The subject of race and ARTs started in the 1980s, when feminists such as Gena Corea (as described in Roberts, 2009) spoke of dystopias in which white women's reproduction was of a higher value in perception than that of women of colour. Corea discussed the idea in her work *The Mother Machine*, predicting that women of colour would be hired as surrogates for white women at low costs. The opposing relationship of white women and women of colour to ARTs has been critiqued by feminist scholars and has been termed "'stratified reproduction'" by anthropologists such as Rayna Rapp (as described in Roberts, 2009). Arguments on the racial disparities caused by ARTs are made by many other scholars such as Chin et al. (2015), Elster (2005), Guendelman and Stachel (2011), Jain (2006), and Quinn and Fujimoto (2016). Dorothy Roberts (2009), rather than placing these groups (white women and women of colour) at opposite spectrums, examines them in relation to the trend towards privatisation.

She argues that population control programmes and ART place infertility in the hands of individuals, thus privatising remedies for social inequity and illness (Roberts, 2009). In contrast to before, women of colour are now a part of the market of reproductive technologies and as such a new understanding of the relationship between race and ARTs is needed. Roberts (2009) examines the relationship between racism, race and ARTs with the intention of illuminating a new dystopia in which neoliberalism, racism and reproduction converge. Following this, she goes on to examine how reproductive technologies are facilitating a resurgence of race (Roberts, 2011: preface), writing that 'fertility clinics solicit egg donations on the basis of race and use race in genetic tests to determine which embryos to implant and which to discard'. Roberts (2011) discusses in her work the phenomenon of 'race-based medicine' and how despite the findings of the Human Genome Project, there has been a resurgence of the use of race, and it is this resurgence through reproductive technologies that this article explores.

Scholars who discuss how ARTs and race intersect also examine the choices surrounding sperm and ova, noting that within these choices there is always a desire to racially match or achieve resemblance in the narratives of clinic staff and patients (Ikemoto, 1995; Krølokke, 2014; Quiroga, 2007; Russell, 2015). Ikemoto (1995) discusses the media attention surrounding reproductive technologies in the early 1990s noting that the media attention focused on Black women selecting white donors and post-menopausal women having babies through ARTs. Yet, despite artificial insemination providing the same opportunities for trait selection, the media gave no attention to that. It was only a problem worth highlighting when Black women choose white ova (Ikemoto, 1995) thereby making racial selection evident. Race, therefore, is only interrogated when colour lines are crossed and not when a racial match is sought out, due to racial matching being seen as an obvious and natural occurrence when using reproductive technologies (Ikemoto, 1995).

Quiroga (2007) argues that the myth of racial purity is maintained by sperm banks through creating careful catalogues of the physical characteristics of sperm donors, which allow for racial matching to take place. She finds that the purpose for matches are three-fold: the first is to increase the chances of the child resembling the social parent. Second, to legitimise the family by creating white Americans' conception of a biological family. Third, to maintain secrecy about the use of an egg donor in the hopes that the child will 'pass' as genetically connected to the social parent (Quiroga, 2007). Russell (2015) furthers this argument, noting that the idea that the race of the child must match that of the intended parents is so natural it does not even constitute a choice. The influence of race and its biologisation in these reproductive technologies is imposed very strongly. In some contexts it was, and still is, standard policy to racially match, or 'ethnically match' as it is sometimes referred to. In the UK, for the Human Fertilisation and Embryology Authority (HFEA) matching the race of the donor and the recipient used to be official practice up until 2014 (Maung, 2018). Clinics, however, continue to racially match and in European countries such as Spain, Norway and Finland, race matching remains standard practice (Maung, 2018). The importance of racial matching is valued tremendously. So much so that until recently, the largest sperm bank in the US shipped semen in colour-coded vials to ease fears of racial 'mix-ups' (Russell, 2015: 605–6).

Interestingly, while the predominant scholarship produced has indicated that racial matching is part of the desired goal in the process of selecting an egg donor, Pande (2021) has discovered through her recent research, *'Mix or Match?' Transnational Fertility Industry and White Desirability*, that this desire to racially match does take place amongst white, heterosexual intended parents, but that further, particularly among same-sex couples there is a trend of seeking not a match, but a strategic 'racial hybridisation' (Pande, 2021). Pande's work examined the transnational fertility industry, following the travel of biomaterial from one nation to another, hence conducting a mobile ethnography. Despite the fact that these same-sex couples who do not identify as white disrupt the myth of racial purity which racial matching perpetuates, what is fascinating is that this strategic mixing will often involve using the genetic material of a white donor in order to 'whiten' future generations (Pande, 2021). Hence, while the myth of racial purity and resemblance is not perpetuated among these couples, the dynamics indicate a racialised manner of selecting donors and a naturalisation of both race and white desirability in the process (Pande, 2021). While Pande's work spans across multiples locations and indicates that not all couples seek the racial match, her work still reinforces the argument this chapter makes, which is that race is central in the process of selecting an egg donor.

Further scholarship has started to emerge which emphasises the importance of race as an analytical tool in examining reproduction and takes feminist anthropologists' 'stratified reproduction' as a central theoretical frame, along with reproductive justice (Valdez and Deomampo, 2019: 551). Given current events indicating the persistence of racism globally, as well as taking seriously the assertion that reproductive politics involves racial politics, there is an increasing focus of the issues on race and racialisation within reproduction (Valdez and Deomampo, 2019).

Scholarship already doing this work includes Deomampo (2019), who examines the racialisation of gametes at a fertility clinic in Hawaii. She discusses how gametes are commodified by being inscribed racial categories, thus making racialisation and commodification interlinked within the fertility clinic. She focuses particularly on Asian Americans, a diverse group where what is said to qualify as 'Asian' differs from one group to the next. The categorising of donor tissue is linked to shared ancestry and similar phenotypical features as a tool in the process of family formation (Deomampo, 2019). The danger being an implication of a 'pure' Asian tissue for the consummation of recipients, a false promise that race is inheritable and therefore biological (Deomampo, 2019). This employment of race transcends mere individual choice Deomampo argues and lends itself to the resurgence of race as biological. The issue being that this reinforcement of race as biology poses the basis for persisting inequalities and instances of racial discrimination. Cromer (2019) similarly, examines these processes of racialising reproductive tissue, but notes that in the US adoption agency for embryo adoption where she conducts her fieldwork, the term 'ethnicity' is used to describe categories that point to race (Cromer, 2019). She argues that this is similar to arguments scholars make when examining embryo transfers and adoption of children. Her research adds a further dimension of exploring these practices of racialisation in US agencies where embryos are adopted. She finds that a commodifying effect, where recipients are able to consume and choose via race-based preference, is produced regardless of staff attempts to neutralise race by employing terms such as 'ethnicity'. Newman (2019), similarly to Deomampo and Cromer, examines the racialisation of reproductive tissue. Her study focuses on the choices for sperm donors made by interracial lesbian couples, finding that should both women desire to be pregnant in the family formation process, they are faced with the question of whether to prioritise biological ties between their children by using the same donor, or prioritise a racial match and select two different donors. Newman (2019) argues that either way, traditional hegemonic constructs of the family as racially homogenous or genetically linked are being perpetuated. It is these hegemonic constructs that this chapter calls into question, using South Africa as its field.

Despite the fact that the first test tube baby conceived in South Africa was in 1983 and the ARTs industry has grown vastly since then, the social science literature has barely scratched the surface of this area. The disadvantage being that the history of South Africa provides a necessary and relevant platform, particularly for the field of ARTs and race. The work of Tessa Moll provides a welcome investigation into race and gamete donation in South Africa. Moll's (2019) article is titled 'Making a match: curating race in South African gamete donation' and discusses insights from her ethnographic research in the office of an embryologist, as well as the larger structures and outcomes of racial 'donor matching' in South African fertility clinics. Moll argues that in the process of gamete donation, race is 'enacted' through what she termed 'curatorship' by fertility staff. This 'curatorship' is the racial classifying and organisation of the donor's information, the result being a biologised understanding of race which is inheritable and enacted by fertility staff, whom she refers to as 'matchers' (Moll, 2019: 589). These 'matchers', in an understanding of shifting relations of power, take up the role of the state in racial classifications in a post-apartheid context. Private fertility clinics hence become a site of power in the making and reproduction of race, particularly modes of whiteness in a neoliberal context of health. Moll (2019) posits the idea that while these power dynamics and the reproduction of whiteness has been echoed by scholars before her, there has been a tendency to neglect those who's race is unknown or 'just-about-white' (Moll, 2019: 598). Moll's work, which points to the perpetuation of a biocentric understanding of race through gamete donation, is the argument this chapter explores, though in the context of interviews and with a lens of neo-eugenics.

Warranted investigation: race matching as a form of neo-eugenics

In exploring the links between racial matching in egg donation, and the concomitant control of bodies using racial markers, which is a fundamental part of neo-eugenics, it is necessary to explore the history of eugenics. This contextual history explores how eugenics has morphed, and frames how race matching becomes a form of neo-eugenics warranting investigation.

In the nineteenth century, scientists such as Herbert Spencer, Gregory Mendel and Charles Darwin focused their work on understanding the internal traits of animals, humans and plants, which contributed to their differences as well as their ability to survive, reproduce and adapt (Allen, 1983, 1997; Black, 2003). From this work erupted ideologies of how to improve the human race, rooted in a belief that there were genetically inherited traits which were responsible for the stratifications within society (Black, 2003). The European theorist, Francis Galton, focused on this work with the aim of quantifying evolutionary processes and coined the term 'eugenics' (Black, 2003; Perkowitz, 2017). Galton wanted the use of government policy to restrict marriages between those with desirable and undesirable traits, thereby restricting and eventually eroding the reproduction of those found to have undesirable traits (Black, 2003). Black argues that Galton made a shift from hoping for political backing to religious backing, with the aim of creating a pure master race by determining which people are fit to procreate together.

Eugenicists often described their ideology using garden metaphors, stating that society is like a garden which is in need of weeding. European and American eugenics focused primarily on race (Dyck, 2014). American and German eugenicists also employed a biological understanding of race in their programmes. At the core of eugenics lay a desire to exert power and control over those deemed undesirable within the national plan, and while eugenics presented itself as a science with the interests of health and nationalism in mind, it was in fact a means of ensuring the maintenance of the myth of racial purity (Dyck, 2014). In the nineteenth and twentieth centuries, western nations embraced eugenics, firmly believing that lower classes and minorities were genetically inferior and that, therefore, their offspring would also have these genetically inferior traits (Black, 2003). Eugenics was strongly spearheaded by scholar and head of Eugenics Record Office, Charles Davenport, and much funding was put into research and implementation. Even prior to this, criminals and those admitted to psychiatric hospitals were already being sterilised as a means of preventing the spread of their 'inferior genes' (Allen, 1997: 80).

This movement reached its peak during the twentieth century, culminating in the Nazi-led Holocaust, which highlighted the scale and severity of the dire consequences of eugenic thinking and its manipulation (Dyck, 2014). The link between eugenics and genocide was popularised in the public mind and for decades to follow eugenics was linked to Nazism. The Holocaust changed the language used with regards to eugenics and the direction of the movement, such that many scholars are convinced that eugenics ended with Nazi Germany after 1945. However, while the formal application of eugenics ended, there was a shift in language and application to accommodate the change in reproductive politics (Dyck, 2014). In the latter half of the twentieth century the discourse changed to birth control, population control, and access to healthcare, disability and reproductive technologies. Discussions about choice and the complexities of genetics gave way to a rising neo-eugenics by the new ARTs and prenatal screening.

While scientists eventually came to the conclusion that eugenics was merely pseudoscientific racism, the truth is that eugenics has not entirely left us. We need look no further than Murray and Herrnstein's (1994) publication of *The Bell Curve*, a controversial piece of work, which makes the argument that Black people are less intelligent than white people. Eugenics, therefore, is never far from reach, and with the advancement of genetic technologies, some scholars have found that a process of neo-eugenics is able to take place. In her article, 'Donor insemination: eugenic and feminist implications', Allan Hanson (2001) points out that one of the concerns of ARTs lies in their use for positive eugenics. As the technologies become safe and affordable, people may wish to 'improve' their offspring by endowing them with desirable traits. Hanson (2001) argues that within the politics of reproduction this is one of the central concerns, the use of reproductive technologies for positive eugenics. While biomedical establishments hail the arrival of the genetic technologies as tools to fight off genetic disease and disability, there is the concern that people may employ these technologies to enhance the intelligence, athletic skill and other characteristics deemed desirable (Hanson, 2001; Sandel, 2004).

In their work, Daniels and Heidt-Forsythe (2012) examine a pool of over 1,500 donors between the years of 2006 and 2008. They discovered in their study what they term a gendered eugenics, in which recipients preferred the tissue of donors that fitted the conception of western ideals of masculinity and femininity. For men these were the donors who mainly matched idealised traits of race, class and masculinity, achieved above average grades, had leaner figures and were above average height (Daniels and Heidt-Forsythe, 2012). For women they discovered there is a preference for tall, thin and racially whiter women, with above-average education for women their age (Daniels and Heidt-Forsythe, 2012). This is not only a phenomenon of western countries using these technologies; in India, where the reproductive market is booming, Sarojini, Marwah and Sanoi (2011) found that the genetic technologies in Asia are being used for sex selection of males.

While reproductive technologies facilitate positive eugenics and the myth of racial purity through the phenomenon of race matching, sterilisation and contraceptives through population control programmes facilitate the negative eugenics of today, lying within a discourse of the idea that having many children is what makes poor people poor (Roberts, 1997). Melinda Gates has stated that contraception is one of the 'greatest antipoverty innovations in history' (Gates and Gates, 2017), and France's President, Emmanuel Macron, has said that African women would choose to reproduce less if they were given access to education and family planning (Wintour, 2018). In South Africa in recent years it was revealed that twenty-two HIV positive women were involuntarily sterilised (Strode et al., 2012). In addition, problematic public discourses about Black women being hyper-fertile and their 'welfare babies' are still prevalent (Roberts, 1997). Amrita Pande (2016: 250), who examines surrogacy in India, has also discussed neo-eugenics, stating that currently, it is 'the new, subtle form of eugenics whereby the neoliberal notion of consumer choice justifies promotion of assisted reproductive services for the rich and, at the same time, by portraying poor people (often in the global South) as strains on the world's economy and environment justifies aggressive anti-natal policies.' Neo-eugenics hence is an interesting term used to describe the manner in which eugenics presents itself today. Eugenics didn't end in 1945, but instead the language and discourse simply changed and it continues to conceal itself behind humanitarian ideals of alleviating poverty and healthcare. Thus I use neo-eugenics and race matching as theoretical frameworks in this chapter, employing and expanding upon Pande's (2016) definition. I see neo-eugenics as the promotion of reproductive technologies for the rich and anti-natal policies for the poor, while also understanding that amongst the use of reproductive technologies is not only the quest for 'better birth', as the term eugenics implies, but also reinforcements of the myth of racial purity with regards to race matching.

Methodology

The focus of my research investigates whether ARTs in Cape Town, in particular egg donation, facilitate a process of neo-eugenics at the stage of selecting a donor through the practice and process of 'race matching'. Research was conducted in the form of ten interviews with nine participants, all staff working in the field of fertility. A few of these individuals had been through the process of egg donation as intended parents and, therefore, had a dual perspective from the position of staff as well as recipient.

The purpose of having chosen staff specifically was to gain the perspective of the agents who naturalise the use of racial categories and at times impose it as the obvious means to choose a donor. In addition, because these staff members interact with both egg donors and, more importantly, recipients/patients/intended parents on a daily basis, their insights were invaluable as they had a broader view of how intended parents choose egg donors and how they engage with race in this process. Interviews were semi-structured and open ended, and explored staff's observations of recipients' desires, what they generally seek and how they engage with race in the process of selecting an egg donor. Of the three fertility clinics and four egg donor agencies in Cape Town at the time of my fieldwork, staff were interviewed from two fertility clinics and three egg donor agencies, thus making the study almost exhaustive. Yet, while the study collected data from almost all fertility clinics and egg donor agencies in Cape Town at the time, the findings of the study are not presented as an all-encompassing truth; to do so would be very reductionist. The study merely presents itself as one of the early works on race and ARTs, specifically egg donation, in South Africa.

The findings: *much ado about race, obviously*

Despite the Human Genome Project's discoveries of the lack of hereditary significance with race, race continues to be the central marker of identity in the process of selecting an egg donor. While the social sciences understand race to be a social construct with no scientific validity, ARTs have allowed for a resurgence of the use of race in the field of science (Roberts, 2011). Racial categories are used in the process of selecting an egg donor, and it is the first marker of identity after gender that is used. Yet history has shown us that not only is race an artificial construct, there are also many people who do not fit into the given categories. I often find myself wondering that if the use of racial categories is truly about finding a donor who resembles the intended parent, why not use a spectrum of skin colour pigments? What is it about race that makes this marker of identity so central in choosing someone of our likeness? The interesting matter at hand is with the way in which donor agents naturalise race and point to its 'obviousness' as a necessary identity category in the process of selecting a donor. The implication being, ultimately, a replication of ideas surrounding the myth of racial purity. A Black woman should want a Black egg donor, and a white woman should want a white egg donor, and unless recipients express a different desire, donor agents will often implement or assume that a racial match is the desired and natural choice. Russell (2015) makes the argument that this naturalisation of race is so eminent that the race of the child does not constitute a choice. Similarly to Russell, my study indicated that the naturalisation of race matching was prevalent amongst egg donor agencies and their staff, and operated in ways that perpetuate a kind of race based neo-eugenic process.

Naturalising race: the categories

There are five racial categories that are employed, similar to the ones used during the apartheid era. White/Caucasian, African/Black, Cape Coloured/Coloured/Mixed Race, Asian and Indian. At one of the agencies they distinguish between Cape Coloured and Mixed Race. Nevertheless, all of the donor agencies consulted pointed out the use of racial categories in the process of identifying an egg donor. Already, there are discrepancies that may be identified in these categories. For example, the synonymous use of 'African' and 'Black', implying that Caucasian or Asian South African people are not African. The fluidity of 'Mixed Race' and Coloured, and the reductionist category of 'Asian'. The concern is that during the apartheid era, the government simply placed very heterogeneous people into reductionist categories without much meaning, such as 'Coloured'. There are Coloured people who originate from Malaysia and make up the 'Cape Malay', there are Coloured people who are descendants of the Khoi and San people, but were placed in the category Coloured, instead of Black due to the light brown pigment of their skin. They were people of African, Asian and mixed descent and due to the colour of their skin were labelled 'off-white', 'half-castes', 'bastards' and then came to make up the identity group, Coloured (Adhikari, 2013). The case with racial categories is not only in its perpetuation of apartheid categories, which were state-given and reductionist in nature, but also in the fact that these categories are not clear cut and that there are many people who can 'pass' for another race they do not identify with. While these categories are important in their use of redressing social injustices of the past, ARTs employs race as though it is a natural and given way of identifying people, despite its reductionist nature. It is employed as though it is the ultimate determinant of what makes a family (Quiroga, 2007; Russell, 2015). This was made evident in my interviews, where donor agents repeatedly pointed to the 'obviousness' of race as a means of identifying donors and recipients.

Naturalising race: obviously

Donor agents, and fertility staff in general, determine that race is the natural and 'obvious' means of identifying an egg donor. In instances where recipients choose an egg donor from a different race, they find it 'confusing', as though the natural and 'obvious' choice is to choose a donor who is of the same race. The phenomenon to deconstruct, therefore, is the way in which donor agents and ARTs at large impose race and perpetuate it as a naturalised and 'obvious' means of identification, despite the fact that race is in fact a reductionist social construct with no genetic validity.

As the gynaecologist I interviewed points out, race was problematic because there were instances where the government could not place racially ambiguous people into a clear-cut category. Race was about a system of oppression that placed human beings in a hierarchy based upon their appearance (Adhikari, 2013; Winant, 2000). Despite this understanding of race as a social construction by fertility staff, there is also an essentialist understanding of race at the same time, presenting a paradox in which race is a social construction yet an integral part of identification of someone in one's likeness concurrently. The interesting part is that race is not an automatic qualifier for how a person appears, yet *the look* (in other words, the practice of immediate categorising of racial identity based on physical appearance – Erasmus, 2017) as an understanding and process of racialisation is the one that donor agents employ. There are many people who identify as Black, but appear Coloured. There are people who identify as Coloured, but are able to pass as white. Which begs the question of the validity and necessity of race as a means of identifying a person in one's likeness. Aside from the ambiguity of race and its social constructiveness, the other matter is that donor agents take it to be natural and expected for recipients to racially match when choosing a donor. Hence, if a recipient desires otherwise, they have to state so, and in some cases explain their choice. The problematic nature of this being a resuscitation of eugenic ideas around the myth of racial purity, in which white people were to reproduce with whites and Black people were to reproduce with Blacks, so as to maintain a pure and superior race (whiteness) (Quiroga, 2007). In addition, race is then presented as a biological phenomenon which one can inherit. These dynamics continue to play themselves out in these ARTs. Donor agents may hold naturalised views about race matching in the process of selecting an egg donor but it is not their sole desire. Even recipients who do not seek assistance in selecting a donor tend to racially match when selecting a donor. This happens for numerous reasons, but the first is said to be a search for resemblance.

Race matching at the desirable centre: resemblance as aim, race is the game

All fertility staff interviewed indicated that the most important aspect in searching for an egg donor was to find someone who resembled the intended mother. Hence, physical characteristics are often the first criteria used by recipients and donor agents to narrow down the search for a donor. Maintaining that most recipients will often desire a donor that has some physical resemblance to the intended mother, Becker, Butler and Nachtigall (2005) write about this phenomenon of 'resemblance' in their work. They point out that often people look for resemblance between parents and their children. Hence, with egg donation, recipients will seek a donor who is physically similar to them, in the hope that the child will look somewhat like they do when they are born and perhaps pass as a biological child and be accepted as such (Becker, et al., 2005; Quiroga, 2007). This is materialised through the use of photographs. In South Africa, despite the fact that egg donation is anonymous, photographs of donors up until the age of ten can be provided. However, due to the fact that the egg donor agents and doctors can see the adult photo of both the recipient/intended parent and donor, recipients will at times ask donor agents to ensure that the final donor chosen is the closest in resemblance.

Although resemblance is the ultimate aim of the majority of recipients when choosing an egg donor, the starting point in selecting a donor who resembles them always starts with race and a process of racialisation that employs *the look* as its epistemology (which is further ensured and made 'accurate' through the use of photographs). Race therefore remains the significant marker of identity in the egg donation process, despite its fluidity, constructive nature and lack of hereditary significance, presenting it as a biological phenomenon for the process of family formation.

From the general to the specific: skin tone

While resemblance is the desired end result in choosing an egg donor, race and then, furthermore, skin tone (particularly in the case of Coloured and Black patients) is used as a tool to facilitate selecting this donor. For white recipients, they often look at the phenotypical features of hair colour and eye colour in their search for a donor. Donor agents note that due to the variation in hair and eye colour that white recipients have, they then also tend to focus on other softer traits such as academics, or musical and sporting talent, while the recipients of colour, due to the fact that many people of colour in South Africa generally have dark hair and dark eyes, take skin tone to be their primary focus.

The effort to try as far as possible to, firstly, match the race and then secondly, match the skin tone indicates the perceived importance and validation of family that comes from being the same colour (Harrison, 2013). The former phenomenon of race matching is one that many scholars on ART and race point to in their work (Ikemoto, 1995; Krølokke, 2014; Quiroga, 2007; Russell, 2015). In addition, there is often a strong reaction that people have when a recipient chooses ova from a donor who is not of the same race (Ikemoto, 1995; Quiroga, 2007). This study found that race matching is also prevalent in Cape Town with Participant 7 pointing to this when asked how recipients engage with race. She stated that, generally, Black recipients choose Black donors and white recipients choose white donors. It is the mixed race couples that may select either. Hence, mixed race recipients have more leeway to experiment racially with their choice. But between the imposed binary of Black and white, it remains expected and practised that Black recipients will choose a Black donor and white recipients will choose a white donor. This dynamic which is created in the process of selecting an egg donor mimics the eugenic practices and ideologies of the myth of racial purity. The latter phenomenon of further matching skin tone is indicative of a desire to further legitimise hegemonic notions of the family through specifically colour matching. Even within the same race there are various shades of complexion. This is pointed out by Participant 2 who says, 'You know, but if you're a family of light skinned black people and then your baby's dark that might be a problem.' Not only is the desire to match colour relevant for further legitimisation but, in addition, there is also the need to note that skin colour creates what is termed 'epidermic capital' in which there are privileges that come with having a lighter complexion (Walther, 2014: 521) – perhaps explaining what Participant 2 further notes, 'a black recipient if they are looking at a donor and she [the recipient] is light in complexion and the donor we show them is dark in complexion, they immediately move on.' Hence, while race and skin tone/complexion are two classifications that at times overlap and intersect (Deomampo, 2016) within the South African context, recipients distinguish between the two, using race first, and then, particularly in the case of patients of colour, skin tone to ensure the closest possible match of skin pigmentation. The aim being two-fold: first, to ensure legitimacy for the family structure and in particular the social parent; and second, specifically for fairer patients of colour, to ensure the epidermic capital that comes with lighter complexions is passed onto the child.

Desires to conceal: stigma, culture and religion

What became very evident in my research was that not only do recipients wish to racially match as a method of seeking resemblance, but that this strong affinity for resemblance derives from the desire to conceal the use of reproductive technologies and, in particular, the body tissue of another person. Donor agents pointed to the cultural stigma surrounding infertility as well as the desire to avoid marginalisation within religious communities.

There is a shame and a stigma that still hinders recipients from wishing to disclose due to cultural reasons. The donor agents make a distinction between Caucasian recipients and Black recipients in terms of disclosure rates. They state that roughly 40% of white clients will opt not to disclose, whereas 90% of Black patients will not disclose.[1] This was attributed to the perception of fertility within

Black families. Indeed, within numerous African cultures children are seen as a blessing, and a woman who cannot have children to carry on the family name is often shunned (Dyer et al., 2004).

The phenomenon of there being a greater stigma towards infertility amongst Black patients indicates a racialised dynamic to the stigma associated with infertility. This stigma is not only racialised but is also globally geographical. The consequences of infertility and the stigma associated with it is higher in the global south than in the global north (Tabong and Adongo, 2013: 1). These racialised and global dynamics to the stigma of infertility are further reinforced by a false perception that the global south does not and cannot have an infertility problem, due to dominant discourse which perceives people of colour, in particular in the global south, as being hyperfertile (Pilcher, 2006). This lading to great suffering for couples, especially women living in these contexts where children are highly valued, given the gendered dynamics that underpin this stigma as well.

The burden of infertility and the blame is often, if not always, placed upon the woman, leading to greater consequences for her. Tabong and Adongo (2013) discuss examples of these consequences, finding that infertility is considered a major reason for divorce and marital instability in Africa and that women who suffer from infertility often fear divorce, abandonment and polygamy. Infertility, hence, can be a source of great shame for families in contexts where children are highly valued. The desire to conceal the use of an egg donors is therefore high because of the desire to conceal the fact that the female is infertile. Recipients find greater comfort in searching for resemblance to hide their struggles with infertility from others due to the marginalisation and oppression that stems from it.

In addition to cultural and social contexts where infertility is stigmatised there is also fear among some of being ostracised/marginalised by religious communities, which underpins concealing the use of donor tissue. The desire to conceal for these couples is not solely based on the stigma attached to infertility, but the doctrines of their faith, which do not allow for the use of donor tissue. They pursue a racial match and a donor who resembles the intended mother to conceal their use of donor tissue as it opposes their faith and they want to avoid marginalisation from their religious communities (see Inhorn, 2011 for similar examples in the Middle East). What is of interest, however, is that even couples who choose to disclose, still often opt to racially match – again, pointing to the role of race in the perceived legitimisation of hegemonic notions of the family.

Fear of the family

Beyond the stigma and cultural beliefs, with the widespread use of ARTs by celebrities and many women as they grow older, the stigma and shame of using these technologies is diminishing (Almendrala, 2017), yet the desire to conceal remains prevalent due to what I term a 'fear of the family'. Families are social units of utmost importance and centrality in our lives. They are the place we learn to bond and are socialised in the ways of our surroundings. It is not far off, therefore, to say that families are generally the most important people in a person's life (Macionis and Plummer, 2008). General expectations about the qualities that family must afford us include love and acceptance. Yet, for the longest time, the family has been conceptualised with genetics and biology in mind.

One of the donor agents I interviewed stated that these ideas (of a genetic link legitimising the family) are greatly pervasive, such that upon discovery that a female may not use her own tissue in the reproduction of a child, there is a grieving process of intense sadness that ensues. Recipients' families place the notion of a genetic link in their conceptualisation of family, and as a result, recipients seek to conceal their use of ARTs, in particular egg donation, out of a fear of their children not being as loved and accepted (Becker et al., 2005). While some participants pointed to shame and stigma,or religious and cultural factors as facilitating a desire to conceal the use of egg donation, all participants made the point that the desire to conceal largely derives from a fear of lack of acceptance and adequate love for the child from other family members. This is partially embedded in the normative kinship model which equates family with a 'blood' or genetic relationship. These genetic links are reinforced in everyday life by phenomenon such as 'resemblance talks'; as friends, family and strangers make comments about how children resemble either of their (heterosexual, biological?) parents (Becker et al., 2005).

Genetics and parenthood are inextricably linked, so strongly that the biological parent is seen as the 'real' parent and the parent that raises the child, is given an alternate name such as 'social parent' or 'adoptive parent', hence giving the impression that they are always second to the biological parent (Hargreaves, 2006: 269). This illustrates a normative conceptualisation of motherhood as being based solely in biology, as opposed to the social process of raising a child. MacCallum and Golombok (2007) find similar arguments in their study of disclosure decisions among mothers of donor conceived children. They discovered that mothers who opted not to disclose, firstly did not do so to protect their child. There was a fear that with knowledge of the lack of a genetic link the family would treat the child differently. Another reason for choosing not to disclose relates to concerns about disapproval, particularly from grandparents who are said to be 'of a different generation' (Shehab et al., 2008). There were other reasons, such as opting not to disclose the use of donor sperm in order to keep the husband's infertility a secret (MacCallum and Golombok, 2007). Similar sentiments were expressed by participants of this study. Race matching and resemblance hence becomes integral to the egg donation process in order to ensure that the use of donor conception remains concealed from family members.

The fear of family rejection is reminiscent of feminist family theories on the family as a site of strength and collective survival as well as oppression and conflict (Allen, 2016). The traditional ideal family centres itself upon the notion of a racially homogenous, heterosexual couple who marry and produces their own biological children, as being legitimate (Hill Collins, 1998). This family provides a private haven from public life and is held together through love and care. It assumes a sexual division of labour in which the woman maintains the home and the man works in the public sphere. This family is seen as biological and natural, stemming from heterosexual love. It serves therefore a 'dual function', as an ideological construction and a fundamental principle of social organization' (Hill Collins, 1998: 62–3). This ideology of the traditional family is a construction and a fantasy that superimposes itself as the ideal, marginalising and delegitimising family structures that do not follow this form. The family, hence, is an important social structure in the lives of individuals, but because of this traditional family ideal that continues to impose itself, the family then becomes a site of oppression for those individuals who do not conform to this constructed fantasy of suburban bliss.

What is interesting and of import is that race takes the central and beginning stage as the marker of identity, which assumptively allows donor agents and recipients to choose a donor in the likeness of the recipient, often leading to a prevalence of racial matching. The concern is that this racial matching is naturalised, seen as obvious and, at times, highly mimics eugenic ideologies about the myth of racial purity and who can reproduce with who. In addition, race is then made to be a biological phenomenon, which legitimises family ties, as opposed to a social construct created with the intention of enforcing power dynamics and oppression.

Conclusion

In conclusion, race plays a central role in the process of selecting an egg donor in Cape Town, South Africa. The ARTs indicate the pervasive way in which race asserts itself in our lives and these technologies reinforce it as though it is a natural biological phenomenon, as opposed to a social construct. Recipients and donor agents reinforce this use of race and often tend towards race matching, the ensuing effect being not only a naturalisation of race, but a resurgence of eugenic ideas around the myth of racial purity.

Racial categories were used to organise donors on the agency websites and when questioned about the use of these racial categories fertility staff pointed to an 'obviousness' of the relevance of race for identifying a donor despite race being a fluid social construction with no hereditary significance. This naturalisation is very prevalent, such that recipients who do not wish to racially match have to make that known to the donor agents in the event that it is the donor agent who will search for a donor for them. The use of race was justified as the best way to seek out a donor that resembles the intended mother. While many recipients seek resemblance between themselves and the chosen donor, the first step in the process of identifying this donor is always race. Race is the central marker of identity within the process of egg donation. The matching of race and the desire to achieve resemblance often stemmed within a desire to conceal the use of reproductive technologies and donor tissue for conception. The desires to conceal stemmed from the stigma regarding infertility, conservative cultural ideals and religion. But the leading factor in the desire to conceal was the recipients' fear of rejection from other family members. Many recipients who seek resemblance in a desire to conceal fear that their child will not be accepted or as loved if family members are aware that donor tissue was used to conceive the child. Race matching therefore becomes a means of attempting to mimic a biological link, to ensure acceptance for the child and legitimisation of the family, further perpetuating hegemonic constructs surrounding race and biology in the family. This process, I have argued, is a resurgence of eugenics.

There are two misconceptions about eugenics that I have observed. The first is that eugenics ended with Nazi Germany. When people think of eugenics they often think of Nazi Germany and the concentration camps that killed those deemed undesirable. They assume that eugenics is a thing of the past, steeped in a time when science was used to push racist political agendas. The second misconception is that eugenics only means 'better birth' and genetic improvement. They think of 'better birth' and today as 'designer babies' along with prenatal testing to screen out traits deemed defective. The issue is, eugenics did not end with the Second World War. Eugenics persisted and changed its discourse to facilitate the political shifts of the climate, manifesting itself presently in population control programmes and reproductive technologies. In addition, while many view eugenics as 'better birth' and a search to genetically improve one's family line, I view it differently. Eugenics is not so much about better birth as it is about the myth of racial purity. The eugenics movement dictated who could procreate with whom to maintain the myth of racial purity, concealing itself in a rhetoric of nationhood and health improvement. Similarly, egg donation mimics this, bringing forth a perpetuation of these ideas. Egg donation perpetuates ideas about the myth of racial purity through racial matching and a naturalisation of race. Similarly to the eugenics movement, it conceals the power dynamics it perpetuates in the discourse of resemblance. ARTs have brought treatment and hope to those struggling with infertility and indicate the advancement of science and technology within the health sector. However, the persisting power dynamics surrounding race and desirability have come to manifest themselves within these technologies, indicating that as time changes, the discourse within medicine and science shifts itself to accommodate the politics of the time. For social justice to be achieved, these power dynamics must be identified and then dismantled to ensure just experiences in society for all.

Notes

1 It is interesting that, despite many more white patients choosing to disclose, there is still often a desire to racially match – indicating that while desires to conceal are a part of the motivations for racial matching, there are still other prevalent factors leading to this phenomenon.

References

Adhikari, M. (ed.) (2013). *Burdened by Race: Coloured Identities in Southern Africa*. Cape Town: University of Cape Town Press.

Allen, G. E. (1983). The misuse of biological hierarchies: the American eugenics movement, 1900–1940, *History and Philosophy of the Life Sciences* 5:2, 105–28.

Allen, G. E. (1997). The social and economic origins of genetic determinism: a case history of the American eugenics movement, 1900–1940 and its lessons for today, *Genetica* 99, 77–88.

Allen, K. R. (2016). Feminist theory in family studies: history, reflection and critique, *Journal of Family Theory and Review* 8, 207–24.

Almeling, R. (2007). Selling genes, selling gender: egg agencies, sperm banks, and the medical market in genetic material. *American Sociological Review* 72, 319–40.

Almendrala, A. (2017). 12 Celebrities who have opened up about IVF and surrogacy. *Life – Huffington Post*. www.huffpost.com/entry/12-celebrities-who-have-openedup-about-ivf-and-surrogacy_n_575a22cfe4b0ced23ca7a74a. Accessed 11 October 2018.

Becker, G., Butler, A. and Nachtigall, R. (2005). Resemblance talk: a challenge for parents whose children were conceived with donor gametes in the US, *Social Science and Medicine* 61:6, 1300–9.

Black, E. (2003). *War Against the Weak: Eugenics and America's Campaign to Create a Master Race*. Westport, CT: Dialog Press.

Chin, H. B., Howards, P. P., Kramer, M. R., Mertens, A. C. and Spencer, J. B. (2015). Racial disparities in seeking care for help getting pregnant, *Paediatric Perinatal Epidemiology* 29:5, 416–25.

Cromer, R. (2019). Making the ethnic embryo: enacting race in US embryo adoption, *Medical Anthropology* 38:7, 603–19.

Daniels, C. R. and Heidt-Forsythe, E. (2012). Gendered eugenics and the problematic of free market reproductive technologies: sperm and egg donation in the United States, *Signs* 37:3, 719–47.

Deomampo, D. (2016). Race, nation and the production of intimacy: trans-national ova donation in India, *Positions: East Asia Cultures Critique*, 24:1, 303–32.

Deomampo, D. (2019). Racialized commodities: race and value in human egg donation, *Medical Anthropology*, 38:7, 620–33.

Dow, K. (2017). 'The men who made the breakthrough': how the British press represented Patrick Steptoe and Robert Edwards in 1978, *Reproductive Biomedicine & Society Online* 4, 59–67.

Dyck, E. (2014). History of eugenics revisited, *Canadian Bulletin of Medical History* 31:1, 7–16.

Dyer, S. J. and Kruger, T. F. (2012). Assisted reproductive technology in South Africa: first results generated from the South African Register of Assisted Reproductive Techniques, *South African Medical Journal* 102:3, 167–70.

Dyer, S. J., Abrahams, N., Mokoena, N. E. and van der Spuy, Z. M. (2004). 'You are a man because you have children': experiences, reproductive health knowledge and treatment seeking behaviour among men suffering from couple infertility in South Africa, *Human Reproduction* 19:4, 960–7.

Elster, N. R. (2005). ART for the masses? Racial and ethnic inequality in assisted reproductive technologies, *De Paul Journal of Health Care Law* 9:3, 719–34.

Erasmus, Z. (2017). *Race Otherwise: Forging a New Humanism for South Africa*. Johannesburg: Wits University Press.

Gates, B. and Gates, M. (2017). Our 2017 annual letter: Warren Buffet's best investment. *Gatesnotes*. www.gatesnotes.com/2017-Annual-Letter. Accessed 17 September 2017.

Guendelman, S. and Stachel, L. (2011). Infertility status and infertility treatment: racial and ethnic disparities, *Reducing Racial/Ethnic Disparities in Reproductive and Perinatal Outcomes* 93–117.

Hanson, F. A. (2001). Donor insemination: eugenic and feminist implications, *Medical Anthropology Quarterly* 15, 287–311.

Hargreaves, K. (2006). Constructing families and kinship through donor insemination, *Sociology of Health and Illness* 28:3, 261–83.

Harrison, L. (2013). The woman or the egg: race in egg donation and surrogacy databases, *Genders Online Journal* 58. www.genders.org/g58/g58_harrison.html. Accessed 9 September 2018.

Hill Collins, P. (1998). It's all in the family: intersections of gender, race and nation, *Hypatia* 13:3, 62–82.

Ikemoto, L. C. (1995). The infertile, the too fertile, and the dysfertile, *Hastings Law Journal* 47:4, 1007–61.

Inhorn, M. (2011). Globalization and gametes: reproductive 'tourism', Islamic bioethics, and Middle Eastern modernity, *Anthropology and Medicine* 18:1, 87–103.

Jain, T. (2006). Socio-economic and racial disparities among infertility patients seeking care, *Fertility and Sterility* 85:4, 876–81.

Kroløkke, C. (2014). West is best: affective assemblages and Spanish oocytes, *European Journal of Women's Studies* 21:1, 57–71.

Lewis, J. (2003). Design issues. In J. Ritchie and J. Lewis, *Qualitative Research Practice: A Guide for Social Science Students and Researchers*, 47–76. London: Sage.

MacCallum, F. and Golombok, S. (2007). Embryo donation families: mothers' decisions regarding disclosure of donor conception, *Human Reproduction* 22:11, 2888–95.

Macionis, J. and Plummer, K. (2008). *Sociology: A Global Introduction*. 4th ed. London: Pearson Education.

Maung, H. H. (2018). Ethical problems with ethnic matching in gamete donation, *Journal of Medical Ethics* 45, 112–16.

Moll, T. (2019). Making a match: curating race in South African gamete donation, *Medical Anthropology* 38:7, 588–602.

Murray, C. A. and Herrnstein, R. J. (1994). *The Bell Curve: Intelligence and Class Structure in American Life*. New York: Simon and Schuster.

Nachtigall, R. D. (2005). International disparities in access to infertility services, *Fertility and Sterility* 85:4, 871–75.

Nahman, M. R. (2016). Reproductive tourism: through the anthropological 'reproscope', *Annual Review of Anthropology* 45:1, 417–32.

Newman, A. M. (2019). Mixing and matching: sperm donor selection for interracial lesbian couples, *Medical Anthropology* 38:8, 710–24.

Pande, A. (2016). Global reproductive inequalities, neo-eugenics and commercial surrogacy in India, *Current Sociology* 64:2, 244–58.

Pande, A. (2021). 'Mix or match': transnational fertility industry and white desirability, *Medical Anthropology* 40:4, 335–47.

Perkowitz, S. (2017). How to understand the resurgence of Eugenics, *Jstor Daily*. https://daily.jstor.org/how-to-understand-the-resurgence-of-eugenics/. Accessed 4 October 2018.

Pilcher, H. (2006). Fertility on a shoestring, *Nature* 442, 975–7.

Quinn, M. and Fujimoto, V. (2016). Racial and ethnic disparities in assisted reproductive technology access and outcomes, *Fertility and Sterility* 105:5, 1119–23.

Quiroga, S. S. (2007). Blood is thicker than water: policing donor insemination and the reproduction of Whiteness, *Hypatia* 22:2, 143–61.

Roberts, D. E. (1997). Race and the new reproduction, *Faculty Scholarship*. Paper 1154. http://scholarship.law.upenn.edu/faculty_scholarship/1154. Accessed 23 January 2017.

Roberts, D. (2009). Race, gender and genetic technologies: a new reproductive dystopia? *Faculty Scholarship*. Paper 1421. http://scholarship.law.upenn.edu/faculty_scholarship/1421. Accessed 23 January 2017.

Roberts, D. (2011). *Fatal Invention: How Science, Politics and Big Business Re-create Race in the Twenty-first Century*. New York: The New Press.

Roberts, E. (2012). *God's Laboratory: Assisted Reproduction in the Andes*. Berkeley, CA: University of California Press.

Russell, C. (2015). The race idea in reproductive technologies: beyond epistemic scientism and technological mastery, *Bioethical Inquiry* 12, 601–12.

Sandel M. J. (2004). The case against perfection: what's wrong with designer children, bionic athletes and genetic engineering, *The Atlantic Online*. www.theatlantic.com/magazine/archive/2004/04/the-case-against-perfection/302927/. Accessed 28 May 2018.

Sarojini, N., Marwah, V. and Shenoi, A. (2011). Globalization of birth markets: a case study of assisted reproductive technologies in India, *Globalization and Health* 7:27, 27.

Schurr, C. (2017). From biopolitics to bioeconomies: the ART of (re)producing white futures in Mexico's surrogacy market, *Environment and Planning D: Society and Space* 35:2, 241–62.

Shehab, D., Duff, J., Pasch, L. A., Mac Dougall, K., Scheib, J. and Nachtigall, R. (2008). How parents whose children have been conceived with donor gametes make their disclosure decision: contexts, influences, and couple dynamics, *Fertility and Sterility* 89:1, 179–87.

Strode, A., Mthembu, S. and Essack, Z. (2012). 'She made up a choice for me': 22 HIV positive women's experiences of involuntary sterilization in two South African provinces, *Reproductive Health Matters* 20:39, 61–9.

Tabong, P. T. and Adongo, P. B. (2013). Infertility and childlessness: a qualitative study of the experiences of infertile couples in Northern Ghana, *BMC Pregnancy and Childbirth* 13, 72.

Valdez, N. and Deomampo, D. (2019). Centering race and racism in reproduction, *Medical Anthropology* 38:7, 551–9.

Walther, C. S. (2014). Skin tone, biracial stratification and tri-racial stratification among egg donors, *Ethnic and Racial Studies* 37:3, 517–36.

Winant, H. (2000). Race and race theory, *Annual Review of Sociology* 26, 169–85.

Wintour, P. (2018). Emmanuel Macron: More choice would mean fewer children in Africa. *The Guardian*. www.theguardian.com/global-development/2018/sep/26/education-family-planning-key-africa-future-emmanuel-macron-un-general-assembly. Accessed 6 December 2021.

Epilogue

Malika Ndlovu

Here and now
Familiar ominous shadows are swirling
Around this beckoning global portal
Dominance-obsessed insatiable forces
Howling like sirens, like threatening winds
Rampant fear and greed agendas ride the waves
Go viral, online, occupying vulnerable minds

Yet if we look or dive beneath the turbulence
Explore beyond the projected plots, the surface
The orchestrated distractions – to pause, slow down
Recognise the recurring crimes, echoes over time
Observing our triggered reactions to old wounds
We can feel the grounding, inward gravitational pull
Towards a conscious centre, a quiet knowing
That amidst all this violation, dying, is also a growing

Here and now
Re-membering ourselves inextricable from each other
From all that breathes, that has its place in the story
We begin collapsing illusions of superiority, exclusivity
Steadily exposing the seen and unseen toxicity
The hidden violence, the unsustainable inequity

Humanity at its earth-and-womb root
Is phenomenal change generator
Every human being, a dream-seed carrier
Imagination, collaboration and co-creation
Not only the quantifiable tangible and visible
Are central to our development, our survival

We come from gene-trees with the capacity to transcend
The audacity to tunnel through oppression and negation
To reveal and express perspectives that tip the world's axis

In the naming, the claiming of what we collectively desire
As we navigate between known and unknown territories
We are birthing visions, vocabularies for a different world
Tilling fertile land beyond binaries, man-made boundaries
Courageously calling in essential healing, urgent re-balancing
Here and now

Index

EU authorised representative for GPSR:
Easy Access System Europe, Mustamäe tee 50,
10621 Tallinn, Estonia
gpsr.requests@easproject.com